# Delusions and Other Irrational Beliefs

# Delusions and Other Irrational Beliefs

Lisa Bortolotti

Senior Lecturer in Philosophy,
University of Birmingham,
UK

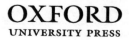

OXFORD
UNIVERSITY PRESS

# OXFORD

UNIVERSITY PRESS

Great Clarendon Street, Oxford ox2 6DP

Oxford University Press is a department of the University of Oxford.
It furthers the University's objective of excellence in research, scholarship,
and education by publishing worldwide in

Oxford New York

Auckland Cape Town Dar es Salaam Hong Kong Karachi
Kuala Lumpur Madrid Melbourne Mexico City Nairobi
New Delhi Taipei Toronto

With offices in

Argentina Austria Brazil Chile Czech Republic France Greece
Guatemala Hungary Italy Japan Poland Portugal Singapore
South Korea Switzerland Thailand Turkey Ukraine Vietnam

Oxford is a registered trade mark of Oxford University Press
in the UK and in certain other countries

Published in the United States
by Oxford University Press Inc., New York

British Library Cataloguing in Publication Data

Data available

Library of Congress Cataloging in Publication Data

Data available

Typeset in Minion by Glyph International, Bangalore, India
Printed in Great Britain
on acid-free paper by the
MPG Books Group, Bodmin and King's Lynn

ISBN 978-0-19-920616-2

Oxford University Press makes no representation, express or implied, that the drug dosages in this
book are correct. Readers must therefore always check the product information and clinical
procedures with the most up-to-date published product information and data sheets provided
by the manufactures and the most recent codes of conduct and safety regulations. The authors
and the publishers do not accept responsibility or legal liability for any errors in the test or for the
misuse or misapplication of material in this work. Except where otherwise stated, drug dosages and
recommendations are for the non-pregnant adult who is not breastfeeding.

To Matteo
In loving memory of Elvira Prandi and Giada Paternoster

# Acknowledgements

Ideas in this book have been slowly developing since I started my PhD in 2000, but most of the writing has been done in the 2008/2009 academic year. First and foremost, I am grateful to the University of Birmingham for granting me study leave from September to December 2008. During this period I visited the Macquarie Centre for Cognitive Science (MACCS) in Australia. My research visit was made possible by the financial support of the Endeavour Programme, funded by the Australian Ministry for Education and Training, and managed by Austraining.

As a 2008 Endeavour Research Fellow, I benefited from the thriving research culture of MACCS and from the many opportunities for discussion with Max Coltheart and Robyn Langdon. I am grateful to all the members of the *Delusion and Hypnosis* reading group for making me feel extremely welcome and helping me understand better what it is that cognitive psychologists do. Amanda Barnier and Rochelle Cox introduced me to the literature on confabulation and hypnosis which had a significant impact on the development of my ideas.

I would not have finished the book if I had not obtained AHRC funding for research leave from January to April 2009 (AH/G002606/1).The AHRC grant allowed me to dedicate all of this time to completing the book, and also funded a short but very productive visit to the Department of Philosophy at the University of California Berkeley, where I benefited from John Campbell's comments on the arguments presented in the book, and from the opportunity to talk to John's graduate students and to Ken Kendler.

I owe a great debt to Eva Picardi, Martin Davies, and Matthew Broome. Eva got me interested in beliefs 16 years ago and I am still interested in them now—she must have done a good job. Martin first introduced me to the literature on delusions, and was the ideal PhD supervisor. He has been a source of encouragement and inspiration in my post-doctoral work. Matthew helped me navigate the psychiatric literature and has been an invaluable collaborator. His influence is apparent in every section of this book. For constant support and encouragement, I thank David Papineau, John Harris, Helen Beebee, and Kim Sterelny. The arguments presented in the book have been tuned in conversation with Matteo Mameli, Hanna Pickard, Dominic Murphy, Jakob Hohwy, Derek Bolton, Rachel Cooper, Edoardo Zamuner, Dan López de Sa, Max Coltheart, Jordi Fernández, Daniel Cohen, Nic Damnjanovic,

Ian Ravenscroft, Phil Gerrans, Amanda Barnier, Rochelle Cox, John Sutton, Peter Menzies, Eric Schwitzgebel, Robyn Langdon, Mark Colyvan, Ken Kendler, John Campbell, and Flavie Waters. Neralie Wise, Matthew Broome, Kirk Surgener, and Rochelle Cox read an early draft of the book and provided detailed and insightful comments which have been very precious to me. I am also grateful to my colleagues and students at the University of Birmingham, where I presented early versions of the book chapters at staff seminars, and I taught a third-year module in the Philosophy of Psychology since 2005 on the relationship between intentionality and rationality.

I received good feedback from the participants in departmental seminars and reading groups where I presented sections of my work at the Open University, the University of Reading, Northampton University, the University of Glasgow, Macquarie University, the University of Sydney, the University of Western Australia, the University of Adelaide, Flinders University, Charles Sturt University in Wagga Wagga, and the European School of Molecular Medicine in Milan. For helpful comments, I am also indebted to the audiences of the following workshops and conferences: the Philosophy of Psychiatry Work-in-Progress Workshop organised by Rachel Cooper at the University of Lancaster in January 2008; the Delusions and Self Knowledge Workshop organised by Finn Spicer at the University of Bristol in February 2008; the Delusion Day organised by Nic Damnjanovic at the University of Western Australia, Perth, in September 2008; the Introspection and Consciousness Workshop organised by Daniel Stoljar, David Chalmers and Declan Smithies at the Australian National University, Canberra, in October 2008; the Memory Day organised by John Sutton and Amanda Barnier at the Macquarie Centre for Cognitive Science in November 2008; the AHRC Workshop on the Concept of Mental Disorder organised by Havi Carel and Rachel Cooper at Warwick University in March 2009; the symposium on psychiatry as cognitive neuroscience at the meeting of the Royal College of Psychiatrists in Liverpool in June 2009; the Joint Session and the annual meeting of the British Society for the Philosophy of Science at the University of East Anglia in July 2009; the symposium on the application of memory biases and distortions to experimental psychopathology at the meeting of the Society for Applied Research on Memory and Cognition in Kyoto in July 2009.

Some of the material in the book comes from systematisation and revision of previous work, and especially the following papers: 'Inconsistency and interpretation' (*Philosophical Explorations*, 2003); 'Can we interpret irrational behavior?' (*Behavior & Philosophy*, 2004); 'Delusions and the background of rationality' (*Mind & Language*, 2005); 'Intentionality without rationality' (*Proceedings of the Aristotelian Society*, 2005); 'If you didn't care, you wouldn't notice' (with M. Broome, *Philosophy, Psychiatry, & Psychology*, 2007); 'Delusional beliefs and reason giving' (with M. Broome, *Philosophical Psychology*, 2008); 'A role for ownership and authorship in the analysis of thought insertion' (with M. Broome, *Phenomenology and the Cognitive Sciences*, 2009); 'Shaking the bedrock' (forthcoming in *Philosophy, Psychiatry, & Psychology*); 'The epistemic benefits of reason giving' (*Theory & Psychology*, 2009); 'Can we create delusions in the laboratory?' (with R. Cox and A. Barnier, *submitted*); and 'Faultless ignorance: strengths and limitations of epistemic definitions of confabulation' (with R. Cox, forthcoming in *Consciousness & Cognition*).

I acknowledge the support of my extraordinary parents, my courageous sister, and my closest friends. They have all borne with grace my extensive travelling and my eremitic tendencies during the preparation of this book. Matteo deserves a special mention as he has always been there to push me one step further when I needed extra confidence. In the last year, we have talked about delusions a lot, and our conversations have helped me clarify my ideas. The book is also dedicated to my grandma and my baby niece. I miss them dearly.

# Contents

# Synopsis

Here is an overview of the book contents.

## Chapter 1: The background

In Chapter one, I describe the aims of the book, offer some background information, and defend a general framework in which the question whether delusions are beliefs has important consequences for our conception of mental illness and for our understanding of the relationship between rationality, intentionality, and self knowledge. I briefly explain how a notion of rationality of beliefs can be developed, by reference to theories of belief ascription and to the relevant epistemological features of beliefs. I also summarise contemporary debates about the definition of 'delusion', the aetiology of delusions, and the analogies and disanalogies between clinical delusions and other superficially similar phenomena (self deception, obsessive thoughts, confabulation, and hypnotically induced beliefs).

## Chapter 2: Procedural rationality and belief ascription

In Chapter two, I examine whether we can legitimately deny belief status to delusions by virtue of their procedural irrationality. I explain what procedural rationality is, and ask whether we are justified in thinking that delusions are procedurally irrational. Then I offer some concrete examples of the arguments against the belief status of delusions based on procedural irrationality (e.g. the bad integration argument) and assess them by reference to different cases of delusions. I argue that there are pervasive and significant failures of procedural rationality both in delusions and in beliefs—this suggests that procedural rationality should not be a constraint on the ascription of beliefs.

## Chapter 3: Epistemic rationality and belief ascription

In Chapter three, I discuss whether delusions should be denied belief status by virtue of their epistemic irrationality. Delusions are often defined in terms of their violation of norms of epistemic rationality, but there are some interesting debates as to whether they are epistemically irrational, and to what extent. I sketch some arguments against the belief status of delusions based on their alleged lack of evidential support, and their resistance to counterevidence. Then I assess these anti-doxastic arguments by reference to different types of delusions. I argue that there are pervasive and significant failures of epistemic rationality both in delusions and in beliefs. As the epistemic rationality constraint on belief ascription has numerous counterexamples, it should be abandoned.

## Chapter 4: Agential rationality and belief ascription

In Chapter four, I assess the argument that delusions are not beliefs because subjects reporting delusions do not act on their delusions in the appropriate circumstances and cannot endorse the content of their delusions with reasons that are intersubjectively good reasons. I emphasise the special role of agential rationality in bridging the traditional divide between theoretical and practical rationality. Then I ask whether we are justified in thinking that delusions are agentially irrational. In the first part of the chapter, I discuss arguments against the belief status of delusions based on their alleged failure to guide action, and assess these arguments by reference to different types of delusions. In the second part of the chapter, I explain the relationship between authorship and agential rationality, and claim that, although most subjects with delusions are agentially irrational, many are the authors of their delusional states. Then I assess the argument that delusions are not beliefs because the subject does not endorse the content of the delusion on the basis of intersubjectively good reasons. In the end, I argue that there are pervasive and significant failures of action guidance and reason-giving in both delusions and beliefs, which undermine agential rationality as a constraint on the ascription of beliefs.

## Chapter 5: Beliefs and self knowledge

In Chapter five, I concentrate on some of the implications of the previous discussion for the debate on the nature of delusions and for belief ascription in general. I maintain that agential irrationality with respect to a thought does not compromise the doxastic nature of that thought, or the subject's first-person authority over that thought. However, if the thought is neither owned nor authored by the subject reporting it, the characterisation of that thought in doxastic terms and the subject's self knowledge with respect to that thought are at risk, as the case of 'inserted' thoughts illustrates. Beliefs that are self ascribed and authored are integrated in a self narrative, and contribute to the construction or preservation of a conception of the self. I end by exploring the consequences of the analysis of self narratives for the status of delusions as irrational beliefs.

## Conclusions

I summarise my conclusions on the nature of delusions and the ascription of beliefs.

# Chapter 1

# The background

In this chapter I offer a very general overview of the topic, methodology, and aims of the book and provide some relevant background to current debates on rationality, on the conditions for belief ascription, and on the nature of delusions.

## 1.1 Introduction to the project

In what conditions is it legitimate to ascribe beliefs to others? The answer to this question is interesting for the following reasons. Belief ascription is an extremely common activity, but the capacities involved in having and ascribing beliefs are not well-understood yet, and there are a number of lively debates, for instance in the areas of animal cognition and psychopathology, about who can be ascribed intentional states and about the extent to which behavioural evidence can support claims about the possession of such states. Questions about belief ascription are no less important in the age of neuroscience: progress with a story about the subpersonal mechanisms underlying belief ascription can be more effectively achieved if we have a better account of the capacities that those mechanisms make possible.

Thus, it is useful to science to identify which capacities interpreter and subject need to have for the interpreter to successfully ascribe beliefs to the subject. A better understanding of the capacities involved in interpretation will be the basis for judgements about which of the systems we habitually interact with are *intentional* systems. These judgements can have repercussions: having beliefs is a necessary condition for autonomous agency. This means that to have a principled way to tell whether an individual can be ascribed beliefs and other intentional states does not only satisfy intellectual curiosity about the criteria for mindedness, but contributes to determining appropriate ethical stances towards other individuals. The debate for and against the doxastic conception of delusions, that is, whether delusions should be conceived of as beliefs, is of course a debate about the criteria for ascribing beliefs. The implications of the nature of delusions for the philosophy of mind and ethics are sometimes explicitly acknowledged in the literature (Bayne and Pacherie 2004b; Frankish 2009) and I shall attempt to bring them to the fore whenever it seems relevant, for they are the fundamental motivation behind the present project.

With the book I also hope to contribute to the debate on the nature of beliefs, and to a better understanding of the relationship between beliefs and behaviour. 'Belief' is a folk-psychological concept that might have correlates at different levels of explanation (scientific psychology, neuroscience, etc.), or turn out to be just a useful construct for the efficient exchange of information and the management of social relationships that characterise contemporary humans. No metaphysical issues about beliefs will be addressed in detail, because I take it that questions about the way in which we ascribe beliefs make sense independent of a complete theory of what beliefs are, over and beyond their role in folk-psychological practices. That said, a good account of how belief ascription works will impose constraints on the type of things that can play the role of beliefs. Think about the following analogy. The story of Cinderella may just be a fairy tale. The question whether Cinderella was happy when the prince found her makes sense within the fairy tale, independent of there being a real-life Cinderella. Whether there existed a girl, out of fiction, who experienced what Cinderella experienced, and inspired the fairy-tale, is a question that we can begin to answer only by comparing what we know about the girl in the fairy tale and the girl in real life who might have been the source of inspiration for the story. If there is no real-life girl who was abused by her step-mother and her step-sisters but then ended up marrying a prince who fell for her at a ball, then maybe Cinderella never existed (out of fiction). But how much of the fairy tale needs to have happened for real in order for Cinderella to have existed, is debatable. Can we say that the real-life girl was Cinderella, if she had only one step-sister instead of two? The same range of options can be assessed with respect to the question whether beliefs exist (out of folk-psychological talk). Telling a coherent story about how belief ascription works is the first step of the process that will lead us to discover what beliefs really are or deny that they can possibly exist. This project does not commit us to either of these possible outcomes. If one day we find entities that satisfy the description of beliefs only to some extent, there will be a choice to make: either beliefs don't exist but something else does, or beliefs do exist but don't behave exactly as we thought they would.

My starting point is to ask whether we have any good reason to think that delusions should be denied belief status on the basis that subjects reporting them fail to meet relevant standards of rationality. The objectives of this investigation are two-fold. In the attempt to show that considerations of rationality should not determine whether a reported state has belief status, delusions are just a convenient test case. The assessment of the arguments we shall consider in order to determine whether delusions are beliefs will contribute to clarifying conditions for the ascription of beliefs in general. For this general purpose of the book, using delusions is not essential. We could have started from any phenomenon that is usually described at the periphery of what counts as a standard typical belief (e.g. religious beliefs, obsessive thoughts, mental representations in non-humans). Delusions help me make salient and relevant the observation that the states we ascribe to ourselves and others and that we call 'beliefs' are very heterogeneous. They can have some typical belief-like features (such as being manifested in action or being used in inferences) without satisfying norms of rationality that some philosophers have regarded as preconditions for mentality, and more specifically, for the possession of beliefs.

But the other objective of the present investigation is to gain a better understanding of what delusions are, and this is a worthwhile project in its own right, as it has ramifications for a number of issues and disciplines. First, agreeing on the belief status of delusions would provide justification for the approach of cognitive neuropsychology, which is explicitly grounded in the assumption that abnormal cognition can be explained as a deviation from the very same processes that characterise normal cognition. The project is also relevant to the assessment of the view that psychotic behaviour and experience are on a continuum with normal behaviour and experience, although clarifying the status of delusions would not be sufficient to endorse or reject continuum theories of psychosis. Second, confirming the belief status of delusions would have consequences for diagnosis and therapy in psychiatry, where the status of delusions as beliefs is so central to differentiating delusional disorders and schizophrenic delusions from other pathologies. Third, the nature of delusions is important to classificatory and taxonomic purposes—the DSM-IV definition of delusions has been widely criticised and attempts have recently been made to improve on it, but one increasingly influential view is that delusions should not be described as beliefs at all, or that their definition should not be entirely based (as it is now) on surface features that are epistemic in kind (such as resistance to counterevidence). Fourth, characterising subjects with delusions as intentional agents capable of forming beliefs and acting on them would impact significantly on current debates about their ethical standing in clinical and forensic settings, and on the suitability of different types of psychiatric treatment. Should delusional reports be listened to with attention? To what extent should choice of treatment be offered to subjects with delusions when several options are available? Should personal autonomy and responsibility be attributed to subjects whose behaviour shows a commitment to the content of their delusional reports?

The argument I am set to undermine in this book is that delusions are not beliefs because they are irrational. Before we can assess this argument (which is rather a family of closely interrelated arguments with varying degrees of plausibility), we need to establish whether delusions are irrational, and to what extent. This is largely an empirical question, once we have a clear sense of the notion(s) of rationality that can be fruitfully applied to beliefs. Then, we need to establish whether there are good reasons to think that the relevant notions of rationality can serve as a precondition for ascribing beliefs. This can be done in several ways, but my strategy will be to see whether non-pathological beliefs satisfy the relevant norms of rationality that have been proposed as preconditions for belief ascription. We can have a combination of outcomes here, depending on the answers we find to these questions. For instance, we can agree that a certain notion of rationality is a precondition for the ascription of beliefs, but find that delusions are not necessarily irrational according to that notion. Or we can discover that delusions are irrational according to a certain notion of rationality, but that, in that respect, typical beliefs are just as irrational as delusions.

In the end, I hope we will have made some progress on two intersecting debates, one on the conditions for belief ascription, and the other on the status of delusions. On the basis of the arguments presented in the following chapters, I shall attempt to persuade you that the view that delusions are not beliefs is unsatisfactory, and that the rationality constraint on belief ascription should be put to rest, with no regrets. This does not mean that we cannot say anything interesting about what makes belief ascription appropriate or useful in the context of the interpretation of other people's behaviour. The analysis of the philosophical and empirical literature on belief rationality will help us identify key features of beliefs, which are not necessarily rationality constraints.

## 1.2 Reflections on methodology

The collaboration of philosophers with psychiatrists and psychologists is very fertile in the investigation about the nature of mental states and about the conditions for their attribution, for reasons that I would like to briefly discuss here. Psychopathology has become of extreme interest to philosophers, but mainstream philosophers rarely stop and think about how they can contribute to a scientific or medical understanding of mental disorders, or about the implications of the experiences of people affected by such disorders for their autonomy and their integration in the moral community. Rather, psychopathology is an endless source of funny quotes, and intriguing examples. One looks for counterexamples to certain general statements about the mind, and often finds fascinating real-life scenarios in the psychiatric literature. A case is mentioned, but the discussion focuses on the mere possibility that the case exemplifies, and not on the details of the case itself. As a result, the case plays the role of a compelling thought experiment. The aim is not to better understand a particular phenomenon but to point to the elements of a conceptual framework that need to be changed for the case to be accommodated. For example, does the possibility of thought insertion falsify the claim that there is immunity from error through misidentification? Do delusions force us to reject the assumption that individuals with beliefs are largely rational?

These questions are important, and tackling them with real-life cases rather than anecdotal evidence, outlandish thought experiments, or references to works of fiction is progress. Thus, an instrumental approach to the literature on psychopathology is not to be condemned. But it would be a disappointment if this exhausted the range of serious intellectual engagement that philosophers can have with the empirical evidence. My main concern is that it encourages a one-way approach to the way in which the empirical literature can interact with the philosophical literature. When philosophers invoke the simplified description of case histories in order to conjure a counterexample, the process starts from questions emerging from theoretical philosophy and ends with answers to those original questions. No genuine dialogue with the other disciplines is initiated, and no philosophical expertise has been put to their service. Psychologists, psychiatrists and philosophers are perfectly able to promote a better, more fertile, interaction between conceptual and empirical issues within the framework of empirically informed philosophy of mind, cognitive neuropsychology, and cognitive neuropsychiatry. Here are some illustrations of how a two-way interaction can help us both make better science and construct more plausible theoretical accounts of the mind:

> Modern neuropsychology has concentrated on the acquisition of empirical data that would support or disconfirm a theoretical position about the form and organisation of mental functions. The underlying construct is thus a model of normal performance in some cognitive domain or other. Such models [...] then provide the theoretical constraints on how the system can fractionate after brain damage. [...] Patterns of impaired and preserved performance in individual cases [...] can be assessed for compatibility with normal models of psychological functioning. Those latter accounts can in turn be revised when data from pathology cannot be accommodated by the current version of the model.

> (Marshall and Halligan 1996, pp. 5–6)

> The approach of cognitive neuropsychology has two main aims. The first is to explain aberrant behaviours and symptoms seen in patients after brain damage in terms of what has been lost (damaged or disconnected) and what remains intact in a model

(or theory) of normal cognitive functioning. The second is to evaluate models of normal cognition in terms of how well they explain the various patterns of spared and dysfunctional cognitive capacities observed in neurological patients.

(Langdon and Coltheart 2000, pp. 185–6)

Research in cognitive neuropsychology has two complementary aims. One is to use data from people with acquired disorders of cognition to constrain, develop, and test theories of normal cognitive structures and processes. The other is to use theories about normal cognition to help understand disorders of cognition that result from stroke or head injury.

(Aimola Davies and Davies 2009, p. 288)

If what these authors say about the purposes of cognitive neuropsychology and psychiatry is true, then the role of the empirically informed philosophers of mind and the philosophers of cognitive science can and should be ambitious. By reaching a better understanding of the cognitive capacities that normal subjects exhibit, philosophers can contribute to building a model of normal performance, and then to reassessing it if it is shown to be incompatible with the incoming data. By working together in developing the theoretical dimensions of this framework, philosophers and cognitive scientists do not just further the project of classifying observed phenomena and highlighting previously neglected conceptual connections between cognitive functions, but can also start understanding mechanisms that are causally responsible for the symptoms of mental disorders. A preliminary account of basic psychological capacities informs models of normal cognition that are useful to the analysis, description and causal explanation of 'disorders of cognition'. In turn, the discoveries we make when we study disordered cognition contribute to the testing and further development of our initial model of normal cognition. Philosophical analysis is instrumental to: (a) working out the implications of the available empirical results; (b) suggesting new avenues for empirical research; (c) drawing some conclusions about ordinary cognition on the basis of what seems amiss in psychopathology by reflecting on which capacities are impaired or compromised in the pathological case; and (d) assessing the relationship between data and interpretation in order to foster a critical attitude towards scientific methodologies and inspire progress.

Philosophers have something to offer to the development of the empirical literature if they work in collaboration with psychologists and psychiatrists in order to gain a better understanding of psychiatric disorders and other relevant phenomena. Collaboration brings fruits, and there are splendid examples of work co-authored by philosophers, psychiatrists, and psychologists in the delusions literature, work that has generated controversies and made substantial progress towards answering key questions. One example of a beneficial contribution that philosophers can make is to attempt to place single findings and interpretations of localised phenomena into a bigger picture which inspires new experimental questions and hypotheses. There are some advantages (and risks) in drawing 'big pictures'. Only when one takes some distance from the specific context in which some interesting data were found, can one identify previously neglected links with other areas of investigation. Moreover, big pictures help identify connections between what scientists and academics do on one side, and the concerns laypeople might have on the other. Views about the legitimacy of ascribing beliefs and preferences to others, for instance, have implications for issues of autonomy and responsibility, and for ethical questions about respectful treatment. It would be much harder to identify links between these ethical issues and neuroscientific phenomena that bear no apparent relation to folk-psychological practices. The fact that big pictures are useful doesn't tell us that they are necessarily accurate representations, or that any explanation at an alternative level of discourse would not be as accurate or as useful. On the contrary, big pictures carry some risks, such as the risk of oversimplification, and therefore should always be accepted critically and with caution.

Minimally, a sound methodology for the development of a philosophical theory about the mind should make sure that the theory to be developed is *compatible* with the relevant empirical data. This methodological approach is applied to the study of memory and in those research projects aimed at identifying benefits and limits of introspective knowledge. We should regard with suspicion a philosophical theory about memory that openly conflicts with things we know about memory from psychology and neuroscience. When it is indeterminate what the available data seem to suggest, either because data pull in different directions, or because they haven't been interpreted yet in a satisfactory way, this indeterminacy is an opportunity to think about ways of reconciling apparently conflicting data and come up with an explanation for the difficulty in providing an acceptable interpretation. There are a number of philosophical myths that a careful consideration of the psychological literature has contributed to displace. For example, the claim that humans are rational is a philosophical myth. Philosophers have often assumed that humans are rational, either because rationality is regarded as a defining feature of humans, or because it is regarded as a precondition for certain other capacities that humans exhibit. That assumption has suffered severe blows as a consequence of the psychological studies on human reasoning, which revealed the extent to which people are prone to making basic mistakes in different types of inferences (deductive, probabilistic, and statistical) and in decision-making. The message is not that the data about reasoning mistakes have *proven* that humans are irrational, but that they have made it obvious that general claims about human rationality cannot be uncritically assumed, but need to be carefully qualified and argued for, on the basis of a properly defined notion of rationality.

My project here can be seen as an instance of the following strategy. Take a well-established principle. Instead of accepting it as an a priori truth and applying it to the case at hand, start thinking about possible counterexamples, situations in which the principle does not seem to apply. If you find convincing counterexamples, question the principle and do not uphold it at all costs, maybe by changing the description of the phenomenon you are observing in an attempt to reconcile it with the principle. Rather, start entertaining the possibility that the principle should be revised, replaced by a more refined principle, or altogether abandoned. The rationality constraint on belief ascription is the view that rationality is a precondition for the ascription of beliefs. Even a cursory familiarity with folk-psychological practices and with scientific psychology would tell us that we frequently ascribe irrational beliefs. Not just that: via the ascription of less than optimally rational beliefs, we can explain satisfactorily and predict accurately the behaviour of ourselves and others in intentional terms ('He has always failed to recognise his mother's kindness: that is why he is so hostile to her'). Should we try and re-describe what we do in order to 'save' the principle? Maybe these irrational things that we seem to ascribe to people are not beliefs, but *something else* cleverly disguised as beliefs. Or maybe these beliefs that we ascribe are not *really* irrational. Or they are not irrational *in the relevant sense*. In this book I consider some of these possibilities, but I'm also open to revising the principle. Instead of establishing that delusions are not beliefs on the basis of the rationality constraint on belief ascription, we should be open to rejecting the constraint *because* delusions and other irrational beliefs get ascribed and play the same role as rational beliefs in underpinning explanation and prediction of behaviour in intentional terms.

It sounds like I am going to talk about delusions instrumentally, as a good example of a phenomenon that can undermine the conceptual link between the intentionality of belief states and rationality. The instrumental move is certainly on the agenda, but I hope that it will not be the end of the story. First, empirical data and empirical theories about delusions will act as *constraints* on philosophical claims about the human mind, but a consistent account of belief rationality, ownership, and authorship of thoughts will be developed in order to make sense in a unified way of available data, and (hopefully) give rise to further empirical work. Second, as I have already hinted, a solution to the debate on the nature of delusions will be proposed. Whether delusions are beliefs is a question that is important not just for philosophers but for any scientist or clinician working in this area. Moreover, the status of delusions matters to people with delusions, and to people who may not be diagnosed with schizophrenic delusions or delusional disorders, but experience delusion-like phenomena and encounter people with delusions in their lives. Any significant contribution to the debate on the nature of delusions and other psychiatric disorders is destined to affect more than just a conceptual dispute about theories of belief ascription. It is going to shape societal and individual attitudes to 'cognitive abnormalities'.

## 1.3 Introducing the rationality constraint

Interpretation happens all the time. On the way to the station, you see a tourist looking intently at the city map and infer that she is lost and does not know where to go. Your friend yawns repeatedly during a theatre performance, and you guess that he finds the play boring. Philosophers of mind want to know how we ascribe intentional states (beliefs, but also desires, intentions, preferences, emotions, etc.), and whether the way in which we ascribe them can tell us something interesting about the nature of these mental states. They are interested both in the principles that make interpretation possible and in the cognitive mechanisms underlying interpretation.

How does belief ascription differ from interpretation, and from theory of mind? 'Interpretation' has a broader meaning than 'belief ascription'. Interpretation is any attempt to make sense of the behaviour of others by ascribing to them intentional states. 'Theory of mind' refers to the set of capacities that humans typically exhibit when they engage in interpretation, and some have argued that individuals who are capable of complex social interactions and can communicate linguistically must possess a theory of mind. There are several tests aimed at establishing whether an individual has a theory of mind (e.g. false belief task). The capacity to ascribe beliefs is one of the capacities involved in the theory of mind, but it is not the only one. Another is being able to interpret other people's emotions by looking at their facial expressions.

One way of describing interpretation is to say that when an intentional state is ascribed to someone, it is ascribed in virtue of causal relations between an *interpreter* (the individual who does the ascribing), the *subject* of interpretation (the individual whose behaviour is observed), and the *environment* shared by the two (Davidson 1975). Interpretation is presented as a dynamic relation between two individuals and the environment in which they are situated. This has implications for intentionality. If we are interpretationists, we will think that all it takes for a subject to have a certain intentional state is for a suitably located interpreter to ascribe that intentional state to that subject in order to explain an observed pattern of behaviour. The attribution of intentional states is contextualised to an interpreter and a shared environment, and intentionality is demystified to some extent: we cannot 'see' or otherwise directly experience what the subject thinks, hopes, or plans, but we can infer the subject's thoughts, hopes, and plans from her observable behaviour.

Now, in most accounts of interpretation, the 'reading-off' process is constrained by some principles that are taken to be constitutive of intentionality. In the case of the ascription of beliefs a rationality constraint is taken to apply.

### 1.3.1 Interpretation and rationality

The rationality constraint on belief ascription says that interpreters cannot ascribe beliefs to a subject exhibiting (patterns of) irrational behaviour. In another (non-equivalent) formulation, the constraint says that interpreters cannot ascribe irrational beliefs. Let me offer some examples. First, let's concentrate on the irrationality of the subject's *behaviour*. An instance of behaviour that appears irrational will not support the ascription of beliefs. If I claim that the Democrats are the best party overall, but then vote for the Republicans, in absence of any other relevant information about my cognitive situation or my environment, an interpreter will not be in a position to ascribe to me the belief that the Democrats are the best party. If I am sincere in my initial claim, and vote under no duress, and without making any unintentional mistake, then I behave irrationally because the belief-like state I have reported fails to be consistent with my subsequent behaviour. Second, let's concentrate on the irrationality of the *belief-like state*. In absence of relevant information that might convince an interpreter that believing that pigs can fly would be rational in exceptional circumstances, I cannot be ascribed the belief that pigs can fly. That belief would conflict with many other things that I believe about what type of animals pigs are, and would fail to be supported by evidence (as I have presumably never seen any flying pigs in real life).

Why is the rationality constraint worth discussing? Having a belief that *p*, minimally, requires taking *p* to be true. If I believe that it will rain tomorrow, I take it that it is true that tomorrow it will rain. Anything in my behaviour that makes an interpreter think that I don't take *p* to be true, also makes the interpreter doubt that I believe that *p*. If I'm explicitly inconsistent when I discuss the weather forecast for tomorrow; if I show indifference to accurate and reliable reports that tomorrow the sun will shine; if I plan a day at the seaside for tomorrow in spite of my conviction that it will rain—something is amiss. Do I really *believe* that it will rain?

There is most certainly a phenomenon that the rationality constraint is designed to explain, which concerns the relationship between the intentionality exhibited by belief states and rationality as defined in terms of (a) the relationship between the belief and other beliefs, or other intentional states (e.g. consistency); (b) the relationship between the content of the beliefs and the evidence available to the subject (e.g. responsiveness to evidence); and (c) the relationship between the belief and the subject's behaviour (e.g. action guidance and reason-giving). There can be a correlation between failures of belief ascription and breakdowns of rationality, but the issue is what this correlation amounts to. Is it a conceptual relation between the ascription of beliefs and rationality, where rationality plays the role of a necessary condition for the ascription of beliefs? Before we decide whether to accept or reject the principle, we need to know what it states. The two formulations of the rationality constraint on belief ascription which I have presented have in turn multiple versions, carrying different degrees of strength, and plausibility. Two things should be immediately noted about the proliferation of rationality constraints. First, one common point to all variations is that rationality is supposed to be a *necessary* condition for belief ascription. If there is no rationality, then belief ascription is impossible or illegitimate.[1] Second, the implications of the view will vary according to the following factors: how rationality is defined, and to what extent the subject's behaviour or belief-like state has to diverge from standards of rationality in order for the ascription of beliefs to be impossible or illegitimate.

### 1.3.2 **Features of beliefs**

It is a real challenge to provide a definition of what beliefs are, let alone an account of the necessary and sufficient conditions for believing that something is the case. But here I would just like to extract from the literature some aspects of belief states that are not controversial and that are central to the understanding of the role of belief talk and belief attributions in folk-psychological predictions and explanation of behaviour. When I *believe* that something is the case, as opposed to *desire* that something is the case, or *hope* that something will be the case, I take my belief to represent how things are. This fundamental difference between beliefs and desires (or wishes, acts of imagination,

---

[1] In chapter 2 we shall see a version of the rationality constraint, the *indeterminacy* argument, according to which it is possible to ascribe beliefs to subjects behaving irrationally, but the content of the ascribed beliefs won't be determinate, thereby compromising explanation and prediction of behaviour in intentional terms.

regrets, plans, hopes, etc.) can be cashed out in terms of the following dimensions: (1) procedural; (2) epistemic; and (3) agential:

1)  Beliefs have relations with the subject's other beliefs and other intentional states.

2)  Beliefs are sensitive to the evidence available to the subject.

3)  Beliefs are manifested in the subject's behaviour.

This rough description, of course, does not exhaust the features of beliefs that might be relevant to distinguishing beliefs from other mental states, and it does not take into account the fact that beliefs differ. One preliminary consideration is that there are significant differences among types of beliefs: some beliefs are occurrent and other beliefs are dispositional. Similar but not equivalent distinctions are between implicit and explicit beliefs, long-lived and short-lived beliefs, and belief contents that are either attended to or not attended to. As these distinctions suggest, beliefs can vary considerably in duration and stability.

> One's repertoire of beliefs changes in nearly every waking moment. The merest chirp of a bird or chug of a passing motor, when recognized as such, adds a belief to our fluctuating store. These are trivial beliefs, quickly acquired and as quickly dropped, crowded out, forgotten. Other beliefs endure: the belief that Hannibal crossed the Alps, the belief that Neptune is a planet. Some of one's beliefs are at length surrendered not through just being crowded out and forgotten, but through being found to conflict with other beliefs, new ones perhaps, whose credentials seem superior. It is this need to resolve conflicts that prompts us to assess the grounds of belief.
>
> (Quine and Ullian 1978, Chapter 2)

When I stop and listen to a bird chirping, paying attention to the chirping, the belief that the bird is chirping is occurrent, and I attend to its content. But the belief that Hannibal crossed the Alps is a dispositional belief of mine. If someone asks me whether Hannibal did anything extraordinary, I will be disposed to answer that he crossed the Alps, but that is a thought that is rarely at the forefront of my mind. In the present discussion I shall confine my attention to beliefs whose content may not be attended to, but which can be conscious and open to introspection. A typical feature of belief states is that they come in degrees, and one can express conviction in the endorsement of the content of the belief to different extent.[2] Here I shall not discuss this feature in any detail, and will confine my discussion of beliefs to beliefs that involve a high degree of conviction. For the purposes of the present project,

---

[2] Thanks to Mark Colyvan for useful discussion on this issue.

I shall assume that there are two relevant states: entertaining $p$ as a hypothesis without accepting $p$ as true; and endorsing $p$ as a belief. If I entertain $p$ as a hypothesis, $p$ has been generated (typically) to explain a salient fact in my experience. The hypothesis that $p$ is subject to evaluation.[3] Before endorsing $p$ as a belief, I shall ask whether the hypothesis is consistent with the beliefs I already have, and whether it can explain the fact satisfactorily, given alternative hypotheses. In the process of evaluating $p$ as an explanatory hypothesis, I'm not committed to its truth. When I endorse $p$ as true after it has been through the evaluation process, then $p$ is something I believe, and I believe it with some conviction.[4]

Stephens and Graham (2004, p. 237) offer another characterisation of the main features of belief, which only partially overlaps with mine. They observe that beliefs involve a *content* claim, a *confidence* claim, a *reason-and-action* claim, and an *affect* claim. First, if something is a belief, it has some representational content, that is, it represents the world to be in a certain way. Second, a belief is characterised by the subject believing with conviction that such representation of the world is true (curiously, this feature includes a variety of elements, the basic 'taking-to-be-true' attitude and an assumption that the subject is convinced and confident in the truth of the belief). Third, the representational content believed to be true is taken into account in reasoning and in action. Fourth, beliefs are accompanied by suitable affective responses and emotions.

The emphasis on the affective dimension of beliefs is important in the analysis of what beliefs involve, and it is a limitation of my rough description of beliefs in (1) to (3) that the relationship between cognitive and affective states is not spelled out more clearly. However, (1) tells us that beliefs are part of a system in which they are connected with other beliefs and intentional states. I suggest reading 'intentional states' in the broadest possible way to include emotional and affective states with intentional content. Moreover, (3) tells us that beliefs are manifested in the subject's behaviour. The behavioural dispositions beliefs give rise to include the disposition to have affective responses that are consistent with the endorsement of the content of the beliefs.

Beliefs should not be idealised. The formulation of the four criteria adopted by Stephens and Graham tend to capture what *rational* beliefs should be like,

---

[3] This process of hypothesis evaluation can happen subpersonally and preconsciously.
[4] There being different levels of commitments to belief states will be discussed also in Chapter 4, where I review Frankish's distinction between level-1 and level-2 beliefs.

and not what actual beliefs are like. Surely, in a rational subject, beliefs command to be followed through in reasoning and action, and have appropriate effects on the subject's emotional responses. But not all beliefs behave that way. The belief that I didn't prepare for the driving test does not necessarily make me feel less angry at the examiner for failing me. The belief that I should be there for my friends when they need me is not consistently acted upon. Although (1) to (3) are not very specific, the point is to offer a description that captures the features that most beliefs, typical beliefs, have in common. This does not mean that we cannot offer a more detailed account of what it is to have a particular type of belief (e.g. a perceptual belief, a religious belief, a belief in a scientific hypothesis, an opinion, and so on), or an account of what it is to be rational with respect to one's beliefs.

As we shall see in the next section, the features of beliefs listed earlier correspond roughly to three notions of rationality for beliefs.

1*) Beliefs are procedurally rational if they are *well*-integrated in a system with other beliefs or intentional states.

2*) Beliefs are epistemically rational if they are *well*-supported by and *responsive* to the available evidence.

3*) A subject is agentially rational if she can endorse beliefs by offering *good* reasons in support of their content, and by acting in a way that is *consistent with* and *explicable by* their content.

The whole purpose of the present project can now be rephrased as the attempt to distinguish the general features of beliefs in (1) to (3) from the conditions for rationality of beliefs in (1*) to (3*). Whereas (1) to (3) are features of belief states that help us distinguish them from other intentional states, (1*) to (3*) are conditions that need to be met by rational subjects with beliefs.

This distinction is not entirely new: Bayne and Pacherie (2005, p. 171) distinguish between a *constitutive* and *normative* conception of requirements for belief ascription. The dimensions of inferential relatedness, sensitivity to evidence, and behavioural manifestability are to be intended as constitutive. They describe what features a mental state should exhibit in order to count as a belief. The requirements of procedural, epistemic and agential rationality are normative. They describe how subjects with beliefs *ought* to behave in order to be rational.

### 1.3.3 **Rationality for beliefs**

The notion of rationality relevant to belief states needs to capture the sense in which rationality is normative, and the sense in which having rational (as opposed to irrational) beliefs brings epistemic benefits. Some friends of the rationality constraint on belief ascription claim that rationality is something in the absence of which observed instances of behaviour can become harder to understand. Other friends of the constraint go further and argue that in the absence of a large background of rationality, there cannot be any beliefs.

Not all beliefs behave in the same way. Some beliefs are almost never reported, and remain in the background, even when they seem to be relevant to our everyday activities. On the train to work, the commuters who drink coffee and read the paper *believe* that the world is not coming to an end in the next ten minutes. But they probably do not attend to that belief, and do not report it. It is a belief that they can be said to have, but that is rarely, if ever, activated and attended to. If I enter the lecture room and start counting chairs, in the end I will come to *believe* that there are 45 chairs in the classroom. That belief will interact with prior beliefs (e.g. the belief that 50 people will attend the lecture), will give rise to new beliefs (e.g. the belief that the chairs will not be enough), and will also lead to action (e.g. it will lead me to grab five extra chairs from another lecture room). Do these two beliefs, that the world is not coming to an end in the next ten minutes, and that there are 45 chairs in the classroom, have anything in common? They do. They tell us how the subjects having these beliefs represent the world, or expect the world to be. They stand in inferential and evidential relations with other beliefs and other intentional states. They are sensitive to how reality is. They have some bearing on what subjects do.

Not all distinguishing features of beliefs will apply to *all* beliefs, or they will apply in significantly different ways. There are beliefs (e.g. beliefs about possible situations that are not actual, or beliefs that lie at the very foundations of our understanding of the world in which we live) that might have no obvious or no clearly identifiable action-guiding potential. Endorsing these belief contents might have pervasive behavioural consequences for the subjects involved, but no specific action can be described *as the effect of endorsing one of those belief contents in isolation from other belief contents.* My taking the bus to go to work this morning shows (in some very loose sense) that I didn't believe that the world would come to an end in the next ten minutes, but the connection between my action and my belief is very remote. Similarly, not all beliefs can be endorsed on the basis of reasons, that is, not all belief contents are candidates for justification via reason-giving. This type of endorsement is expected in the case of beliefs about one's future career or choice of partner, which often reflect decisions that have been deliberated about. However, the content of perceptual beliefs is not an obvious candidate for endorsement via reason-giving. I believe there are 45 chairs in the room, because I have counted 45 chairs. No further reasoning seems appropriate in this context.

These distinguishing features of beliefs are the bases for identifying criteria of rationality for beliefs. Table 1 summarises three influential notions of rationality for beliefs discussed in philosophy, psychology, and the social sciences.

**Table 1.1** Three notions of rationality for beliefs and believers[5]

| Procedural Rationality | Epistemic Rationality | Agential Rationality |
|---|---|---|
| Beliefs ought to be well-integrated with the subject's other beliefs and intentional states. | Beliefs ought to be well-supported by and responsive to the evidence available to the subject. | The subject ought to be disposed to provide reasons for her beliefs and act on them in the relevant circumstances. |

## Procedural rationality

Procedural rationality concerns the way beliefs interact with and relate to one another. The basic thought is that a belief should be well-integrated with the other beliefs and the other intentional states of the same subject. If I say that I prefer rice pudding to chocolate mousse, and chocolate mousse to cheesecake, you would expect me to prefer rice pudding to cheesecake. Otherwise, my preference-set is inconsistent. The violation of principles of deductive and inductive logic, of probability theory and of decision-theory is often taken to be an instance of procedural irrationality.[6] In the literature there are many versions of procedural rationality. The idealised version is known as the *standard picture of rationality* (Stein 1996, p. 4). According to the standard picture, for a subject to be rational is to have beliefs that conform to the best available standards of correct reasoning. In the psychological literature, versions of the standard picture have been used to assess human performance in reasoning tasks:

> We are interested in the sense of 'rationality' in which a thought or action is rational if it conforms to the best available normative standards. Thus we define rational behavior as what people should do given an optimal set of inferential rules.

> (Thagard and Nisbett 1983, p. 251)

> On some conceptions of rationality, a rational subject is one whose reasoning conforms to procedures, such as logical rules, or Bayesian decision theory, which produce inferentially consistent sets of propositions.

> (Gerrans 2001a, p. 161)

---

5 The descriptions below will be discussed and improved upon in the course of the following chapters.
6 For other descriptions of procedural rationality, see Bermúdez (2001) and Gold and Hohwy (2000).

According to the dictates of *minimal rationality,* for a belief-like state to be minimally rational is to conform to standards of correct reasoning that are feasible in light of the limitations of human cognitive capacities.

> For our purposes, the normative theory is this: The person must make all (and only) feasible sound inferences from his beliefs that, according to his beliefs, would tend to satisfy his desires.

> (Cherniak 1986, p. 23)

Not everybody agrees with the claim that the standards of good reasoning that make up procedural rationality should be derived from logical principles. Gigerenzer and colleagues (2000), Harman (1999), and Goldman (1993), for instance, have argued that human thought should have independent normative standards, standards that reflect cognitive capacities and limitations. I take it that these authors would agree that it makes sense to talk about how well or badly beliefs are integrated in a system, but the difference would be that in their accounts normative standards of procedural rationality would not necessarily be modelled on formal principles of logic, statistics, probability, and decision-theory.

## Epistemic rationality

Epistemic rationality concerns the relation among beliefs and the available evidence, and depends upon a subject's capacity to form new beliefs that are firmly grounded on the available evidence and to update existing beliefs when relevant evidence becomes available. A subject with beliefs is epistemically rational when her beliefs are not just sensitive to evidence, but *responsive* to it. Ideally, hypotheses should not be endorsed if there is no convincing evidence in their support, and beliefs should not be maintained with conviction if there is overwhelming evidence against them. For instance, my behaviour is epistemically irrational, if I continue to believe that the daily horoscope is a reliable guide to what happens to me, in spite of being aware of its inaccurate predictions. Gerrans (2001a, p. 162) lists some questions that are relevant to epistemic rationality: What counts as good evidence? How far should we search for further evidence? How should we decide which of two equally plausible hypotheses we should adopt? Bermúdez (2001, p. 468 and p. 474) characterises epistemic rationality as governing the way in which beliefs relate to evidence and the way in which they should be changed in response to changes in the structure of evidence.

## Agential rationality

Agential rationality is about what a subject does with her beliefs. It is a complex notion because it brings together the theoretical and practical dimensions of intentional agency. There are two aspects of agential rationality that I shall consider in this project: whether a subject is in a position to give intersubjectively good reasons for the content of a reported belief, and whether she manifests her endorsement of the belief content by acting on it in the relevant circumstances. Examples of agential irrationality are a reported opinion that the subject cannot justify with good reasons, or a belief that is behaviourally inert, in spite of having potential for action guidance. Suppose I say to you: 'My job is pointless and I want to quit', but when you ask me why, I cannot think of any reasons. This would not necessarily be a failure of rationality if it occurred for other types of beliefs or intentional states whose content is not expected to be deliberated about or justified, but in this case the belief I reported was an evaluative judgement. Thus, endorsement via reason-giving was expected of me as a rational subject with beliefs. Let's further elaborate the example. In spite of claiming that my job is pointless, I don't show any change of attitude towards my job. I go to work every day with a smile on my face, and I neither resign nor look for other jobs. This behaviour badly *matches* my initial report. What I do is not explicable by or compatible with what I say.

Stephens and Graham (2004, p. 237) deploy a notion that is very close to what I called agential rationality when they explain that subjects with beliefs tend to act in a way that is compatible with their beliefs: 'Believers take account of the truth of the content or proposition in reasoning and action. Beliefs guide the believer's decisions about what she might or ought to think or to do.' A sophisticated elaboration of the notion of authorship of mental states, which is interestingly linked to the notion of agential rationality, has been developed by Richard Moran (2001) and challenged in the literature on the introspection effects and the limitations of self knowledge.[7]

### 1.3.4 The rationality constraint on belief ascription

The rationality constraint on the ascription of beliefs has some initial plausibility. Interpreters often experience puzzlement and disconcert when confronted with irrational behaviour, and such behaviour often defies explanation and makes prediction of future behaviour arduous. Moreover, the notions of rationality for beliefs we described above match to some extent the features that distinguish belief states from other mental states, and from meaningless utterances; both the core features of beliefs and the notions of belief rationality share a procedural, an epistemic and an agential dimension. Thus, it is not much of a stretch to claim that when the standards of rationality for beliefs

---

[7] The relationship between the agential dimension of beliefs and knowledge of the self will be explored in Chapter 5.

are not satisfied, reported states or utterances cannot be ascribed as beliefs—or, in a weaker version, that belief ascription becomes harder when there is no background of rationality.

One might immediately reply to this point that the examined notion of rationality is a *regulative ideal*, telling us how beliefs should be, and is not meant to define or describe how beliefs are. But systematic failures to satisfy the demands of rationality arguably compromise the very project of ascribing beliefs: a wooden construction connecting the two banks of the river is not a safe bridge if it swings in the wind exposing pedestrians to the risk of falling, but a wooden construction that fails to connect the two banks of the river isn't a bridge at all.[8] To what extent must a belief-like state conform to the standards of rationality in order to be worthy of belief status? Is any deviation from the norms an instance of irrationality that compromises belief ascription? Or can some deviation from the norms be tolerated? Answers to these questions will depend on the preferred version of the constraint.

## Ideal rationality constraint

According to this version of the constraint, when an individual's report does not conform to the norms of rationality, it does not qualify as the report of a belief. In such cases, the observed behaviour is explained or predicted by reference to the physical constitution or the design of the individual making the report rather than by reference to the intentional features of the observed behaviour.[9] Let me offer an example by reference to a failure of procedural rationality: I believe that all mammals breastfeed, and that horses are mammals, but I do not believe that horses breastfeed. According to the ideal rationality constraint, when I say: 'Horses do not breastfeed', I am not reporting a belief, and an interpreter should not predict my future behaviour on the basis of the attribution of this belief.

> … Any attempt to legitimize human fallibility in a theory of belief by fixing a permissible level of error would be like adding one more rule to chess: an Official Tolerance Rule to the effect that any game of chess containing no more than *k* moves that are illegal relative to the other rules of the game is a legal game of chess.
>
> (Dennett 1979a, p. 21)

## Background argument

According to this version of the constraint, an individual's behaviour can be described in intentional terms even if it fails to satisfy the requirements of ideal

---

[8] Thanks to Laura Schroeter for a helpful discussion of this very point.

[9] For arguments supporting this view, see Dennett (1979a,b); Dennett (1998c); Dennett (1998d). For an argument against this view, see Cherniak (1986) and Campbell (2009).

rationality. For belief ascription in particular, it is sufficient that the exhibited behaviour is *largely rational*. If deviations from norms of rationality are too widespread, then the ascription of beliefs is compromised. There is a limit, even if difficult to identify, to how irrational the behaviour of an individual with beliefs can be.[10] Let me offer an example by reference to epistemic rationality. In general, my beliefs about how much people weigh are updated on the basis of the most recent measurements on an accurate scale. If until yesterday I believed that Peter weighs 70 kilos, and today his weight is measured at 68 kilos, I shall acquire the belief that Peter has lost weight and now he weights 68 kilos. But suppose that when it comes to my own weight, my beliefs are not revised in the same way. When the scale indicates that I have lost weight, I come to believe that I have lost weight. When the scale indicates that I have gained weight, I do not come to believe that I have gained weight. Rather, I form the belief that the scale does not provide accurate measurements. Is this a case of epistemic irrationality? The belief that I have not gained weight, when the available evidence suggests that I have, constitutes a deviation from epistemic rationality. But my other beliefs about people's weight are not similarly irrational. My failure of rationality is local, and, moreover, explicable by reference to motivational factors (I don't *want to* even consider the possibility that I have put on weight, because the thought would be distressing for me). In this case, the background argument does not necessarily demand the suspension of the attribution of beliefs to me.

## 'Sliding scale'

According to this approach, no pre-established threshold of rationality guarantees that behaviour is characterized via the ascription of beliefs. If the subject deviates from norms of rationality, the state that will be ascribed to her will not be a *full* belief, but a *partial* belief. Let me offer an example by reference to agential rationality. If I claim that giving money to organisations that promote education in developing countries is preferable to adopting a child at a distance, but can give no reason for my claim, the interpreter can doubt whether I believed what I reported, or I had some other attitudes to the content of that report which did not require me to be able to support it with reasons. Another way of describing the situation is that it is *indeterminate* whether I believe that giving money to organisations that promote education in developing countries is preferable to adopting a child at a distance. Notice that the degree to which the reported state is, in fact, a belief does not

---

[10] For arguments supporting this view, see Davidson (1985a,b); Heal (1998). For arguments against, see Bortolotti (2005a) and Campbell (2009).

indicate the subject's level of confidence in the believed state of affairs, but the extent to which her behaviour can be legitimately characterised by the ascription of beliefs. On this view, 'belief' is not an on/off concept but admits of degrees.[11]

Overall, the background argument seems to be the most attractive version of the rationality constraint on belief ascription, for the following two reasons. As opposed to the ideal rationality constraint, it does not need to deny that there are instances of irrationality in intentional behaviour, and it can also provide an explanation for these deviations: they are *exceptions* to the *rule*. Over the sliding scale approach, the background argument has the advantage that it can answer the question whether an instance of behaviour is intentional in a more straight-forward way, thereby making applications of the intentionality test to policy and ethics easier. The sliding scale approach acquires some credibility and plausibility when we think about the question whether non-human animals or radically impaired humans behave intentionally. A graded account might be useful in those cases. In the literature on non-human animal cognition, notions such as proto-concepts and proto-beliefs have been used to characterise mental representations that lack the conceptual sophistication and the number of inferential connections that mental representations in typical humans have (e.g. Loewer 1997). For the purposes of my present discussion, I shall mainly refer to the background argument when I talk about the rationality constraint on belief ascription, and assess whether it can account for the intentional characterisation of delusions as irrational beliefs that constitute an 'exception to the rule'.

## 1.4 **Introducing delusions**

In this section I shall approach two questions: what delusions are and how we differentiate them from other apparently similar phenomena. As part of the point of the whole book is to argue that (most) delusions are beliefs, this is just intended as a preliminary introduction to the debate about the nature of delusions, and to the distinction commonly made in the philosophical literature on delusions.

According to the *Diagnostic and Statistical Manual of Mental Disorders*, delusions are false beliefs with certain epistemic features:

> **Delusion.** A false belief based on incorrect inference about external reality that is firmly sustained despite what almost everyone else believes and despite what

---

[11] For an example of this strategy, see the interpretation of Cherniak's minimal rationality constraint on belief ascription in Stich (1990).

constitutes incontrovertible and obvious proof or evidence to the contrary. The belief
is not one ordinarily accepted by other members of the person's culture or subculture
(e.g. it is not an article of religious faith). When a false belief involves a value judgment, it is regarded as a delusion only when the judgment is so extreme as to defy
credibility.

(DSM-IV 2000, p. 765)

Delusions are a symptom of a number of psychiatric disorders (such as
dementia, schizophrenia, delusional disorders, and many more) and there is
no consensus on the mechanisms responsible for their formation. Thus, most
accounts of what delusions are refer to the observable features of delusions
rather than to their causes. A surface feature would be, for instance, that
delusions resist counterevidence. The surface features by which delusions are
defined are epistemic features, that is, features that make reference to epistemic notions such as belief, knowledge and rationality. In the rest of the book
I am going to focus on the surface features of delusions that are epistemic, and
on the relationship between the epistemic features of delusions and the
epistemic features of beliefs. We detect delusions on the basis of their surface
features, as we detect beliefs. So my strategy seems sensible. This does not
mean, of course, that aetiology does not matter to a satisfactory account of
delusions.

Epistemic accounts have two limitations. First, by epistemic features alone
the phenomenon of delusions cannot be demarcated from other similar phenomena. As we shall see, delusions share some surface features with confabulation, obsessive thoughts and self deception. Second, the degree to which cases
of delusion fit the epistemic account varies considerably. Just like 'belief', the
term 'delusion' is applied to cases that differ in surface features, such as rigidity
or persistence. Not all subjects with delusions have insight into the implausibility of their delusion or are disposed to defend the content of their delusion
with reasons.

It is unlikely that a unified theory of delusions will be forthcoming […]. One would
none the less hope that theories of normal belief formation will eventually cast light
on the both the content of delusions and on the processes whereby the beliefs came
to be held.

(Marshall and Halligan 1996, p. 8)

The conditions listed in current epistemic accounts are neither necessary
nor sufficient for delusions. It is possible that, when we have more and better
evidence about underlying mechanisms, aetiological considerations can be
included in definitions of delusions and partially solve these problems. We
might be able to identify a criterion demarcating delusions from beliefs,

or decide that the general term 'delusion' is unhelpful as it groups together phenomena with significantly different causal histories. But even if we believe that aetiological considerations will improve current criteria for classification and diagnosis, we need to start from surface features, and work our way backwards.[12]

## 1.4.1 Definitions of delusions

All parts of the DSM-IV definition of delusion have been challenged and counterexamples have been found.

> Delusions are generally accepted to be beliefs which (a) are held with great conviction; (b) defy rational counter-argument; (c) and would be dismissed as false or bizarre by members of the same socio-cultural group. A more precise definition is probably impossible since delusions are contextually dependent, multiply determined and multidimensional. Examplars of the delusion category that fulfil all the usual definitional attributes are easy to find, so it would be premature to abandon the construct entirely. Equally, in everyday practice there are patients we regard as deluded whose beliefs in isolation may not meet standard delusional criteria. In this way a delusion is more like a syndrome than a symptom.
>
> (Gilleen and David 2005, pp. 5–6)

> 1. Couldn't a true belief be a delusion, as long as the believer had no good reason for holding the belief? 2. Do delusions really have to be beliefs—might they not instead be imaginings that are mistaken for beliefs by the imaginer? 3. Must all delusions be based on inference? 4. Aren't there delusions that are not about external reality? 'I have no bodily organs' or 'my thoughts are not mine but are inserted into my mind by others' are beliefs expressed by some people with schizophrenia, yet are not about external reality; aren't these nevertheless still delusional beliefs? 5. Couldn't a belief held by all members of one's community still be delusional?
>
> (Coltheart 2007, p. 1043)

Here I won't go into the details of these debates, but present some useful distinctions introduced in the literature which will be relevant to the discussion in the rest of the book. Let me add that almost all of the distinctions are contentious, and that disagreement on the correct use of some terms used in descriptive psychopathology can be found even across textbooks and in the practice of experienced clinicians (McAllister-Williams 1997).

Standard definitions of delusions in purely epistemic terms (e.g. those definitions according to which delusions are false beliefs which resist

---

[12] For a sophisticated and historically informed discussion of the difficulties of classifying mental disorders, I recommend Bolton (2008), Murphy (2006), Cooper, R. (2007) and Samuels (2009).

counterevidence, are not shared etc.) fail to acknowledge that having a delusion has significant repercussions on the life of the subject reporting the delusions, and on the life of the people around her. There are some exceptions. McKay, Langdon and Coltheart (2005a, p. 315) propose a definition which makes explicit reference to disrupted functioning:

> A person is deluded when they have come to hold a particular belief with a degree of firmness that is both utterly unwarranted by the evidence at hand, and that jeopardises their day-to-day functioning.

Freeman (2008, pp. 24–6) also stresses the multi-dimensional nature of delusions, and lists among the key features of delusions not just that delusions are unfounded, firmly held, and resistant to change, but also that they are preoccupying and distressing, and that they interfere with social functioning. As Garety and Freeman (1999, p. 115) observe, preoccupation and distress with the content of a report affect diagnosis: 'the presence of distress, preoccupation or action accompanying the belief also increases the probability that it will be described as delusional'. It is worth noticing that distinct dimensions of delusions correlate with other variables – for instance, conviction in reports of the delusion correlates with the presence of certain reasoning biases (e.g. jumping to conclusions), and distress correlates with anxiety.

Providing a definition of delusions in terms of epistemic features *plus* disruptive functioning is an attractive move. Another option is to define delusions in terms of epistemic features alone, and then distinguish between *everyday* delusions and *psychotic* delusions (Hamilton 2007). Disrupted functioning would be part of the description of the psychotic delusions alone, which come to the attention of mental health professionals and are the object of diagnosis and treatment. Everyday 'delusions' would be false beliefs that resist counterevidence, etc. *minus* the distressing effects on the subject's health, social and professional life. Candidates for this label could be beliefs with very implausible content which may be accepted in a certain subculture (e.g. 'God spoke to me'). Elements of continuity exist between psychotic delusions and other epistemically irrational beliefs which do not disrupt social functioning: both are reports that 'reality has failed to constrain' (McKay *et al.* 2005a, p. 316). Moreover, epidemiologists have found that demographic, social and environmental risk factors for schizophrenia, such as victimisation, use of cannabis and urbanicity, are also interestingly correlated with the occurrence of non-clinical experiences that are similar to the experiences reported by subjects with delusions (Rutten *et al.* 2008). In an article for the New York Times, Brendan Maher said that 'the standard of rational, deductive thinking does not apply to normal thought' and that 'many or most people privately hold strange beliefs that could be diagnosed as delusional if brought to the attention of a clinician' (Goleman 1989).[13]

The delusions that cause disruption and come to the attention of mental health care professionals were divided into *functional* and *organic*, although the distinction is now regarded as obsolete. The term 'delusion' is used to refer both to disorders that are the result of brain damage, usually damage to the right cerebral hemisphere, and to disorders with no known organic cause. The former were called 'organic' and the latter 'functional'. Now the consensus is that there is a biological basis for all types of delusions (e.g. an underlying neuropathy that explains their surface features), but in some cases we are not able to identify it with precision yet. Some studies have reported very little difference between the phenomenology and symptomatology of delusions traditionally divided in organic and functional (Johnstone *et al.* 1988). Persecutory delusions ("Everybody hates me") were often described as functional, and are characterised by the belief that one is followed and treated with hostility by others who intend to cause harm. Mirrored self misidentification ("It is not me in the mirror") is an organic delusion, and it is caused by brain damage, which can ensue after a stroke or in the early stages of dementia. It is characterised by the subject thinking that the person she sees when she looks in the mirror is not herself but a stranger (Breen *et al.* 2001).

Delusions are generally either *monothematic* and *circumscribed*, or *florid* and *polythematic* (see Davies and Coltheart 2000). These distinctions are relevant to the question whether delusions are procedurally and agentially irrational. The level of integration between delusions and the subject's other intentional states and the manifestability of the endorsement of the delusion in observable behaviour vary considerably depending on whether the delusion is limited to one specific topic (monothematic) such as mirror reflections of oneself, or it extends to more than one topic (polythematic), where the topics can be interrelated, such as the hostility of others and their intention to cause harm. A subject who systematically fails to recognise her image in the mirror and comes to think that there is a person identical to her following her around has a monothematic delusion that does not necessarily affect other areas of her reasoning and may have no serious consequences for her behaviour. A subject who believes she is surrounded by alien forces controlling her own actions and slowly taking over people's bodies might have a number of different delusional beliefs that are interrelated and affect her interpretation of most events

---

[13] Chapters 2 to 4 will offer some examples of beliefs which do not differ in kind from delusions with respect to their epistemic features.

occurring in her life. Naturally, things are never so simple. Monothematic delusions might be more or less circumscribed. They are circumscribed if the delusional state does not lead the subject to form other intentional states whose content is significantly related to the content of the delusion, neither does it have pervasive effects on behaviour. Monothematic delusions can be elaborated, if the subject draws consequences from her delusional states and forms other beliefs that revolve around the theme of the delusion. The same distinction applies in principle to polythematic delusions, though polythematic delusions tend to be elaborated rather than circumscribed.

Depending on whether the delusion is defended with reasons, and whether the subject can offer grounds for the reported delusional state, delusions can be *primary* (true delusions) or *secondary* (delusional ideas) The traditional way of distinguish primary from secondary delusions relied on the notion that primary delusions 'arise out of nowhere'.

> A primary delusion is one that arises without any discernible precipitating factor. The delusional idea(s) appears to emerge *de novo* into the patient's mind. In contrast, a secondary delusion is a manifestation of delusional thinking that is linked to some particular precipitating factor. [...] Whilst the distinction between primary and secondary delusions might make some sense phenomenologically, it does raise difficulties. To claim that primary delusions just arise out of nowhere in the patient's mind tends to put them beyond the range of experimental investigation.
>
> (Miller and Karoni 1996, p. 489)

The notion of primary delusions has been found problematic by other authors too (see Delespaul and van Os 2003, p. 286). But the idea that delusions may be supported with reasons to a greater or lesser extent is still being explored by using different methodologies. Bortolotti and Broome (2008) talk about delusions whose content is defended with reasons as *authored* by the subject, where reasons do not need to be intersubjectively good reasons. Aimola Davies and Davies (2009) distinguish between *pathological beliefs* (for which the subject cannot offer any justification), and *pathologies of belief* (for which the subject can provide justification).

Not everybody thinks that what needs explaining in the phenomenon of delusions is their being false or irrational beliefs. Some distinguish between delusional mood as an *affective* component of behaviour, and delusional interpretation as a *cognitive* component of behaviour (e.g. Campbell 1999; Berrios 1991; Sharfetter 2003, pp. 278–9). Others regard the *experiential* and *phenomenological* character of delusions as more important than the *doxastic* one (e.g. Sass 1994; Gold and Hohwy 2000) or prefer to describe delusions as failures of reasons for action rather than as purely cognitive failures (Fulford 1993, 1998). Another view is to conceive delusions not as representations, but as attitudes towards representations (e.g. Currie 2000; Currie and Jureidini 2001; Stephens and Graham 2006). Let me add that, although some of the experiential, phenomenological and metarepresentational accounts of delusions are critical towards standard doxastic conceptions, they do not necessarily deny that the phenomenon of delusions involves the formation, endorsement or mainte-nance of beliefs. Rather, the central idea as I understand it is that, even if subjects of delusions report false or irrational beliefs, paying attention only to the subjects' first-order cognitive states and to the doxastic dimension of their pathology can lead to a partial and incorrect view of the phenomenon of delusions. For instance, Gallagher (2009) argues that an explanation of the delusion as a mere cognitive error would be inadequate, and introduces the terminology of *delusional realities*, modes of experience which involve shifts in familiarity and sense of reality and encompass cognition, bodily changes, affect, social, and environmental factors. He compares delusional realities to the alternative realities we experience on an everyday basis (e.g. when we identify with a fictional character while reading a book or watching a movie). Such modes of experience require belief possession and are implicated in the formation of beliefs.

## 1.4.2 Delusion formation

There are many different theories of delusion formation. One preliminary distinction is between motivational or psychodynamic accounts (e.g. Bentall and Kaney 1996) and neuropsychological accounts (e.g. Frith 1992). Motivational accounts hold that some or all delusions are caused by motiva-tional factors. For instance, delusions of persecution would be developed in order to attribute negative events not to the subject but to some malevolent other. The delusion would play the role of a *defence* mechanism to protect self esteem. Other delusions would be formed in an attempt to reduce anxiety. Here are two examples of a motivational explanation of Capgras delusion, the delusion that a dear one has been substituted by an impostor. A subject who does no longer love his wife but cannot accept the feelings of guilt towards her develops the belief that the woman living in his house is not his wife but some-one who pretends to be his wife. A young woman believes that her father has been replaced by a stranger looking just like him in order to make her sexual desire for him less socially sanctionable. Motivational accounts of some delu-sions that are monothematic and have a known organic cause have been strongly criticised because their neuropsychological bases seem to be sufficient to explain their occurrence. But motivational accounts of other delusions (e.g. those involved in persecution and anosognosia, the denial of illness) are still very popular.

According to neuropsychological accounts, delusions are the result of a cognitive failure or a combination of cognitive failures. Such failures can be due to an abnormal perceptual experience (Maher 1974), an abnormal experience accompanied by a milder dysfunction such as reasoning biases (Garety and Freeman 1999; Garety et al. 2001) or a breakdown of certain aspects of perception and cognition including a deficit in hypothesis evaluation (Langdon and Coltheart 2000). Another account which is neuropsychological in nature and applied to some schizophrenic delusions is that by Frith (1992), who claims that such delusions are due to a deficit that manifests in the failure to monitor one's own or other people's intentions. I shall come back to some of the differences between the various neuropsychological accounts shortly.

In most perceptual and cognitive deficit accounts, an abnormal event is responsible for the formation of the delusion. The man with Capgras delusion who thinks that his wife has been replaced by an impostor would form this belief because he has reduced autonomic response to familiar faces, and this affects his capacity to recognise the face of the woman in front of him as his wife's face, even if he can judge the face identical to that of his wife. But this abnormal event (reduction of autonomic response leading to a failure of facial recognition) is not the only factor responsible for the formation of the delusion according to influential two-factor theories (which I shall describe in the next section). These theories also postulate a deficit at the level of hypothesis evaluation to explain why the thought that one's wife has been replaced by an impostor is adopted as a plausible explanation of the abnormal event. There are alternative views about what the 'second factor' may be. Some suggest that the 'second factor' contributing to the formation and maintenance of the delusion is not a deficit, but the presence of exaggerated attributional or data-gathering biases, such as the tendency to 'jump to conclusions' on the basis of limited evidence (Garety and Freeman 1999). Others argue that it is a problem with mental time travel, and the capacity to develop a coherent self narrative (see Gerrans 2009; Kennett and Matthews 2009).[14]

Neuropsychological accounts of delusions offer very satisfactory accounts of organic delusions, as one can often identify with some precision the damaged region of the brain and the causal link between the damage and the formation of the delusion. Neuropsychological accounts of so-called functional delusions are also being developed and explored. For some delusions, hybrid accounts have been proposed, where motivational and neuropsychological factors both

---

[14] I shall discuss reasoning biases at greater length in Chapter 3, and come back to the relationship between delusions and self knowledge in Chapter 5.

contribute to the formation of the delusion (e.g. McKay *et al.* 2007). It is worth mentioning that not all neuropsychological accounts of delusions agree that the delusion is due to an abnormal experience. Another useful distinction, introduced and developed in the philosophical literature on delusions, is between rationalism and empiricism about delusion formation. *Empiricists* argue that the direction of causal explanation is from the experience to the belief. Delusions involve modifications of the belief system that are caused by 'strange experiences', in most cases due to organic malfunction (Bayne and Pacherie 2004a; Davies *et al.* 2001). These accounts are also referred to as bottom–up (from experience to belief):

> *Bottom-up etiology thesis:* The proximal cause of the delusional belief is a certain highly unusual experience.

> (Bayne and Pacherie 2004a)

*Rationalists* about delusion formation argue that delusions involve modifications of the belief system that cause strange experiences. This thesis, where the direction of causal explanation is reversed, has been proposed for monothematic delusions such as Capgras (Campbell 2001; Eilan 2000; Rhodes and Gipps 2008) and for delusions of passivity, in which the subject experiences her movements, thoughts or feelings as controlled or generated by an external force (Sass 1994; Graham and Stephens 1994; Stephens and Graham 2000). These accounts are also called top–down (from belief to experience):

> On what I will call a rationalist approach to delusion, delusion is a matter of top-down disturbance in some fundamental beliefs of the subject, which may consequently affect experiences and actions.

> (Campbell 2001, p. 89)

The sharp dichotomy between rationalists and empiricists is an obvious simplification, as in some models of delusion formation top–down and bottom–up processes can co-exist. The subject's prior expectations affect the way in which the signal is processed and gives rise to the unusual experience. Then, the unusual experience goes through reality testing and is responsible for the formation of the delusional belief (see Hohwy and Rosenberg 2005 and Hohwy 2004). Moreover, there are significant differences in doxastic and non-doxastic explanations of delusions which have a largely empiricist flavour. For some (Bayne and Pacherie 2004a; Langdon and Coltheart 2000; Davies *et al.* 2001), the delusion is *the belief* caused by the experience, and theories of delusion formation need to explain where the processes of normal belief formation went wrong. For others (Gold and Hohwy 2000; Parnas and Sass 2001; Gallagher 2009), the delusion is *the experience*, from which doxastic states might ensue, and this is reflected in the way in which theories of delusion formation need to account for the experiential and phenomenological character of delusions.

As we anticipated when we described the possible neuropsychological bases for the formation of delusions, empiricists who identify the delusion with a belief-like state can be further subdivided into those who think that the unusual experience is sufficient for the formation of the delusion (one-factor theorists), and those who think that the unusual experience is only one factor in the formation of the delusion (two-factor theorists). In some descriptions of empiricist views, it is assumed that the delusion is a *rational* explanation for the unusual experience. This is not necessarily the case. For some one-factor theorists (Maher 1974), the delusion is a *reasonable hypothesis* given the strangeness of the experience, or the strange experience is in a sensory modality or at a processing stage where further reality testing is not available (Hohwy and Rosenberg 2005). But other one-factor theorists (e.g. Gerrans 2002a) argue that, although it may be reasonable to articulate a delusional hypothesis, it is not rational to maintain it in the face of counterevidence. For some two-factor theorists (Davies *et al.* 2001), the delusion is formed in order to explain a puzzling experience or a failed prediction, but the presence of the experience is not sufficient for the formation of the delusion, and the *explanation is not rational*. The explanation is due to a mechanism affected by reasoning deficits. For other two-factor theorists (Stone and Young 1997), the delusion is a *rational response*, overall, because the biases that contribute to its formation are not different from those that characterise ordinary belief formation, and no specific reasoning deficit needs to be involved.

To sum up, we have reviewed three main positions as to whether reasoning is impaired in subjects with delusions: (1) it is not impaired at all; (2) it is impaired due to a hypothesis evaluation deficit, and possibly reasoning biases; (3) it is impaired due to reasoning biases only. A fourth option is to recognise that subject with delusions behave irrationally, but ascribe the reasoning impairment to a failure of performance rather than a failure of competence (Gerrans 2001a and 2002a; Hohwy 2007). It is not completely transparent how the distinction between competence and performance should be explained, but one straight-forward reading of it is that a failure at the level of reasoning competence is a permanent deficit which compromises inferential mechanisms, whereas in performance failures no permanent deficit needs to be involved.[15]

---

[15] The differences and similarities between these accounts are briefly addressed in Chapter 3, where we ask whether delusions lack evidential support.

Different ways of conceiving the relationship between experience and belief lead to another distinction, between explanationists and endorsement theorists. According to the *explanationist* account (Maher 1999; Stone and Young 1997), the content of experience is vaguer than the content of the delusion, and the delusion plays the role of one potential explanation for the experience. For instance, in the Capgras delusion, I see a stranger who looks like my father (experience), and I explain the fact that the man looks like my father by coming to believe that he is an impostor (delusion). In persecution, I perceive a man's attitude as hostile (experience), and I explain his looking at me with hostility by coming to believe that he has an intention to harm me (delusion).

According to the *endorsement* account (Bayne and Pacherie 2004a; Pacherie *et al.* 2006), the content of the experience is already as conceptually rich as the content of the delusion. The delusion is not an explanation of the experience, but an endorsement of it: the content of the experience is taken as veridical and believed. In Capgras, the experience is that of a man being an impostor, and when the experience is endorsed, it becomes a delusional belief with the same content. In persecution, the experience is that of man having an intention to harm me, and when it is endorsed, it becomes a delusional belief with the same content. For either account, there are two options: either there is a conscious experience that gives rise to the delusion via a personal level process, or there is an event below the level of consciousness that gives rise to the delusion pre-consciously via a subpersonal process. Some suggest that for some delusions (e.g. the primary ones) the latter option is most likely (e.g. Aimola Davies and Davies 2009, p. 286). Others (e.g. Coltheart 2005b) maintain that the typical case is the case in which the process of delusion formation starts with an event that the subject is not aware of (e.g. lack of autonomic response).

## 1.4.3 The two-factor theory

Max Coltheart proposes that there are two main factors involved in the formation of monothematic and polythematic delusions:

(a) There is a first neuropsychological impairment that presents the patient with new (and false data), and the delusional belief formed is one which, if true, would explain these data. The nature of this impairment varies from patient to patient.

(b) There is a second neuropsychological impairment, of a belief evaluation system, which prevents the patient from rejecting the newly formed belief even though there is much evidence against it. This impairment is the same in all people with monothematic delusions.

(Coltheart 2005b, p. 154)

Two-factor theories can be characterised in terms of the following steps (Davies *et al.* 2001; Coltheart 2007):

◆ Neuropsychological impairment leading to an abnormal event (this can be an abnormal experience that is consciously attended to, or a failed prediction not attended to by the subject). The cause of this abnormal response will depend on the type of delusion considered.

◆ Hypothesis generation (as explanation of the experience or endorsement of the content of the experience). This step is performed in accordance with the *principle of observational adequacy*, that is, the hypothesis generated needs to be such that, if true, it could explain the experience or failed prediction.

◆ Impairment of hypothesis evaluation, probably due to frontal right hemisphere damage. This is manifested in failure to reject hypotheses that are not supported by the available evidence and failure to reject hypotheses that are implausible given the beliefs previously accepted by the subject. The hypothesis should be assessed on the basis of how it fits with other things the subject believes (*principle of conservatism*) and on the basis of the probability of the hypothesis given the evidence, and of the evidence independently of the hypothesis (*principle of explanatory adequacy*).

◆ Acceptance of a hypothesis, which becomes a belief and is attended to and reported, and can be subject to further (personal-level) evaluation in the face of counter-evidence. When it is endorsed, the hypothesis is usually regarded as more plausible, more probable, and more explanatory than relevant alternatives.

This influential view of the neuropsychology of delusions (Langdon and Coltheart 2000) appeals to general mechanisms of belief formation, in terms of hypothesis generation and evaluation. Already Kihlstrom and Hoyt (1988, p. 96) write that subjects with delusions have 'non-optimal hypothesis-testing strategies', but Langdon and Coltheart offer a more detailed account of the normal mechanisms responsible for the formation and assessment of beliefs, and then suggest what might be going amiss in the case of delusions. Ramachandran and Blakeslee (1998) defend an explanation of some delusions which is in part compatible with Langdon and Coltheart's two-factor account. They endorse the thesis of *hemispheric specialisation*, which postulates that the two hemispheres of the brain have different tasks. The left hemisphere generates new hypotheses that are consistent with things previously known and believed, whereas the right hemisphere evaluates the generated hypotheses on the basis of their fit with reality. The left hemisphere is conservative, whereas the right one has a 'discrepancy detector' and tends to initiate belief revision when necessary.

Let me offer some examples of how the two-factor account would explain a variety of delusions. In the case of delusions with bizarre content such as alien control, when people believe that their thoughts and actions are controlled by an external force, the account would look like this:

◆ [First deficit] Perceptual 'aberration' due to cognitive impairment (necessary to explain the content of bizarre delusions but not sufficient to explain the presence of a delusion).

- ◆ Attributional biases affecting the generation of hypotheses (neither necessary nor sufficient to explain the presence of a delusion, but possibly relevant to explain the content of the delusions).
- ◆ [Second deficit] Permanent deficit of hypothesis evaluation which prevents the subject from discounting those hypotheses that are implausible given previously acquired beliefs or improbable given the data (necessary to explain the presence of the delusion, but not sufficient to explain its content).

In the case of delusions of reference, when people come to believe that they are the object of attention, or certain neutral events are particularly significant to them, the account would look like this:

- ◆ [First deficit] Mechanisms that direct the subject to new or relevant stimuli are dysfunctional. This causes an 'aberrant quality of salience' (necessary to explain the content of the delusion but not sufficient to explain the presence of a delusion).
- ◆ [Second deficit] A permanent deficit of hypothesis evaluation which prevents the subject from discounting those hypotheses that are implausible given previously acquired beliefs or improbable given the data (necessary to explain the presence of the delusion, but not sufficient to explain its content).

Take an account of the formation of delusions of paranoia as another example (Combs and Penn 2008, p. 192). An event occurs, such as this: a co-worker passes by without speaking. Abnormalities in emotion perception cause the subject to focus her attention on non-essential areas of the face of her co-worker when scanning it visually, and to fixate longer on facial features that might be neutral or give ambiguous signals in terms of emotion expression. The limited 'evidence' gathered by the subject is then interpreted excessively negatively in terms of threat and negative emotions. These characteristics in emotion perception combined with data-gathering biases such as jumping to conclusion lead the subject to hypothesise that her co-worker is angry. Further, attributional biases due to deficits in theory of mind cause the subject to form the hypothesis that the co-worker is angry *with the subject*, and this hypothesis is then endorsed as a paranoid belief about possible harm: 'My co-worker is trying to harm me'.

Langdon, McKay and Coltheart (2008a, p. 229) suggest that 'attentional biases to threat related material in the environment might be sufficient to set the persecutory train of thought rolling', and that motivational factors, as well as neuropsychological ones, can be responsible for the content of the delusion. It is possible that in some cases social perception issues are due to low self-esteem. But attentional biases can be aggravated or simply accompanied by other impairments: auditory impairments, which might give the impression to the subject that other people are whispering; memory impairments, which might lead the subject to attribute the alleged disappearance of valuable objects to malevolent others; failures of inner speech monitoring; ideas of reference; and so on.

Other cases can also be accounted for by similar models of belief formation (see McKay *et al.* 2005a; Barnier *et al.* 2008). In the case of everyday delusions (e.g. jealousy), we would have no 'first' and 'second' deficit, but a single deficit: there would need to be no 'perceptual aberration'. Rather, experiential information would be misinterpreted due to attentional biases that affect the generation of hypotheses (these biases do not need to be abnormal). The permanent deficit of hypothesis evaluation would prevent the subject from discounting those hypotheses that are implausible given previously acquired beliefs or improbable given the data. In the case of delusion-like states induced by hypnosis (e.g. 'it's not me in the mirror'), the experiential information would be misinterpreted due to hypnotic suggestion. The strength of the hypnotic suggestion would prevent the subject from discounting those hypotheses that are implausible given previously acquired beliefs or improbable given the data.

The deficit of hypothesis evaluation would be responsible for the failures of procedural and epistemic rationality that have been noticed in the behaviour of subjects with delusions. Delusions are not formed in a way that conforms to the dictates of procedural rationality, because the adopted (delusional) hypothesis has not been assessed on the basis of whether it coheres with accepted beliefs and prior knowledge. Further, the subject does not assess the adopted (delusional) hypothesis on the basis of its 'fit' with experience other than the failed prediction which constitutes the 'first factor' in organic delusions (Langdon and Coltheart 2000, pp. 211–3). The mechanisms of belief evaluation determining the procedural and epistemic rationality of delusions operate at the subpersonal, pre-conscious level unless the subject's attention is required. But it is after the subject has accepted the delusional hypothesis and is aware of its content that the behaviour typically associated with delusions can be observed. When the subject is confronted with apparent counterevidence and is asked to justify her delusion, other questions about procedural and epistemic rationality, and new questions about agential rationality become relevant. The subject can be unusually resistant to modifying or doubting the content of the delusion, and can mention reasons which are not regarded by others as good reasons, and which haven't actually had a causal role in the adoption of the delusional hypothesis.

It is important to distinguish between the processes of hypothesis generation and evaluation that can happen at the subpersonal, pre-conscious level and the behaviours typical of subjects with delusions that are manifested in the subjects' attachment to the delusional state and in their level of commitment to the content of the delusion (these are the features of endorsement we discussed with respect to the notion of agential rationality). The process of hypothesis generation is triggered by an event that is not necessarily conscious and can be described as a falsified prediction.[16] According to a predictive model of perception, there is a pre-conscious system that is constantly making predictions such as: 'When I see a person with this particular face, I will get an autonomic response'; 'When I try to move my arm, it will move'. When predictions are confirmed, no search for explanations is triggered. When predictions are falsified, the system generates a hypothesis which, if true, would successfully account for the unpredicted event. This hypothesis is then evaluated on the basis of its probability given the occurrence of the event. If no alternative hypotheses fare as well as the hypothesis just generated, the hypothesis is adopted. If there are rival hypotheses that seem to be equally plausible, further evaluation needs to take place, and this is likely to happen at conscious level. The subject assesses multiple hypotheses in order to establish which hypothesis should be adopted as a belief. What happens at the personal-level concerns conscious and reflective processes by which the accepted hypothesis, now a belief, is re-assessed in the light of new information and either confirmed or revised. Considerations relative to epistemic and procedural rationality can apply also at this stage, and considerations relative to agential rationality matter to the type of commitment that the subject makes to the belief—whether the belief can be justified with reasons or otherwise manifested in a range of behavioural dispositions.

My approach in the rest of the book will be more congenial to empiricists who endorse some version of the two-factor theory of delusion formation. I am not going to take a stance in the debate between whether the trigger of the delusion is a conscious experience or a pre-conscious failed prediction. It seems plausible to say that neither the event nor the relationship between the event and the generation of the hypothesis *need* to be something the subject is aware of, or something she attends to. It is also plausible that the processes of hypothesis generation and evaluation can be attended to in special circumstances, and this probably depends not just on the type of event to be explained, but also on individual differences and differences in the epistemic features of the context in which false prediction and hypothesis evaluation take place.

There is some indication that the pre-conscious processes of hypothesis evaluation and the conscious processes of belief re-assessment can be quite independent. Brakoulias and colleagues (2008) have found that cognitive behavioural therapy is efficacious in the treatment of subjects with delusions

---

[16] I am grateful to Max Coltheart for explaining this aspect of his model in detail in personal communication.

when their symptoms are stable and subjects are not undertaking trials of anti-psychotic medication. In particular, the rigidity of the delusion decreases, and also the preoccupation with the themes of the delusion and the conviction in the delusion are progressively reduced by cognitive behavioural therapy. Further, Gamble and Brennan (2006, pp. 63–4) report promising results of cognitive behavioural therapy—not only do subjects with delusions often appreciate the active engagement with the content of their delusion (Fowler *et al.* 1995) and become more willing to collaborate as a result, but they are invited non-confrontationally to question their assumptions, which contributes to their reviewing the endorsement of the delusional content. Drury and colleagues (2000) followed a number of patients who were randomly assigned to either cognitive therapy or a recreational and support group for several years. They found that cognitive therapy had comparatively more significant benefits for the capacity of patients to control their illness. That said, anomalies in probabilistic reasoning, theory of mind tasks and attributional biases are neither modified nor eliminated in the course of cognitive behavioural therapy. This result seems to lend support to the view that there are reasoning biases and deficits affecting hypothesis generation and evaluation which are not specific to the content of the delusion, and might contribute to making subjects delusion-prone although no conclusive data are yet available.[17] These biases or deficits cannot be wiped out by challenging the delusion epistemically, although subjects can be invited to re-assess the plausibility of the delusion once it is formed, with encouraging results.

Although I am not competent to address issues about therapy, arguments for and against the efficacy of cognitive behavioural therapy are relevant to the debates about the intentionality and rationality of delusions. If delusions were not belief-like and if subjects with delusions had lost the capacity to reason competently, it would be difficult to justify the cognitive probing of delusions. By arguing for the doxastic nature of delusions, I hope that the present investigation will offer theoretical support to any evidence-based attempts to treat subjects with delusions as intentional agents and largely competent reasoners.

Ultimately, arguments supporting the doxastic conception of delusions can be equally appreciated by rationalists and empiricists; explanation and endorsement theorists; one-factor and two-factor theorists. This is because the aim is not to answer questions such as where delusions come from and what processes cause them, but questions such as how delusions are manifested, once they are formed, and how they affect the cognitive and epistemic situation

---

[17] For a discussion of these issues, see Broome *et al.* (2007).

of the subjects reporting them. Do they affect the intentionality of the subject's reports? Do they necessarily lead to irrational behaviour? Do they allow self knowledge? Even though delusion formation is not our main subject here, some aetiological issues will be addressed again if relevant to answering questions about the ontological and epistemic status of delusions, and some of the claims about the epistemic surface features of delusions will have implications for the development of aetiological theories.

### 1.4.4 Delusions and self deception

I suggested that we cannot distinguish delusions satisfactorily from other similar phenomena on the basis of epistemic features alone. People may express beliefs that, say, resist counterevidence not only when they report a delusion, but also when they are self-deceived or prejudiced, when they confabulate, or when they have obsessive thoughts. What is the relationship between delusions and these other phenomena?

There is no consensus on whether self deception and delusion significantly overlap. Self deception has been traditionally characterised as driven by motivational factors. As we saw, delusions used to be described as generated in a psychodynamic way and the explanation of delusions relied almost exclusively on motivation. Now the preferred accounts of delusions are neuropsychological in nature, and involve reference to perceptual and cognitive impairments, but motivational factors can still play an important role in the explanation of some delusions, by partially determining the specific content of the reported delusional state. Thus, one plausible view is that self deception and delusion are distinct phenomena that may overlap in some circumstances. There are three arguments for the view that delusions and self deception can overlap.

One view is that (some) delusions are extreme cases of self deception and that they share a protective and adaptive function (see Hirstein 2005).[18] One example is the Reverse Othello delusion which involves believing incorrectly that one's partner is faithful. The belief can be regarded as a defence against the suffering that the acknowledgement of the loss of one's partner would cause (see example in Butler 2000 as cited and discussed by McKay *et al.* 2005a, p. 313). Another example is offered by Ramachandran, who discusses anosognosia, the denial of illness, and somatoparaphrenia, the delusion that a part of the subject's body belongs to someone else. Ramachandran (1996) reports the case of a woman (FD) who suffered from a right hemisphere stroke

---

[18] For a critical assessment of this view with respect to delusions and anosognosia in particular, see Davies (2008) and Aimola Davies *et al.* (2008).

which left her with left hemiplegia. FD could not move without a wheelchair and could not move her left arm. But when she was asked whether she could walk and she could engage in activities which require both hands (such as clapping), she claimed that she could. Ramachandran advances the hypothesis that behaviours giving rise to confabulations and delusions are an exaggeration of normal defence mechanisms that have an adaptive function, as they allow us to create a coherent system of beliefs and to behave in a stable manner. In normal subjects, the left hemisphere produces confabulatory explanations aimed at preserving the *status quo* ('I'm not ill'; 'My arm can move'), but the right hemisphere does its job and detects an anomaly between the hypotheses generated by the left hemisphere and reality. So, it forces a revision of the belief system. In patients such as FD, the discrepancy detector no longer works, and the effects are dramatic. In a conversation reported by Ramachandran (1996), FD even claims to see her left arm pointing at the doctor's nose, when her arm lays motionless. That the delusions reported by people with anosognosia involve motivational aspects is very plausible. But whether we believe that these delusions are an exaggerated form of self deception will depend on how we characterise self deception.

In order to explain the second and third views according to which delusions and self deception partially overlap, we need to make a short digression and describe two opposed philosophical accounts of self deception. The core issue is what it is that makes one self-deceived. The traditional position is that self deception is due to the *doxastic conflict* between the false belief one acquires ('My arm can move') and the true belief one denies ('My arm is paralysed'). The rival position is that self deception is due to a *biased treatment of evidence*: there would be a bias against considering or gathering evidence for the true belief. The subject never acquires the belief that her arm is paralysed, because evidence that points in that direction is neglected. Does FD believe that her arm is paralysed when she claims that she can touch the doctor's nose? Or, for a more mundane case, do I believe that my poor performance in the driving test was due to lack of practice, when I blame the examiner for being too strict?

In the delusions literature, the doxastic conflict account of self deception prevails. The subject has two contradictory beliefs, but she is aware of only one of them, because she is motivated to remain unaware of the other (McKay *et al.* 2005a, p. 314). This account derives from Donald Davidson's theory of self deception (e.g. Davidson 1982 and 1985b). When I deceive myself, I believe a true proposition (that I failed the driving test because I did not practise enough) and act in such a way as to cause myself to believe the negation of that proposition (that I failed the test not because I didn't practise enough but because the examiner was too strict). This description of the phenomenon is problematic for two reasons. First, it involves accepting that subjects can believe a proposition and its negation at the same time. Second, it invites us to believe that subjects can withhold information from themselves, which seems counterintuitive. The solution some traditionalists offer for these puzzles consists in postulating mental partitioning. According to Davidson, a subject can have two mutually contradictory beliefs as long as she does not believe their conjunction. The idea is that each of those beliefs is in a different compartment or partition of the subject's mind, and this prevents the subject from recognising and eliminating the inconsistency.[19]

A more revisionist solution to the puzzles (which leads to endorsing the so-called *deflationist* account of self deception) emphasises the differences between *deceiving another* and *deceiving oneself*. In the latter case, when the deceiver and the deceived are the same individual, the 'deception' need not be intentional, and the deceiver need not believe the negation of the proposition that she is causing the deceived to believe. If I want to deceive my mother about the reason why I failed the driving test, the conditions for my deceiving her is that I know that I failed the test because of lack of practice, but I intend to make her believe that that is not the case. However, what I do when I deceive others is different from what I do when I deceive myself and genuinely come to believe that I'm not responsible for failing the test. Al Mele argues that the conditions for self deception are as follows. First of all, my belief about why I failed the test is false. Second, I treat the evidence relevant to the truth of my belief in a motivationally biased way. Third, this biased treatment of the evidence is what causes me to acquire the belief. And finally, the evidence available to me at the time of acquiring the belief lends better support to the negation of content of my belief than to the content of my belief (Mele 2001, pp. 50–1). The ways in which the treatment of evidence can be motivationally biased are varied: one might misinterpret the available evidence, focus selectively on those aspects of the available evidence that support one's belief, or actively search for evidence that supports one's belief, without also searching for evidence that disconfirms it (Mele 2008). In the course of the explanation of these different scenarios, it becomes obvious that the motivationally biased treatment of the evidence is not just relevant to the acquisition of the false belief, but also to its maintenance.

The second view about the relationship between delusions and self deception is that, when they overlap, they do so because they both involve a

---

[19] I shall discuss partitioning at some length in Chapter 2, as it is supposed to offer a solution for the phenomenon of believed inconsistencies, which are a violation of procedural rationality.

motivationally biased treatment of evidence. If we agree with deflationists that the motivationally biased treatment of the evidence is the key feature of self deception, then people with delusions can be said to be self-deceived if they treat the evidence at their disposal in a motivationally biased way, or if they search for evidence in a motivationally biased way. This does not seem to be generally the case, but it is useful to distinguish between different types of delusions. Delusions of misidentification (at least according to neuropsychological accounts) do not seem to be akin to self deception, given that there is no fundamental role for motivational biases in the explanation of how the subject comes to hold or retain the delusional belief. A different analysis might be called for with respect to other delusional beliefs, such as jealousy or persecution.[20]

The third view about the potential overlap of delusions and self deception is that it is the delusions literature (which shows that doxastic conflict is possible) that can help us vindicate the traditional account of self deception. Some delusions seem to be a good illustration of doxastic conflict and should alert us to the fact that there is no puzzle in the thought of entertaining at the same time two contradictory beliefs. Neil Levy argues that the conditions for self deception set by the traditional approach are not necessary for self deception, but that the case of FD described by Ramachandran (1996) is living proof that a subject can, at the same time, believe that her arm is paralysed, and believe that she can move her arm. Moreover, it is the belief that her arm is paralysed that causes her to acquire the belief that her arm is not. This is Levy's analysis of the typical person with anosognosia:

1) Subjects believe that their limb is healthy.
2) Nevertheless they also have the simultaneous belief (or strong suspicion) that their limb is significantly impaired and that they are profoundly disturbed by this belief (suspicion)
3) Condition 1 is satisfied *because* condition 2 is satisfied; that is, subjects are motivated to form the belief that their limb is healthy because they have the concurrent belief (suspicion) that it is significantly impaired and they are disturbed by this belief (suspicion).

(Levy 2008, p. 234)

If this analysis is correct, then at least one case of delusion (e.g. anosognosia) involves the doxastic conflict that is typical of self deception. The most controversial aspect of this analysis concerns condition (2). Is the belief that their limb is impaired truly available to people affected by anosognosia? One could

---

[20] For a more detailed discussion of this point, see the papers by Al Mele and Martin Davies in Bayne and Fernández (2008).

argue that, given that they probably have a deficit in the discrepancy detector of the right hemisphere of the brain, they have no awareness of the impairment they deny (see also Hirstein 2005). But Levy's reply is that availability comes in degrees. He suggests that, given that people with paralysis and anosognosia often avoid tasks that would require mobility when costs for failure are high, and given that they can acknowledge some difficulties in movement (and say 'I have arthritis' or 'My left arm has always been weaker'), it is plausible that they have some awareness of their impairment—although they may lack a fully formed and conscious belief about it.

In sum, the debates I have summarised here show that there is no consensus on the reasons why self deception and some delusions overlap, and that the disagreement is often driven by different accounts of the conditions for self deception, and different theoretical accounts of the formation of delusions. If significant overlap can be convincingly argued for, it is only for a limited sample of delusional states (e.g. anosognosia, Othello syndrome, and persecution), and not for delusions in general.

## 1.4.5 **Delusions and obsessive thoughts**

Common examples of obsessive thoughts are: a constant concern about being contaminated by germs; preoccupation with feeling of inadequacy; the thought that one is responsible for harming others. Obsessive thoughts are often accompanied by compulsive behaviour which is motivated by such thoughts. For instance, fear of contamination might lead the subject to wash her hands every few minutes. Traditionally, delusions and obsessive thoughts have been sharply distinguished, but the reasons offered for the distinction vary. In the classic textbook of psychiatry by von Krafft-Ebing (2007), originally published in 1879, the distinction is characterised in terms of the dichotomy between content and form. Delusions are pathological because they have wildly implausible content, whereas obsessions are pathological because they are recurrent and insistent, independent of the plausibility of their content. This distinction makes sense if we compare delusions with bizarre content (e.g. the substitution of a loved one by an alien) to obsessive thoughts with fairly mundane contents (e.g. contamination). However, we know that some delusions have mundane content and some obsessive thoughts can be bizarre. In terms of form, an apparent reason for the distinction is that subjects with obsessive-compulsive disorder cannot always be said to *believe* the content of the obsessive thought with the conviction, persistence, and fixity that characterises delusional reports. For instance, obsessions about objects being dirty or contaminated might be impossible for the subject to ignore when they appear, but might be short-lived and perceived as feelings rather than thoughts.

In another textbook, Elkin (1999) argues that the difference between delusions and obsessions lies in the subject's *insight* into the irrationality of the reported thoughts. In obsessions, subjects 'are aware of the strangeness of their symptoms and have an intact sense of reality' (p. 96). It is recognised, though, that in acute phases of neurosis the subject with obsessive thoughts can lose her insight into the irrationality of her thoughts, and that the subject with delusions can appreciate that the content of her delusion is implausible and predict other people's incredulity. Stephens and Graham (2004) summarise the elements of continuity and discontinuity between obsessions and delusions in the following passage, with special attention to differences in form:

> Somewhat similar to obsessive-compulsive thoughts, delusions involve an imprudent or unproductive allocation of a subject's psychological resources in the management and control of her own thinking and attitudes. Delusions therein prevent the subject from dealing effectively with self and world. Unlike obsessive subjects, however, delusional subjects identify with the representational content (at the lower order) of their delusions. They do not experience the content as intrusive or as occurring contrary to their will or control. Obsessive subjects recognize that their obsessions disrupt and diminish their lives and they struggle, perhaps with very limited success, to contain the behavioral damage. Delusional subjects, by contrast, lack insight into the nature and personal cost of their lower order attitudes.
>
> (Stephens and Graham 2004, p. 240)

Matters are complicated by the fact that often subjects with obsessive thoughts also present psychotic behaviour and report beliefs that cannot be easily distinguished from delusional states. When such cases are presented, authors tend to reach different conclusions from their observations (see Solyom *et al.* 1985, Fear and Healy 1995, Insel and Akiskal 1986, and O'Dwyer and Marks 2000). For instance, Fear and Healy argue that subjects should be given a dual diagnosis of obsessive-compulsive disorder and delusion, whereas Insel and Akiskal opt for a single diagnosis of obsessive-compulsive disorder with psychotic features. O'Dwyer and Marks present some cases in some detail: in two cases subjects with ritualistic behaviour prompted by obsessive thoughts also reported beliefs that had a lot in common with those reported by people with delusions of paranoia and persecution; in another case, a subject whose obsessive thoughts and compulsive behaviour primarily concerned mirrors also believed that his friends and family had been replaced by doubles. Given that in these cases insight into the irrationality of the obsessive thoughts is often lost, and beliefs with bizarre content are reported with some consistency, the issue is how to diagnose their condition. It seems unsatisfactory to say that such subjects have both obsessive thoughts *and* delusions, because from the narrative provided by the authors, it is obvious that the delusion-like states and the obsessive thoughts are intimately linked. O'Dwyer and Marks (2000) argue that these subjects should not be treated differently from subjects with obsessive-compulsive disorder, and add that subjects did respond well to treatment aimed at ritual prevention. In the end, they side with Insel and Akiskal (1986), and observe how other conditions can also come with delusion-like states: subjects with anorexia sometimes report incorrigible and inaccurate beliefs about the size and shape of their bodies.

In their conclusions, authors discuss the implications of diagnosis for treatment. They claim that it is pragmatically beneficial for subjects with obsessive-compulsive disorder and delusion-like states to be given a single diagnosis that does not include psychosis, as such a diagnosis would 'lead to a lifetime of antipsychotic medication and a reluctance to consider other, more effective, interventions' (p. 283) such as behavioural therapy. Considerations about stigmatization and availability of treatment drive the diagnosis in such controversial cases. This is because delusional disorders are routinely treated with antipsychotic medication and behavioural therapy is not encouraged. If delusions are continuous with other irrational beliefs, at least in their epistemic features if not in their wider effects on subjects' lives, then there is no reason to assume that antipsychotic medication will work, and cognitive behavioural therapy won't. The increasing literature on the beneficial effects of cognitive behavioural therapy for reducing the rigidity of the delusion and the preoccupation of the subject with the content of her delusional states should contribute to making a wider range of treatment options available to subjects with delusions.

## 1.4.6 Delusions and confabulations[21]

As one of the official criteria of delusional disorder is that memory is intact, whereas confabulation is traditionally presented as an effect of a disturbance of memory, it would seem that the delusion and confabulation are clearly distinct (see Kopelman 1999).

> Confabulations are false memories produced without conscious knowledge of their falsehood.
>
> (Fotopoulou 2008, p. 543)

> An extreme form of pathological memory distortion is confabulation, i.e. the production of fabricated, or distorted memories about one's self or the world, without the conscious intention to deceive.
>
> (Fotopoulou et al. 2008a, p. 1429)

---

[21] The ideas presented in this Ssection have benefited from many constructive suggestions by Rochelle Cox.

However, delusions are not only present in delusional disorders and can be found in other psychiatric conditions which involve memory impairments (e.g. dementia and schizophrenia). Moreover, one can find broader definitions of confabulation in which memory impairments do not play any significant role. This makes it a really arduous task to determine the extent to which delusions and confabulations are distinct. If we take the broader definitions of confabulation seriously, confabulation does not need to be a pathological phenomenon. It is simply characterised by the subject telling a story which involves elements of inaccuracy or is not well-supported by the evidence available to the subject. Nonetheless, the story is genuinely believed by the subject narrating it, and sometimes defended with some conviction, argued for, and acted upon. It is interesting to explore the relationship between the broadly conceived phenomenon of confabulation and that of delusion, because some of the broader definitions of confabulation are almost identical to definitions of delusion:

> Confabulations are typically understood to represent instances of false beliefs: opinions about the world that are manifestly incorrect and yet are held by the patient to be true in spite of clearly presented evidence to the contrary.
>
> (Turnbull *et al.* 2004, p. 6)

> Jan confabulates if and only if: (1) Jan claims that p ; (2) Jan believes that p; (3) Jan's thought that p is ill-grounded; (4) Jan does not know that her thought is ill-grounded; (5) Jan should know that her thought is ill-grounded; (6) Jan is confident that p.
>
> (Hirstein 2005, p. 187)

> In the broad sense confabulations are usually defined as false narratives or statements about world and/or self due to some pathological mechanisms or factors, but with no intention of lying.
>
> (Örulv and Hydén 2006, p. 648)

> Confabulations are inaccurate or false narrative purporting to convey information about world or self.
>
> (Berrios 2000, p. 348)

Even these broad accounts are open to challenges. Criticising definitions according to which confabulation involves falsity, DeLuca (2004) observes that confabulations are not always incorrect. Rather, they can be actual memories or representations of actual events that are 'temporally displaced': the reported event really happened, but not *when* the subject claims it happened. Falsity is disputed in the official definition of delusions as well, as the content of some delusional report can be true (e.g. a spouse's infidelity). What seems to be relevant to the detection of the phenomena of confabulation and delusion is not whether the reported state is true, but whether its content conflicts with other things the subject believes, or it is held with a level of conviction that is not explained by its plausibility or the evidential support available for it.

Kraepelin (1904) proposed a distinction between simple and fantastic confabulation, where the difference consists in whether the *content* of the confabulation is bizarre. Others suggest distinctions between spontaneous and provoked, and between persistent and momentary confabulation (Schnider 2001; Kopelman 1987, 1999, 2007), where the *form* of the confabulation is at issue.

> In 'spontaneous' confabulation, there is a persistent, unprovoked outpouring of erroneous memories, as distinct from 'momentary' or 'provoked' confabulation, in which fleeting intrusion errors or distortions are seen in response to a challenge to memory, such as a memory test.
>
> (Kopelman 1999, pp. 197–8)

It is not clear what the weight of the distinction is, and whether spontaneity should be judged on the basis of purely *verbal* behavioural dispositions, or should take into account the dispositions subjects have to act on their confabulations (see Schnider *et al.* 1996).

> The line drawn between spontaneous *versus* provoked often appears to be quite an arbitrary decision. For example, is action critical to earning the title of spontaneous confabulator or is it simply enough for there to be unprompted confabulations in free conversation?
>
> (Metcalf *et al.* 2007, p. 25)

There have been attempts to establish correlations between the three most common distinctions; fantastic/simple, spontaneous/provoked, and persistent/momentary. For instance, from Kopelman's description, one would infer that spontaneous confabulations are severe, persistent and more likely to be bizarre and preoccupying than provoked ones. But Hirstein (2005) challenges this claim and argues that spontaneous confabulations are not always more severe than provoked ones.

Another possible way of justifying the importance of these distinctions in terms of surface features is to refer to differences in aetiological mechanisms that would correspond to differences in features. Kopelman, Ng and van Den Boruke (1997) argue that a frontal dysfunction is necessary for spontaneous confabulation whereas provoked confabulation is present in healthy subjects when there are memory gaps to be filled or more generally where a request for information cannot be met. But not all the available case studies support this hypothesis (see Nedjam *et al.* 2000, pp. 570–1), and another possible challenge to the neural bases of the distinction comes from the observation that there can be a progression from minor distortions to bizarre tale-telling (Dalla Barba 1993b; Glowinski *et al.* 2008). The dissociation between attributes of confabulation that were meant to be grouped together (e.g. fantastic/spontaneous due to frontal dysfunction) and the arbitrariness of many of the criteria of classification for confabulations lead us to think that we are far from a satisfactory definition of the phenomenon.

When confabulation is encountered together with delusions, many distinguish between *primary* and *secondary* confabulations. The term 'secondary confabulation' denotes a derivative phenomenon. It occurs when subjects with delusions or primary confabulation attempt to justify the content of their previous reports or explain away internal inconsistencies. In most cases, secondary confabulations are provoked by external challenges and are due to further elaboration of the content of an initial delusional or confabulatory report. Secondary confabulations are common in the reports of people with clinical delusions. In Capgras delusion, which involves the belief that one's relatives have been replaced by impostors, individuals will point out subtle physical differences between the 'impostors' and their relatives. For example, a woman suffering from Capgras delusion said that the impostor differed from her son in that her son 'had different coloured eyes, was not as big and brawny, and her son would not kiss her' (Frazer and Roberts 1994, p. 557). This Capgras patient offered *post-hoc* reasons for her belief that the impostor was not her son by reference to physical and behavioural differences between her son and the impostor. Bisiach, Rusconi, and Vallar (1991) described an 84-year-old woman who developed somatoparaphrenia (the belief that one's limb belongs to someone else) after a right hemisphere stroke. In the experimental session, this woman claimed that her left arm belonged to her mother. When asked what her mother's arm was doing there, she replied 'I don't know. I found it in my bed'. Halligan and colleagues (1995) described a 41-year-old man, patient GH, who also developed somatoparaphrenia after a right hemisphere stroke. GH believed that his left hand, arm, leg and foot did not belong to him. GH explained (after he no longer had the delusion): 'I came to the conclusion that it was a cow's foot. And in fact I decided that they sewed it on. It looked and felt like a cow's foot, it was so heavy'.

There are some cases in which subjects experience both delusions and 'false' memories (e.g. pathological lying and dissociative disorders), and it is not obvious whether their confabulatory behaviour is primary or secondary. A highly intelligent woman who had typical symptoms of schizophrenia (thought broadcast and thought insertion) maintained for more than 20 years a delusion of erotomania (Kopelman *et al.* 1995). The delusion seemed to originate from the 'memory' of meeting a famous conductor on a fruit-picking farm in the 1970s. The subject reported that, as a result of the meeting, the conductor fell in love with her and followed her around when she moved cities. He intended to marry her, although he was putting that off. She also thought that they were sharing the same brain, and that he could transmit his thoughts to her. The 'false memory' of the encounter during fruit-picking has the features of a primary confabulation, but it is not easy to determine whether it is the memory that gave rise to the delusion, or whether the memory was fabricated to justify the delusion of erotomania when it was challenged by third parties, as a secondary confabulation.

A number of independent studies showed that subjects with delusions of different types are more likely to engage in confabulation, or confabulate to a larger degree than healthy controls: this seems true for Alzheimer's disease (Lee *et al.* 2007) and for persecutory delusions (Simpson and Done 2002). It is worth pointing out that the epistemic faults of confabulation are usually emphasised in the definitions of the phenomenon, but that confabulation can also have some pragmatic benefits, and indirectly, epistemic ones. For instance, in the context of dementia, confabulations have been viewed as a response to memory gaps that allows the subjects to maintain a positive personal identity and interact socially. In this productive exercise the content of the confabulations behaves very much like the content of typical beliefs, in that it is supported by evidence by the subject, it is related to the subject's own past experiences (the *life history context*) and to current and salient events (the *immediate context*), and it is acted upon (Örulv and Hydén 2006, p. 654). In many case studies of confabulation, subjects seem to create a positive personal identity for themselves, often containing a germ of truth. But the features associated with the presentation of the self can be vaguely contradictory and not very detailed, as if they were variations on the same script.

There are two main views of the relation between delusions and confabulation. One is that delusions and (spontaneous and fantastic) confabulations can co-occur and exhibit very similar surface features, but should be kept distinct until more is known about the underlying mechanisms responsible for their formation.

> There is a strong case for keeping the notions of confabulation, delusional memory, and delusion conceptually separate. Although delusional memories share many characteristics with spontaneous confabulation, they differ in that delusional memories appear to be thematic and unrelated to executive dysfunction, whereas confabulations are fluctuating and multifaceted as well as virtually always related to executive dysfunction [...] Furthermore, it is very important to distinguish between delusional memory, which is rare and by definition a memory phenomenon, and delusions in general, which are common and not necessarily related to memory. In general,

empirical evidence suggests that delusions occur independently of any memory or executive dysfunction.

(Kopelman 1999, p. 203)

The alternative view is that delusions and confabulations present no significant differences in surface features (at least, not when confabulations are persistent), as they can lead to action and be defended with arguments (Berrios 2000). On the basis of these similarities, delusions and confabulation have been placed on a continuum and have been explained on the basis of the same neuropsychological model (Johnson *et al.* 1993; Metcalf *et al.* 2007).

There is no consensus on detailed accounts of what causes confabulation, and multiple deficit models are preferred to single deficit one. There are some motivational accounts, and a variety of cognitive neuropsychological accounts, which seem to focus on one of the following aspects: poor source monitoring (e.g. something imagined is reported as something remembered); a deficit in retrieval strategies (e.g. inability to access relevant memories); or confusion of the temporal order of remembered events (e.g. inability to determine chronology). Not dissimilar from the two-factor account we described for delusions (Langdon and Coltheart 2000), a two-deficit, three-factor theory has been advanced to explain the presence of confabulation and unify some of the considerations made by previous authors about possible neuropsychological causes of the phenomenon. It is unlikely that there is *one* factor-one deficit responsible for *all* pathological cases of confabulation (see Hirstein 2005, p. 21). Confabulation is observed in a variety of pathologies that are likely to differ in neurobiological terms (typically amnesic syndromes including Korsakoff's syndrome, and then accidents involving the anterior cerebral artery, traumatic brain injury, neglect, delusions of misidentification, dementia, and anosognosia). Thus, in the terms of a factor theory, factor one could be instantiated by a number of impairments, among which deficits in strategic memory retrieval or disrupted storage of autobiographical memories, or impeded access to one's experienced past. (Metcalf *et al.* 2007, p. 39).

Personal biases and motivational factors would then intervene as factor two. The explanation for the selectivity of the confabulation, the fact that subjects confabulate on specific topics, is likely to come from factor two, consisting of personal biases and motivational factors. Examples of confabulation that would fit this account can be found in Turnbull and colleagues (2004). The importance of motivational factors in the preference that confabulators usually have for an explanation of the events that is more pleasant than reality is controversial. Turnbull and colleagues (2004, p. 12) consider an interpretation of the data on 'positive' confabulation according to which confabulation 'might occur *in order to* improve the patient's emotional state—such that it protects, or defends, the patient against low mood'. This interpretation would be supported by case studies in which damage caused by illness is mistakenly attributed by the subject to a work-related injury in order to create the illusion of greater control on life events (Weinstein 1991), but cannot be generalised as there are 'negative' or 'neutral' confabulations as well. One more modest hypothesis is that subjects tend to manifest a positive bias in confabulation only when the information is self-referential and presented as relevant to themselves rather than to a third party. The bias would be just an exaggerated form of a self-serving bias which is present in the memories of normal subjects (Fotopoulou *et al.* 2008). Factor three would be similar in all cases of confabulation and delusions (e.g. a failure to inhibit explanatory hypotheses or memories that are implausible or ill-grounded), and could incorporate considerations about defective source monitoring or confusion in the temporal order of memories. In line with this description of factor three, Fotopoulou and Conway (2004, p. 28) report that patients with damage to ventromesial prefrontal cortex are described as 'unable to suppress, monitor, and verify the thoughts and memories that enter consciousness'.

Not all factors would have to be present in the causal account of all types of confabulation. As there can be delusion-like beliefs, in the normal population, so there are instances of confabulatory behaviours that are especially observed when the fabricated or distorted memory or narrative has a defensive function (e.g. protects the subject from self-blame) or is due to source monitoring (e.g. caused by fantasies being taken for facts). Some studies have shown that young children are prone to confabulation (Ceci 1995). For 10 consecutive weeks, children were invited to pick a card with the description of an event and asked whether the event happened to them (e.g. 'got finger caught in a mousetrap'). Then, a different adult interviewed the children discussing both new events, and the events the children had thought about in the previous weeks. The results were very significant: 58% of the children participating produced at least one false narrative, claiming that the fact they had previously imagined really occurred to them, and 28% produced false narratives for most of the events. The most surprising result for the experimenter was the level of detailed information that they provided, and the internal coherence of the narrative. When the tapes of the interviews were shown to professional child psychologists, they were not able to distinguish the true from the false narratives, as the children displayed emotion that was relevant to the narrated facts. When parents told their children these events had not happened, they protested that they remembered them. Here is an example of such a narrative:

> My brother Colin was trying to get Blowtorch from me, and I wouldn't let him take it from me, so he pushed me into the woodpile where the mousetrap was. And then

my finger got caught in it. And then we went to the hospital, and my mommy, daddy, and Colin drove me there, to the hospital in our van, because it was far away. And the doctor put a bandage on this finger.

(Ceci 1995, p. 103)

The participants in the study were pre-schoolers, but other studies have shown that vivid 'memories' of events that never took place can be 'implanted' in adults too. Hyman colleagues (1993) illustrates this in an experiment where college students were asked about personal events that happened during their childhood. Their parents had provided a list of past events and some relevant information to the experimenters. An event that never happened was added to the list before interviewing the students. In the first interview, students did not recall the made-up event, but in a later interview 20% of the participants 'remembered' something about it. A student told the experimenter about a hospitalisation that never happened to her: 'Uh, I remember the nurse, she was a church friend. That helped.'

Confabulatory behaviour can be observed in normal subjects (see Burgess and Shallice 1996; Kopelman 1987; Schacter *et al.* 1995) and is related to the reporting of delusions, the development of self narratives, and the attainment of self knowledge.[22] Given that delusions and confabulations can both be continuous with the behaviour of normal subjects reporting and defending attitudes, and are both defined primarily in epistemic terms, it seems reasonable to leave open the possibility that they significantly overlap in a wide range of cases.

### 1.4.7 Delusions and hypnotically induced beliefs[23]

I hinted at the possibility of delusions and confabulations being observed in non-pathological samples. A good illustration of this phenomenon is offered by beliefs induced by hypnotic suggestions. Are delusion-like states induced by hypnosis significantly similar to delusions observed in clinical settings? Kihlstrom and Hoyt (1988, p. 68) suggested that 'hypnosis may serve as a laboratory model for the study of a wide variety of psychopathological conditions, including delusional states'.

Here are some examples of research that has used hypnosis to model delusion-like experiences. First, in 1961, Sutcliffe explored whether hypnosis could

---

[22] We shall say more about these relations in Chapters 4 and 5.

[23] I worked on the material presented in this section with Amanda Barnier and Rochelle Cox, and I thank them for directing me to the relevant literature on psychopathology and hypnosis.

be used to create a sex-change delusion (a form of identity delusion) in some highly hypnotisable individuals. Building on his work, McConkey and colleagues found that in response to a hypnotic suggestion for a sex-change delusion, highly hypnotisable individuals changed their name, described themselves differently, and selectively processed information that was consistent with their suggested sex (Burn *et al.* 2001; McConkey *et al.* 2001; Noble and McConkey 1995). Second, Zimbardo, Andersen, and Kabat (1981) explored whether a lack of awareness about a suggested change in perception (hearing loss) would produce paranoia. They gave highly hypnotisable participants a suggestion to experience deafness after hypnosis. Half of the participants then received an additional instruction not to be aware of the deafness suggestion (source amnesia suggestion) and half received no additional instructions. After hypnosis, two confederates in the same room as participants engaged in a whispered conversation with each other. Both groups of participants reported difficulty in hearing, but those who were unaware of the source of their deafness (i.e. those who received the source amnesia suggestion) became paranoid about the confederates' conversation and reported more irritation, agitation, hostility, and unfriendliness than participants who had not received the source amnesia suggestion. Third, Cox and Barnier (2009a; 2009b) used hypnosis to model identity delusions by giving subjects a hypnotic suggestion to become a same-sex sibling or a close friend. In response to the suggestion, highly hypnotisable participants changed their name, described themselves differently, and generated autobiographical information from the perspective of their suggested identity. Importantly, the suggested identity delusion was resistant to two challenges—a *contradiction* and a *confrontation*. During the contradiction, participants were asked what they would say if their mother walked into the room and said they were not their suggested identity. During the confrontation, they were asked to open their eyes and look at themselves on a monitor. These two challenge procedures did not breach the delusional experiences of many highly hypnotisable subjects.

In addition, Barnier and her colleagues (2008) observed striking analogies between the behaviour of clinical patients and hypnotic subjects in the way they report the delusional belief, react to the surrounding environment, and respond to challenges. They compared the behaviour of patients in clinical cases of mirrored self misidentification studied by Nora Breen and colleagues (e.g. Breen *et al.* 2000) and that of subjects who received a hypnotic suggestion that they would see a stranger in the mirror. In clinical case 1, patient FE believed his reflection was another person, not himself, who was following him everywhere. In clinical case 2, patient TH also believed that his reflection was another person, not himself. Both FE and TH attempted to converse with their reflected image and were perplexed when the person in the mirror did not reply. In the comparison between the behaviour of these two clinical cases and the hypnotic subjects (Barnier *et al.* 2008), the following manifestations were studied: how the experience of seeing a stranger in the mirror is described; whether an explanation for that experience is articulated, and what form it takes; whether secondary confabulations are generated to justify the experience; whether the characterisation or explanation of the experience is resistant to challenges and apparent counterevidence; and whether the characterisation or explanation of the experience is consistent throughout the experience or whether there are elements of confusion and uncertainty in the subjects' reports.

In response to a specific suggestion, most hypnotic subjects do not recognise their reflection in the mirror, describe the person in the mirror as having different physical characteristics from themselves and refer to their own reflection in the third person. When their suggested delusion is challenged, those who experience the delusion continue to maintain that they do not recognise their reflection in the mirror. Finally, after the hypnotist cancels the suggestion, they express relief at no longer seeing a stranger and they may even engage in personal grooming behaviours in front of the mirror (which were noticeably absent while they reported seeing a stranger in the mirror). These findings suggest many parallels between the features of clinical mirrored self misidentification and its hypnotic analogue. Both are characterised by strong conviction that the person they see in the mirror is not them. One important similarity is that hypnotised individuals, like clinical patients, maintain their mirrored self misidentification delusion in the face of challenges. Even when presented with evidence and rational counterarguments contrary to their beliefs, clinically deluded individuals continue to believe that they are seeing a stranger. When clinical patients TH and FE are challenged by the examiner (Nora Breen) appearing in the mirror alongside them, TH does not recognise her and, although FE does recognise her, he continues to claim that his own reflection is a stranger. When asked to imagine what their family and friends would say about the person in the mirror, hypnotic subjects maintain their belief that they are seeing a stranger. On some occasions, they claim that their family and friends would have no trouble distinguishing them from the stranger. In behavioural challenges, hypnotic subjects argue that the stranger is simply copying their actions, and they easily generate quite sophisticated reasons to maintain and justify their (temporary) delusions. For instance, when asked to touch their nose and to explain what the person in the mirror was doing, one participant said 'she's outside and wants to come in so she's imitating me so I'll feel closer to her'.

Hypnotised individuals, like their clinical counterparts, often express discomfort at seeing the stranger in the mirror staring back. Clinical patient TH used curtains to cover all of the mirrors in his house and he said that whenever he lifted up the corner of a curtain he could see the stranger peering out at him. Similarly, one hypnotised participant commented, 'I was poking my head around as if I was sort of looking at someone secretly.' Clinical patient FE mentioned that the stranger made him feel a bit sick because he moved about so freely with him. Similarly, a number of hypnotic subjects made comments such as 'I felt kind of weird seeing someone just stare at me that close', and 'I didn't trust the other person.' Another striking similarity between clinical and hypnotic delusions is the fact that they give rise to secondary confabulations. In an attempt to recreate somatoparaphrenia in the laboratory, Cox and Barnier gave subjects a hypnotic suggestion to feel like their arms did not belong to them and asked them to describe their arm. One subject (a young woman) said that it was not her arm, but rather the arm of an old man. She scrunched up her face in apparent disgust and said he arm was 'old' with 'old knuckles'. Hypnotic subjects responding to the suggestion that they would see a stranger in the mirror also reported physical differences between themselves and the image in the mirror and often attempted to provide explanations as to whom the person was, or why she tried to copy their behaviour (Barnier et al. 2008).

One obvious difference between clinical and hypnotic delusions is that the former are more persistent. For the most part, hypnotic effects, including hypnotic delusions, are confined to the hypnotic setting. In contrast, clinical delusions persist over time, and often in the face of much stronger and relentless challenges (e.g. constant challenges from family and friends). But based on the similarities we considered, an argument can be made that hypnosis is methodologically useful in the study of delusions (Bortolotti, Cox, and Barnier submitted). It is very challenging to investigate clinical delusions, and in particular the way in which patients defend the content of their beliefs with tentative arguments, construct complex confabulatory explanations, and resist apparent counterevidence. Similarities in the surface features of clinical and hypnotic delusions do not necessarily imply that there are also similarities in underlying mechanisms, although there are some analogies between the two-factor theory of delusion formation and influential accounts of the formation of hypnotic delusions. As we saw, according to the two-factor theory of delusions (Langdon and Coltheart 2000; Davies et al., 2001), delusions are 'breaks' in the way the healthy human mind processes information about self and the world. The first break (factor one) explains the generation of a false hypothesis (e.g. it is not me in the mirror). The second break (factor two) explains why the person fails to reject the hypothesis as implausible given background beliefs, and improbable given the available evidence. These breaks are often, but not always, neuropsychological in origin (Coltheart, 2007; Davies, et al. 2001). But there are other ways to break normal information processing (McKay et al. 2005a; McKay et al. 2007). One such way is with hypnosis (Barnier 2002; Kihlstrom and Hoyt 1988). Hypnotic suggestions can 'break' normal cognitive processing, both to generate false hypotheses (factor one) and to disrupt their normal evaluation (factor two), turning these effects on and off with no lasting consequences (Johnson 2006; Kihlstrom 1988).

There is an extensive literature from the last 30 years on the 'instrumental' use of hypnosis to model pathological phenomena such as auditory hallucinations, functional amnesia, functional blindness, and conversion hysteria (Cox and Bryant 2008). From this and the broader hypnosis literature, there is substantial evidence that hypnotic suggestions create compelling, but temporary breaks in basic cognitive processes (e.g. perception, action, memory) of the kind argued to be involved in delusions and confabulations as factor one (Cox and Bryant 2008; Oakley 2006). For instance, Oakley and colleagues used hypnotic suggestions to create temporary paralysis in healthy subjects, similar to paralysis in somatoparaphrenia. The behaviour, experiences and, notably, brain activation (measured by positron emission tomography) of hypnotised subjects mapped those of a clinical patient diagnosed with hysterical paralysis (Oakley et al. 2003). Similarly, Barnier used hypnotic suggestion to create temporary, partial amnesia of autobiographical events, similar to amnesia in confabulations. Memory disruptions of hypnotised subjects mapped those of clinical patients diagnosed with functional amnesia (Barnier 2002; Barnier et al. 2004). These patterns represented genuine cognitive disruptions, not merely compliance or faking on the part of hypnotised people.

In addition to these factor one-like impairments, hypnosis reduces critical thinking and distorts reality monitoring, akin to the proposed factor two. Hypnotised people will focus on suggested experiences and ignore contradictory information or challenges. For instance, when a male subject received a hypnotic sex-change suggestion to become female, he ignored what he really looked like when he viewed himself on a video-monitor (Burn et al. 2001; Noble and McConkey 1995). Also, hypnotised people attribute as much reality to suggested events as they do to real events. For instance, they believe that a ball they are holding is heating up when this event has been hypnotically suggested to them, no less than they believe it when the ball has chemicals inside it that actually do heat it up (McConkey, 2008). Thus, specific suggestions in hypnosis produce controllable disruptions and distortions to recreate the impact of factor one and factor two in delusions.

To sum up, clinical and hypnotic delusions are sufficiently similar in their surface features to support the claim that hypnosis can be used to study the behavioural manifestations of delusions in the laboratory. However, the aetiology of deluded beliefs across clinical and hypnotic cases may be quite different. In clinical cases the aetiology often includes a neuropsychological impairment; there may be no such impairment in hypnotic delusions. Whereas the neuropsychological impairment presumably produces a 'bottom–up' disruption to cognitive processing (e.g. a disruption in primary perception for faces), hypnotic delusions are created by strategic, 'top–down' processes (e.g. a disruption due to hypnotic ability, social factors, and motivation).

## 1.4.8 Delusions and irrational beliefs

In the literature on delusion, the question whether delusions are beliefs is hotly debated (e.g. Berrios 1991; Bell *et al.* 2006; Hamilton 2007; Frankish 2009; Currie 2000; Currie and Jureidini 2001; Currie and Ravenscroft 2002; Bayne and Pacherie 2005; Gallagher 2009; Sass 1994). Most of the authors who deny belief status to delusions have a negative and a positive thesis. The negative thesis is that delusions are not beliefs (and they mostly use one version of the rationality constraint on belief ascription to prove their point). The positive thesis is an alternative account of what delusions are. For instance, one might argue that delusions are acts of imagination mistakenly taken to have belief status (Currie and Ravenscroft 2002); empty speech acts with no intentional import (Berrios 1991); mental states that appear to have content, but lack the necessary rational connections with the subject's other mental states and thus cannot be beliefs (Cooper, R. 2007); or a sign that the subject has constructed an alternative reality for herself (Sass 1994). Let's concentrate on varieties of the negative thesis. Examples of how the rationality constraint has been used to challenge the belief status of delusions can be found in Campbell (2001) and in Currie and Jureidini (2001).

> The strategy we are proposing for at least some delusions is one that seeks to protect the idea of essentially rational belief from attack by arguing that the delusions in question are not beliefs at all.

> (Currie and Jureidini 2001, p. 161)

How people argue against the view that delusions are beliefs on the basis of the rationality constraint on belief ascription depends on their chosen notion of rationality. The relevant notion of rationality needs to be such that (a) it is plausible as a necessary condition for belief ascription, and (b) delusions do not satisfy it. Negative arguments often make the claim that delusions infringe all three notions of rationality, procedural, epistemic, and agential. For instance,

Currie and Jureidini (2001, p. 161) argue that delusions are more plausibly imaginings than beliefs, because delusions are not action-guiding ('when imaginings masquerade as beliefs, you can have conviction without action-guidance'), because delusions 'fail, sometimes spectacularly, to be integrated with what the subject really does believe', and because they are not sensitive to empirical data available to the subject. As we saw, the structure of the most common objections to the doxastic conception of delusions is very simple: there is a rationality constraint on belief ascription and, if delusions are irrational (in the relevant sense), then they cannot be beliefs.

I identify five main arguments against the doxastic conception of delusions. These arguments can, of course, be used in combination, and it is possible for a belief-like state to deviate from norms of procedural, epistemic and agential rationality all at once.

- *Bad Integration.* If delusions violate norms of procedural rationality, by being badly integrated with the subject's beliefs or other intentional states, then they are not beliefs.
- *Lack of Support.* If delusions violate norms of epistemic rationality, by being formed on the basis of insufficient evidence, then they are not beliefs.
- *Unresponsiveness to Evidence.* If delusions violate norms of epistemic rationality, by resisting revision in face of counter-evidence, then they are not beliefs.
- *Failure of Action Guidance.* If subjects with delusions violate norms of agential rationality, by failing to act on the content of their delusions in the relevant circumstances, then they are not ascribed beliefs.
- *Failure of Reason Giving.* If subjects with delusions violate norms of agential rationality, by not endorsing the content of the delusion on the basis of good reasons, then they are not ascribed beliefs.[24]

Assessing each of these arguments requires assessing both empirical and conceptual claims. Let's take the bad integration objection to the belief status of delusions as an example. In order to see whether the argument is convincing, I need to examine an empirical claim about delusions first: Are they procedurally irrational? Then, I need to assess a conceptual claim, the claim that being procedurally irrational is an obstacle to belief ascription, to the point that reported states cannot be ascribed as beliefs at all, if they fail to satisfy the standards of procedural rationality. If both claims are supported by evidence or argumentation, then the *bad integration* objection succeeds: no procedurally irrational state can be ascribed as a belief; delusions are procedurally irrational; therefore, delusions cannot be ascribed as beliefs.

---

[24] These arguments are ubiquitous in the literature on the nature of delusions, although the terminology varies. Bayne and Pacherie (2005) discuss versions of these five arguments.

We shall carefully review this and the other arguments against the doxastic conception of delusions in the rest of the book, and hopefully develop a convincing account of delusions as irrational beliefs by challenging applications of the rationality constraint on belief ascription. Other strategies have been adopted in order to support the continuity between delusions and other beliefs. A large contingent of philosophers and psychologists insist that there is continuity between delusions and other beliefs. Richard Bentall gathered and commented upon a vast amount of empirical data about the temporal variations in delusions reported by people affected by psychopathologies, and the presence of delusion-like beliefs in the normal population.

> [...] [E]vidence against a categorical distinction between delusions and normal beliefs has been supplemented by recent studies which have shown that quasi-delusional ideas are surprisingly common in normal population samples.

> (Bentall 2003, p. 294)

Brendan Maher (1974) suggested that subjects form delusional explanations in the same way in which they form ordinary beliefs. Their explanations sound weird, because the event they need to explain is an abnormal perceptual experience. The anomalous character of delusions lies exclusively in the perceptual experience—reasoning is unimpaired. Maher's account is attractive, but significantly different from mine. He concludes that delusions are continuous with beliefs because both delusions and beliefs are *rational*. I won't deny that delusions are irrational, but argue that they are irrational in a way that is not qualitatively different way from the irrationality of other mental states that we are happy to regard as typical beliefs.

There are other two arguments against the doxastic conception of delusions that I will not consider in detail in the rest of the book, but that I should mention here. The first is that beliefs need to be true or plausible (*substantive* or *content* rationality constraint), and delusions aren't. The second is that, in order to have beliefs, one needs to be able to attribute beliefs to oneself and others (the *theory of mind* constraint), and subjects with delusions have an impaired theory of mind. These arguments deserve a much more comprehensive treatment than the one I can offer here, but let me just explain why I have chosen not to discuss them at greater length in the book.

The substantive rationality constraint is either about truth, or about plausibility. If it is about truth, it is an interesting constraint, but does not seem to be about rationality as such, as it does not involve reasoning competence. Further, any truth constraint on the ascription of beliefs would have to explain why we do not seem to have any significant difficulty in interpreting people who report false beliefs. If the constraint is about plausibility, then it collapses into arguments that I will discuss in much more detail in Chapters 2 and 3. When we say that we cannot have a radically false belief, we may want to say either that the belief content needs to be plausible *given* the content of the other beliefs the subject has (which is a notion captured by the norm of good integration within the scope of procedural rationality) or that the belief content needs to be probable *given* the evidence available to the subject (which is a notion captured by the norms of good evidential support and responsiveness to evidence within the scope of epistemic rationality).

The theory of mind constraint has been widely endorsed in the literature on belief ascription (Davidson 1975, 2001; Carruthers 1989, 2005) but the conceptual link between having beliefs and being able to ascribe beliefs to oneself or others remains difficult to motivate (in its unqualified formulations), more difficult to motivate, in fact, than the rationality constraint. Why should we accept that a subject has the capacity to possess beliefs only when she has the capacity to ascribe beliefs to others? Some philosophers defend the theory of mind constraint on belief ascription because they suppose that, in order to have mental states that are genuinely conscious, or to have mental states that can play a holistic causal and conceptual role in one's mental economy, one needs to be able to distinguish between fact and representation, objectivity and subjectivity, and one can do so only if one has the concept of 'belief'. This is a counterintuitive move, because the capacity to ascribe beliefs to others requires the capacity to have beliefs *about beliefs*, which seems to be a more sophisticated capacity than the capacity to have beliefs in the first place. It may be plausible to claim that in order to have *some* beliefs (such as beliefs about mental states, or beliefs about unobservable theoretical entities) one needs the capacity for second-order beliefs, but it is not plausible to generalise this claim to *all* beliefs (including basic perceptual beliefs). Even if we were convinced by the conceptual claim that subjects can have beliefs only if they can ascribe beliefs to others, we would then need to assess the empirical claim that subjects with delusions have an impaired theory of mind. The literature suggests that subjects with delusions do not perform as well as other subjects with respect to certain theory of mind tasks and that theory of mind is impaired in schizophrenia (Brüne 2005; Pickup 2008; Harrington *et al.* 2005). Moreover, Frith's metarepresentational account of the positive symptoms of schizophrenia suggests that impaired monitoring of intentions plays an important role in the occurrence of hallucinations and delusions. Nonetheless, no specific link between failures in theory of mind and delusions has yet been firmly established: it is possible that good performance in theory of mind tasks requires capacities that are impaired in subjects with schizophrenia, independent of the occurrence of delusions. For instance, some correlations have been found between poor performance in theory of mind tasks and low IQ or biased probabilistic reasoning (Garety and Freeman

1999, pp. 121–2). Future research will hopefully shed some light on the empirical connections between these phenomena.

## Summary of chapter 1

In this chapter I have introduced debates about the nature of beliefs and delusions to which the other chapters will more substantially contribute. I started with what I take beliefs to be, that is, intentional states that typically hang together with other beliefs in a system, are sensitive to evidence and give rise to behavioural dispositions. Then, I presented the rationality constraint on the ascription of beliefs: irrational behaviour does not support the ascription of beliefs. In order to clarify the implications of the constraint, I distinguished three aspects of rationality that apply to beliefs or believers: procedural, epistemic and agential. Finally, I introduced the notion of delusions. Although I did not settle with a definition of what delusions are, I offered a description of the epistemic features of delusions and of the relationship between delusions, self deception, confabulation, obsessions, and hypnotically induced beliefs. How these conditions are identified is informative about the way in which the concept of 'delusion' is used. Delusions are characterised in terms of their epistemic features, but the failures of rationality observable in subjects with delusions are not sufficient conditions for something to be a delusion.

With the notions of belief, rationality, and delusions already sketched, and the rationality constraint on belief ascription clearly formulated, I could frame the debate on the nature of delusions: following the rationality constraint on belief ascription, delusions are denied belief status, because they present elements of procedural, epistemic, and agential rationality. I listed five objections to the doxastic conception of delusions which we shall discuss in the rest of the book. The main problem with these objections (as we shall see) is that they assume an idealised conception of beliefs, and blind us to the possibility that we are all procedurally, epistemically, and agentially irrational in systematic and (sometimes) disturbing ways.

# Chapter 2

# Procedural rationality and belief ascription

It is only when beliefs are inconsistent with other beliefs according to principles held by the agent himself -in other words, only when there is an inner inconsistency- that there is a clear case of irrationality. Strictly speaking, then, the irrationality consists not in any particular belief but in inconsistency within a set of beliefs.
(Donald Davidson, *Incoherence and Irrationality*)

If someone says that he has discovered a kind of belief which is peculiar in that there is no obligation to resolve or even to be concerned about inconsistencies between these beliefs and beliefs of any other kind, then the correct response to him is to say that he is talking about something other than belief.
(Currie and Ravenscroft, *Recreative Minds*)

In this chapter I assess an argumentative strategy against the doxastic conception of delusions which is based on the procedural rationality constraint on belief ascription. The stronger version of the argument is that delusions cannot be beliefs because they are procedurally irrational. The norm of procedural rationality delusions are supposed to infringe is that of good integration, that is, delusions are badly integrated with the subject's beliefs. There is also a weaker argument I consider. Even if the delusion is procedurally irrational, it is possible to regard the delusion as a belief, but as a belief with indeterminate content. The problem is that ascribing beliefs with indeterminate content might not support explanation and prediction of the subject's behaviour in intentional terms.

Here is what the strong version of the *bad integration* objection to the doxastic conception of delusions looks like:

i) In order for *b* to be ascribed as a belief to a subject, *b* needs to be well-integrated with the subject's beliefs.

ii) Delusions are badly integrated with a subject's beliefs.

Thus, delusions cannot be ascribed to a subject as beliefs.

In Section 2.1, I consider instances of the *bad integration* objection to the doxastic conception of delusions, and ask an empirical question, whether delusions really are procedurally irrational with respect to the norm of good integration. The main purpose will be to assess premise (ii) of the bad integration argument.

In Section 2.2, I turn to the question whether ordinary beliefs satisfy the demands of procedural rationality, and come to a conclusion about whether procedural rationality is a legitimate constraint on the ascription of beliefs. The main purpose will be to start assessing premise (i).

In Section 2.3, I explore the possible differences between the procedural irrationality of delusions and that of ordinary beliefs. Are delusions procedurally irrational in a qualitatively different way? Does this justify denying belief status to them, but not to ordinary (procedurally irrational) beliefs? The aim here is to complete the assessment of premise (i) and some relevant modifications of it.

In Section 2.4, I discuss a weaker formulation of the procedural rationality constraint that represents a more plausible challenge to the intentional treatment of delusions, although it does not lead to a straight-forward rejection of their belief status.

In the end, I invite you to give up the idea of a procedural rationality constraint on the ascription of beliefs, and thus reject the bad integration objection against the doxastic conception of delusions.

## 2.1 Bad integration in delusions

According to the procedural rationality constraint on belief ascription, we cannot ascribe beliefs to subjects who make obvious mistakes in deductive reasoning, or fail to obey basic inferential rules governing the relations among beliefs and other intentional states. This constraint (see for instance Dennett 1979) has been very influential in the philosophy of mind, but also in psychology, anthropology, and sociology. Although it is possible for a belief system to have some internal tension, most philosophers resist the thought that subjects capable of having beliefs can have dissonant attitudes simultaneously activated and operative, at the forefront of their minds.

Suppose that Tim, a company manager in a job hiring committee, sincerely believes that physical appearance should not be a consideration in the selection of applicants, because it is irrelevant to their capacity to contribute to the company's success as junior accountants. But in the final meeting of the committee, when members need to decide whether to make an offer to one or the other of two applicants with equivalent qualifications and experience and who performed equally well in the interview process, Tim argues that the most attractive of the two applicants should be offered the job, because 'she presents herself better'. Can an interpreter ascribe to Tim the belief that physical appearance doesn't matter? There might be many understandable reasons why people report or defend attitudes that are in conflict with one another, or report an attitude that is not reflected in subsequent behaviour.[1] But invariably dissonance creates a problem for the interpreter. Subjects with delusions are often charged with having incoherent belief systems, or dissonant attitudes. These are cases in which subjects with delusions endorse conflicting statements in the same stretch of conversation, where one statement implies the falsity of the other. In those circumstances, it is tempting to say that the subject's reports are too badly integrated with the subject's beliefs to be themselves reports of beliefs, or that the subject is using words and uttering sentences without appreciating their meaning.

However, critics of the rationality constraint have started from the observation that subjects whose behaviour is not procedurally rational are often ascribed beliefs, and have turned these observations into counterexamples to those theories of belief ascription that explicitly rely on a procedural rationality constraint.[2] In order to reply to these objections, some philosophers (Davidson 1982; Davidson 1985a; Davidson 1985b; Heal 1998) have adopted the background argument, a strategy which I briefly sketched in Chapter 1 and I will examine here in much more detail. According to the background argument, only within a belief system that is largely (procedurally) rational can belief status be granted to belief-like states that fail to meet the standards of (procedural) rationality.[3] Dissonant beliefs and beliefs that result from mistakes in deductive reasoning or bad inference may be characterised as beliefs, but only against a general background of (procedural) rationality. According to one influential characterisation of the background argument, due to Donald Davidson, there are two main requirements that a subject must satisfy in order to count as a believer: (1) she cannot explicitly violate a fundamental norm of (procedural) rationality, such as that of coherence, and (2) she cannot fail to recover from a violation of a norm of (procedural) rationality once this violation is made explicit to her.

---

[1] I shall discuss attitude-behaviour inconsistencies in Chapter 4.

[2] Classic objections to the rationality constraint on belief ascription in its idealised form can be found in Stich (1981), Lukes (1982), and Cherniak (1986).

[3] Similar considerations can apply to cases of epistemic or agential irrationality, but here I shall focus on procedural rationality as it is the most fundamental notion of rationality according to Davidson.

## 2.1.1 **Bad integration and meaning**

Delusions seem to violate the requirements of the background argument. Not only can delusions fail to cohere with the subject's beliefs, but they may also constitute an *explicit* violation of fundamental norms of procedural rationality.

> Rationality is a normative constraint of consistency and coherence on the formation of a set of beliefs and thus is prima facie violated in two ways by the delusional subject. First she accepts a belief that is incoherent with the rest of her beliefs, and secondly she refuses to modify that belief in the face of fairly conclusive counterevidence and a set of background beliefs that contradict the delusional belief.
>
> (Gerrans 2000, p. 114)

> Delusions do not seem to respect the idea that the belief system forms a coherent whole and that adjustments to one belief will require adjustments to many others.
>
> (Young 2000, p. 49)

McKay and Cipolotti (2007) refer to the case of LU, a subject with Cotard delusion, who reported that she was dead. She was asked about how she knew whether someone was dead. She answered that dead people are motionless, and don't speak. Then she was asked to explain why she could move and speak, and she acknowledged the tension between her thoughts about dead people and her thought that she was dead. Yet, she did not give up the delusion that she was dead. In the long term, the cognitive probing caused her to doubt her delusion, and a week after her initial assessment she no longer reported she was dead.

The most direct way to argue that subjects with delusions fail to satisfy the demands of procedural rationality is to show that they are inconsistent. In interviews with patients this seems to be often the case.

> In the course of the same interview, she clearly stated that her husband had died suddenly four year earlier and had been cremated (this was correct), but also that her husband was a patient on the ward in the same hospital.
>
> (Breen *et al.* 2000, p. 91)

The patient described by Breen and colleagues suffers from reduplicative paramnesia (the delusion that a place has been duplicated) and is committed to two conflicting reports that cannot both be true. The death of the subject's husband 4 years earlier implies that he cannot be in the hospital where she is. This is a very serious case of bad integration. Similarly, a woman with a long history of schizophrenia and with reverse intermetamorphosis (the delusion that one has transformed into another person) reported to be a man, first her father, then her grandfather, and finally her father again, during the same session (Breen *et al.* 2000). Some attempts at self-identification were defended with reasons and made with abundance of details about relevant family relations and occupation; at other times the subject just appeared confused.

> RZ found it difficult to maintain the delusion when she was interviewed and asked persistent questions about her identity. During the course of the interview she switched identity from her father to her grandfather and then back to her father. At another point her delusional identity broke down completely, and she said 'I'm just confused. It feels like they've taken my brain out and I don't even have a brain'.
>
> (Breen *et al.* 2000, p. 98)

Further evidence of bad integration is available in subjects with delusions, in terms of dissonance among attitudes or lack of mutual support between the reported delusions and the subject's beliefs. For instance, people suffering from anosognosia (denial of illness) deny that their limbs are paralysed, and yet they may recognise that they have difficulties in carrying out everyday tasks such as lifting bags or climbing stairs (Berti *et al.* 1998; House and Hodges 1988; Aimola 1999). Although the two attitudes are not strictly speaking inconsistent, they are badly integrated with one another—e.g. subjects may have no plausible explanation for the acknowledged difficulties they face.

These interesting cases can prompt two objections to the doxastic conception of delusions based on bad integration. First, they invite us to reflect upon the relationship between rationality, meaning and belief. A subject cannot be said to have a belief about death unless she masters the concept of death.[4] And when a subject deviates from rationality, reporting apparent beliefs about death that an interpreter would regard as wildly implausible, one explanation is that the subject does not master the concept of death and thus does not have genuine beliefs about death. In the Cotard case described earlier, the irrationality of the subject's report might lead the interpreter to suppose that the speaker lacks a proper grasp of the concept of death, and thus she cannot be said to have beliefs about death. Second, these cases suggest that delusions are not like beliefs, because they are maintained even when they are incompatible with other beliefs. For any subject with beliefs, the argument goes, awareness of two beliefs in open conflict with each other prompts a reaction: suspension of judgement until further evidence is available, revision or rejection of one of the clashing beliefs. But this does not seem to happen to subjects with delusions. They are typically resistant to restoring conformity to the norms of procedural rationality even after 'Socratic tutoring'.

---

[4] This is a point often rehearsed in the literature on the possibility of animal beliefs: Fido cannot have beliefs about squirrels because he is not a competent user of the concept 'squirrel'.

Campbell describes the rationality constraint approach to beliefs in a way that highlights the role of meaning considerations:

> It is often said that rationality on the part of the subject is a precondition on the ascription of propositional attitudes such as beliefs and desires. One simple reason for thinking that rationality is critical here is that unless you assume the other person is rational, it does not seem possible to say what the significance is of ascribing any particular propositional state to the subject.

(Campbell 2001, p. 89)

> The problem with ascribing irrationality is that if she really knows the meaning of the words she is using, how can she be reasoning so wrongly? Surely a grasp of meaning does provide you with a capacity for correct reasoning using the term.

(Campbell 2001, p. 90)

Delusions are often described as disturbances of meaning, and the Cotard delusion, with its very bizarre content, is an excellent example of how we might come to doubt that the person reporting the delusion understands the meaning of the words she uses. An account of the Cotard delusion identifies the source of the strange report in an anomalous perceptual experience due to a neurological deficit to the affective component of visual recognition. As a result, the subject does not seem to experience familiarity with anything around her, and instead of supposing that something is amiss with the external environment, she postulates that she has undergone a drastic change such as depersonalisation or death (Young and Leafhead 1996; McKay and Cipolotti 2007). Young and Leafhead (1996) suggest that subjects with Cotard have an internalising attribution style, that is, a general tendency to attribute the responsibility of events to themselves rather than to external factors or other people. McKay and Cipolotti (2007) found some empirical confirmation that impairments in processing faces and the internalising bias are observed in subjects with Cotard. An alternative view is that both the lack of affect and the strange explanation for it are due to psychotic depression: Gerrans (2000) argues that the presence of an internalising bias is not sufficient to explain the formation of the delusion, and claims that 'the delusion is a rationalisation of a feeling of disembodiment based on global suppression of affect resulting from extreme depression' (p. 112).[5]

If LU knows what 'death' means, and she knows that dead people don't feel anything, don't move and don't talk to the living, then she should not believe

---

[5] Berrios and Luque (1995b) reconstruct the conceptual history of the disorder and observe that initially Cotard syndrome indicated merely a subtype of depression. Only recently has it been identified as a separate condition with its own neurological correlates.

that she is dead. Rather than ascribing to her the belief that she is dead, an interpreter is likely to conclude that she doesn't know the meaning of 'death' or that she fails to master the concept on this occasion. But in the case of LU (and many other subjects with delusions) there seems to be no problem with the subject's understanding of the concept of death. She correctly answers questions about death and concedes that dead people don't move and don't talk. Apart from her conviction that she is dead, there would be no reason to believe that her concept of death differs from that of her interpreter.[6] What surprises us about LU is that she refuses to change her mind about whether she is dead after she is reminded of what 'death' means and what people look like when they are dead. Subjects with delusions not only report states that conflict with their beliefs, but tolerate such conflicts. One reason why the interpreter might withhold the ascription of beliefs to LU (when it comes to claims about her death) is that she is expected to reject the thought that she is dead if she knows what 'death' means. There are some case studies indicating that, at least initially, subjects with delusions fail to take action in the face of dissonant attitudes, or endorse attitudes that do not match their subsequent behaviour.

In Currie (2002) and Currie and Ravenscroft (2002), the phenomenon of delusions that are not well-integrated with the subject's beliefs is turned into an explicit argument against the doxastic conception of delusions. Subjects with delusions can appear indifferent to the existing dissonance between their delusions and their beliefs. But subjects are not indifferent to dissonance among their beliefs, and attempt to reduce dissonance, if they are made aware of it. This must mean that delusions are not beliefs. In this chapter, we examine in some detail the claim that subjects with belief must be disposed to restore coherence in their belief system when they are made aware of existing conflicts.

This debate can help us choose between competing theoretical accounts of the nature of delusions, but is also relevant to clinical practice and psychiatric treatment. If disruption of shared meaning and imperviousness to revision were central aspects of delusional thought, they would have implications for the effectiveness of cognitive probing for subjects with delusions, or for the effectiveness of any therapy that relies on there being successful communication between patient and therapist. If subjects were not completely insensitive

---

6 The issue of shared versus private meaning in the context of delusional reports deserves more attention, and we shall come back to the view that delusions involve a renegotiation of meanings in Chapter 4.

to the game of arguments and counterarguments with respect to the content of their delusional states, challenges and attempts at Socratic tutoring would make no contribution to the breaching of the delusion.

The importance of preserving or restoring integration among attitudes is one of the bases of cognitive behavioural therapy. For instance, Nelson (2005) describes aspects of procedural rationality as core concepts for cognitive therapy:

> The thoughts we have about a situation and the way we interpret it are inextricably linked to our beliefs about ourselves and the world.
>
> (Nelson 2005, p. 1)

> Contradictory beliefs can coexist if undetected, but once a situation occurs that brings this conflict into awareness, then it is usual for either or both the beliefs to be modified to return harmony to the system.
>
> (Nelson 2005, p. 8)

Here is an example. One of the main strategies used to challenge a woman's belief that she is evil and ease her sense of guilt includes making her aware that she has conflicting attitudes (Nelson 2005, p. 165). On the one hand, she knows that those who are evil want other people to suffer and don't do nice things; on the other hand, she believes that she does nice things, such as sharing food with others. Drawing the subject's attention to the dissonance between the things that she believes relies on the assumption that subject is disposed to reduce or eliminate dissonance when she becomes aware of it. The strategy can be more or less effective depending on the type of delusion, and the individual case history. Literature on the use of cognitive behavioural therapy for subjects with persecutory delusions suggests that the conviction in the content of the delusion and the preoccupation with the delusion can be reduced significantly as a result of these challenges, but the outcome does not often include a reassessment of the delusional states or a satisfactory elimination of dissonance (Garety *et al.* 2008; Kingdon *et al.* 2008).

Let us explore issues of procedural rationality in two types of delusions: monothematic and circumscribed delusion such as the Capgras delusion, and polythematic and elaborated delusions such as persecutory delusions. In both types of delusions, we shall find violations of procedural rationality.

## 2.1.2 Dissonance and double-bookkeeping

Subjects with Capgras delusion and with delusions of persecution can be charged with procedural irrationality. Typically, people with Capgras delusion claim that their spouses or close relatives have been replaced by impostors. Stone and Young (1997) argue that the delusion arises when the affective component of the face-processing module is damaged, leaving recognition unimpaired. The subject sees the spouse's face and recognises it as a face identical (or almost identical) to that of the spouse, but experiences it as the face of a stranger. Coltheart (2005b) maintains that the lack of autonomic response to the familiar face is not something the subject is aware of, or she attends to. But the failed prediction that the face with those features will generate an autonomic response needs an explanation and hypotheses are generated and tested to account for that. According to two-factor theories of delusions, a reasoning bias or deficit is also necessary for the acceptance and the maintenance of the hypothesis that the face seen is that of a stranger, an impostor. The Capgras delusion is monothematic, that is, it is often confined to the alleged substitution of the spouse or close relative with a clone, an alien or a robot that looks identical (or almost identical) to the original person. Possible causes are brain injury or stroke. But the delusion can appear together with other pathologies such as paranoia and obsessive thoughts (e.g. in schizophrenia), and can be one of the first symptoms of a degenerative disorder such as Alzheimer's disease.[7]

Are subjects with Capgras procedurally irrational? Individual differences in subjects' reports do not support a general answer to this question. There is some evidence that subjects with Capgras attempt to integrate their delusional state with other things they know or experience. A subject asked to explain why the 'impostor' had the ring he gave to his wife replied that the ring was not the same one, just a very similar one. Another subject with Capgras delusion asked why he had not reported the disappearance of his wife to the police candidly answered that the police would have never believed that his wife had been replaced by aliens. To some extent, these subjects integrated their delusional states in their system of beliefs. But the attempts to integrate the delusion with beliefs and other intentional states are not always successful. In some cases, subjects can go on with their lives substantially unchanged and show very little concern about their unusual situation or the alleged disappearance of their spouses. In these latter cases, the delusion does not necessarily interact with the subjects' beliefs, or with their emotions. The radical circumscription of the delusion is a clear sign of bad integration.

In the case reported by Lucchelli and Spinnler (2007), a man with progressive loss of memory and first signs of obsessive-compulsive disorder started claiming that his wife had been replaced by a double. In the description of the

---

[7] For accounts of the Capgras delusion, see Gerrans (2000); Langdon and Coltheart (2000); Davies and Coltheart (2000); Bayne and Pacherie (2004a); Fine *et al.* (2005).

case offered by the patient's wife, we see integration and circumscription co-existing: at times, Fred acts as if he is worried about the disappearance of his wife Wilma and actively looks for her (names are fictitious); at other times, he treats the double in a kind and even flirtatious way. These effects on behaviour give us some insight into whether Fred's delusion that his wife has been replaced is well-integrated with his beliefs about what to do when someone disappears, whether doubles have bad intentions, and so on.

> Fred started to behave toward her as if she were not the real Wilma, but another woman who, as he himself stated, bore the same name, had the same physical appearance and the same voice, wore the same clothes, lived in the same house, but nevertheless was a different Wilma. In some cases the disappearance of his 'real' wife upset him: he repeatedly asked where she was, obviously worried about her. On one occasion, despite his wife's strong protests, he left the house and went looking for her in the streets; when he came back after a few hours, he looked relieved to find her at home and anxiously asked where she had been and why she had not told him she was going out. On another occasion, he urged her to go with him to the police to report Wilma's disappearance. Most of the times, however, he seemed quite pleased to see her as the 'double' Wilma and addressed her in a very gentle way. His wife described his manner as 'courting as when we were dating'.
>
> (Lucchelli and Spinnler 2007, p. 189)

Do we observe the same inconsistencies in subjects with polythematic delusions? Polythematic delusions tend to have wider repercussions on the subjects' lives and frequent in subjects with schizophrenia. According to an influential account of the formation of persecutory delusions, these are caused by 'a disturbance of the psychological processes mediating the formation and maintenance of normal social beliefs' (Blackwood *et al.* 2001, p. 527). The accepted view is that ordinary social beliefs seem to be formed in two stages. First, the subject gathers some data about the social environment that is relevant to her situation and her conception of herself. Second, the subject makes hypotheses on the basis of the data and infers what other people's intentions towards herself are. The process of formation of social beliefs might also involve background information about autobiographical experience concerning past social situations and relationships with others. In subjects with persecutory delusions the two stages of belief formation are affected by attentional and attributional biases, which might reflect a combination of neuropsychological deficits and motivational factors. When the subject gathers data about the surrounding social environment, she tends to focus on *threat-related stimuli*. When the subject appeals to background information, she tends to think of herself as responsible for events with a positive outcome (*self-enhancing bias*), and she tends not to take blame for events with a negative outcome (*self-protective bias*). These attributional biases are supposed to have a defensive function, that is, the subjects 'protect themselves from feelings of personal inadequacy by blaming disappointments on malevolent others' (Bentall *et al.* 2001, p. 1150) so as to preserve their self-esteem. The hypothesis is that, together with the attentional bias, self-enhancing and protective biases contribute to the formation of persecutory delusions – although data do not always seem to support this hypothesis.[8]

The subject with persecutory delusions typically believes that some individual, organisation or force, is trying to harm her in some way. The threat could be to damage the subject's reputation, to injure her body, to drive her mad or to bring about her death. A young psychology student thought he was the Messiah and that the CIA wanted to prosecute him for treason. In another famous case, the German judge Schreber believed that his physician was transforming him into a woman in order to sexually abuse him. The persecutors are often individuals the patient knows, or influential religious or political groups and organisations.

Sass describes the world of experience of a subject affected by persecutory delusions by reference to Schreber's autobiography.

> A [...] feature Jaspers considered to be characteristic of schizophrenia is what he called the 'delusional atmosphere' or 'mood' - an overwhelming but almost indescribable transformation of the perceptual world that often precedes or accompanies the development of delusions. In that peculiar state of mind the perceptual world seems to have undergone some subtle but all-encompassing change: unfamiliar events and objects may seem like copies or repetitions of themselves; perceptual phenomena may seem tremendously specific and deeply meaningful, but without the patient being able to explain why.
>
> (Sass 1994, p. 5)

The distinction between mono- and polythematic delusions should not be taken too rigidly. In some circumstances the delusion that a close relative is an impostor is accompanied by suspiciousness towards the alleged impostor which can have the features of a full-blown delusion of persecution.

> She claimed that her son had been replaced by two impostors, which over the next week became four. This delusion also included her daughter-in law and her granddaughter. She said of her son, 'There's been someone like my son's double which isn't my son... I can tell my son because my son is different... but you have got to be quick to notice it.' She renamed one of her son's alleged impostors 'John Yates' and said this one wished to rape her.
>
> (Young *et al.* 1993, p. 696)

---

[8] See Freeman *et al.* (2008) for recent accounts of persecutory delusions.

Both mono- and polythematic delusions can be badly integrated with the subject's beliefs. To make this point, I shall summarise a first-personal account of persecution (Payne 1992) that appeared in the *Schizophrenia Bulletin*. After a history of depression and alcoholism, RP started having vivid visual hallucinations and experiencing 'TV broadcasting'. People at the TV station were forcing her to watch certain movies. She made drawings of strange monsters and she hid them for fear of being watched. She became aware of a magical force being around her and compelling her to do things. For instance, the 'force' made her walk alone at 2 or 3 am in her dangerous neighbourhood, so that she could be killed. During her walks, she felt she was in another dimension. The world started being populated with Alien Beings who revealed themselves to RP alone, and soon after took over her body and 'removed her from it'. They took her to a faraway place with beaches and sunlight, and placed an alien in her body to act like her. She felt she did not exist and she could not make contact with her kidnapped self. The Aliens started taking over other people as well, removing them from their bodies and putting Aliens in their place. RP thought she was the only one to have the power to realise what was happening. The Alien Beings were in control of RP by now and giving her a complex system of rules, among which was the rule of not telling anybody about them. If she had told someone, they would have killed her. She started feeling that she had power over the behaviour of animals and that other people could read her mind. She was sure people were always talking about her.

In this case, there is a plethora of delusions, including people's substitution, alien control and persecution. RP's delusional beliefs are part of a general narrative: from the first-person account of her delusions, one gets the impression that all events happening in her life were interpreted by her in the light of her conviction that the force and the Alien Beings were persecuting her. RP's delusions, as it appears from her full-length report, play the role of beliefs in her cognitive and practical life. For instance, her most important decisions, whether to keep in touch with her family, change job or move to another city, were made on the basis of her delusional states and the fear and anxiety that they were causing her. This shows that RP's persecutory delusion was not circumscribed, but does not show that it was well-integrated with her other attitudes. The very report of her delusional states shows some instances of bad integration: it is not at all clear, for instance, how the TV people, the force and the Alien Being were related to one another; and it is not consistent for RP to claim that *she* wanted to communicate with *her real self* which had been disembodied.

Thus, the application of the procedural rationality constraint on belief ascription poses a challenge for the doxastic conception of both mono- and polythematic delusions. However, challenging the belief status of delusions is never a comfortable move. On the one hand, subjects with delusions seem to behave as if they truly believed the content of their delusions. The subject with Capgras who reports to believe that the woman living with him is an impostor and starts showing hostility to her, if not aggression, behaves in a way that suggests that he genuinely believes his report. Similarly, subjects with persecutory delusions follow through the consequences of their conviction that malevolent others are trying to harm them, and live in great anxiety and distress. On the other hand, these delusions are not well-integrated within the subjects' belief systems, and can be significantly dissonant with other attitudes. Subjects with Capgras often exhibit covert recognition of the pre-sumed impostors and can learn to tolerate presence of such impostors in their lives. Subjects with persecutory delusions express belief-like states that do not amount to a plausible explanation of their experiences and conflict with one another.

### 2.1.3 Delusions as imaginings or alternative realities

If we are attracted to the conclusion of the bad integration argument against the doxastic conception of delusions, we have to start looking for an alternative account of what delusions are. Greg Currie (2000) argues that the presence of significant dissonance between the delusion and the subject's beliefs should alert us to the possibility that at least some delusions are *imaginings*. There is no requirement for the content of one's imaginings to be consistent with the content of one's beliefs—which means that, if delusions are imaginings, then their bad integration with the subject's beliefs does not constitute an infringe-ment of procedural rationality. Currie suggests that a subject's delusion is due to the subject imagining that something is the case and misidentifying her own attitude as a belief. Let's suppose that Jim suffers from persecutory delusions. He *imagines* that everybody hates him, but he misidentifies his imagining *as a belief*. Jim takes himself to believe that everybody hates him and (some of the time) acts as if he had this belief.

What is responsible for the abnormality of Jim's delusional state? It might be perfectly acceptable for Jim to imagine that everybody hates him. Jim is at fault not because he imagines that everybody hates him, or because he forms the irrational belief that everybody hates him, but because he is not a good interpreter of himself. As Currie puts it, there is something amiss in Jim's metarepresentational capacities. (The account of delusions developed along these lines by Currie and colleagues is referred to in the literature as the *metarep-resentational* account of delusions). Notice that Currie's suggestion is not incom-patible with an attempt to characterise the pathological features of delusions in doxastic terms. According to Currie, there is a belief involved in the delusion (Jim's meta-belief that he believes that everybody hates him). Jim believes that he believes that everybody hates him without in fact having any good reasons for believing that he has that belief. Jim's behaviour can be explained and predicted via the ascription of a belief, the meta-belief that he believes that everybody hates him, whereas he just imagines that this is the case. On this account, there is a false and ill-grounded belief involved in the delusion: it is a special kind of belief, a belief about what one believes. Currie concedes that, when a subject believes that she believes that something is the case, often she also ends up having the first-order belief. Returning to my fictional example, Jim might end up believing that everybody hates him as an effect of his believing that he has that belief. On the basis of these considerations, even those delusions that might be plausibly characterised as imaginings misidentified as beliefs can be seen as having a doxastic character and involving false and ill-grounded beliefs.[9]

There are strong elements of continuity between the doxastic and the metarepresentational account of delusions, in that they both identify the pathological nature of delusions in the acceptance of a false and ill-grounded belief. However, there are also elements of discontinuity between the two theses, and I would like to focus on those now. The (positive) thesis that delusions are imaginings, in Currie's account, derives most of its plausibility from the (negative) thesis that delusions are not beliefs. In developing one of these arguments, Currie and Ravenscroft (2002) observe that beliefs and imaginings are different in their origins.

> Our beliefs are formed in response to perceptual information, or by inference from other beliefs we already have. Imaginings can be generated quite independently of these things; what we imagine usually contradicts what we believe and what we perceive.

> (Currie and Ravenscroft 2002, p. 173)

The formation of delusions, then, would be due to the subject's inability to regard the imagined state as autonomously generated. Although this claim is plausible, especially in the context of schizophrenic delusions, the argument relies on a narrow and idealised picture of beliefs. Whereas there are beliefs that come from perceptual experience, testimony, or inference from other beliefs, there are also beliefs that come from reflection on other cognitive and affective states, including imaginings, likes and dislikes, emotions, dreams, raw feelings, and so on. What determines whether a mental state is a belief is a question whose scope exceeds our ambitions here, but here is a suggestion. In order to determine

---

[9] For a different way of making a similar point, see Bayne and Pacherie (2005, p. 179).

whether the mental content 'everybody hates me' is the content of a belief, what matters most is whether such content is endorsed, manifested in behaviour and sensitive to evidence. How the content comes to be entertained by the subject who then reports it is not the only relevant consideration, and might not be a consideration at all, depending of the preferred theory of belief (e.g. whether the type of input matters to the type of attitude the subject has towards a certain mental content). For our purposes, it is sufficient to acknowledge that there is nothing incoherent about the thought of a belief content that is as 'autonomously generated' as the content of an act of imagination.

In another argument for the view that delusions are not beliefs, Currie and Ravenscroft appeal explicitly to a constraint of procedural rationality. They argue that there is a minimal constraint that applies to all beliefs, and this is *consistency*.

> Imaginings are never beliefs because beliefs are subject to the consistency constraints that do not control imaginings [...] we take the consistency constraint to be a minimal constraint on belief of any kind.

(Currie and Ravenscroft 2002, p. 176)

> [If delusions were imaginings], it would be intelligible how it is that people with delusions often do not follow out the consequences of their delusions very far, or try to resolve tensions between their delusions and their other beliefs.

(Currie and Ravenscroft 2002, p. 178)

Other arguments against the view that delusions are beliefs are also based on some version of the procedural rationality constraint on belief ascription. Shaun Gallagher argues that delusions are manifested pre-cognitively, as alternative realities affecting the quality of the totality of the experiences of the subject. The motivation for this view is compelling. In philosophical accounts of delusions not enough attention is paid to the non-cognitive or pre-cognitive features of delusions, and especially to their capacity to cause pervasive disruption in the subject's lives.

> The delusion may not be about external or everyday reality, but may be tied to an alternative reality, in the same way that events that take place in a play are tied to a fictional reality.

(Gallagher 2009, p. 256)

Delusions may not always be true descriptions of reality but if they were not meant to be about reality, then delusional reports would be different from belief reports, and delusions would never motivate action in the actual world. There are two possible cases: either subjects with delusions are aware of inhabiting an alternative reality when they report their delusions, or they aren't.

If they were aware of it, then they would report delusions as they would tell fictional stories (e.g. 'It is *as if* my mother had been replaced by a double'). Subjects who act on their delusions seem to juxtapose what Gallagher would call their *actual reality* with their *delusional reality*, and their endorsement of the delusional reality has all the features of a doxastic attitude. We might feel a bit jumpy after watching a horror movie, because we do not make a smooth transition from the reality of the fiction in which we were absorbed during the movie, and our everyday life. But this is always a temporary displacement. Delusional realities, as Gallagher calls them, seem to intrude the actual reality of the subjects in a more persistent and inevitable way, which would be explained if we characterised the delusion not just experientially, but also in doxastic or metarepresentational terms.

Subjects with delusions are not aware of inhabiting an alternative reality, and believe that their experiences are actual and compelling. Delusional states involve representations of reality: either they manifest as beliefs, albeit false or irrational, or they manifest as something else which is mistaken as beliefs. One of the main reasons Gallagher offers to endorse his account of delusions as alternative realities is that it can allegedly explain the phenomenon of 'double-bookkeeping'. We already saw an example of double-bookkeeping in a case report of a Capgras patient who would reject his wife as an ill-intentioned impostor on some occasions, and treat her kindly on other occasions.

> [M]any schizophrenics are preoccupied with their delusions, but nonetheless treat these delusions with a certain distance or irony. In the MR [Multiple Realities] hypothesis, the possibility of gaining distance from or taking an ironic attitude towards the delusion can be explained to the extent that the subject is able to consider the delusion from the perspective of everyday shared reality. That is, they may be unable to maintain distance as they are caught up in the delusional reality, but to the extent that they can shift back to everyday reality, they may be able to feel the strangeness of the delusion. This may also explain why a patient can view doctors and nurses as poisoners (in delusional reality) but happily eat the food they give her (in everyday reality), or why a patient who treats people as phantoms or automatons (in delusional reality) still interacts with them as if they were real (in everyday reality).

> (Gallagher 2009, p. 260)

Considerations of procedural and agential rationality push Gallagher to reject the standard doxastic account of delusions: if delusions are beliefs, why do subjects maintain an ambivalent attitude towards the content of their delusions? Gallagher assumes that, if delusions were beliefs, there would be no significant dissonance between the content of the delusions and the content of the subject's beliefs, and there would be no inconsistency between the content of the delusion and the subject's behaviour. He acknowledges that some ordinary beliefs also fail to cohere with other beliefs and with behaviour, but argues that those failures of integration can be explained either by reference to 'Davidsonian fragmentation' or by reference to the 'failure of a cohesive introspective or narrative capacity' (Gallagher 2009, p. 250). Delusions, instead, cannot be 'excused' in this way.

In the rest of the chapter I shall offer reasons to resist the arguments against the doxastic account of delusions by Currie and Ravenscroft, and by Gallagher. I shall not confine my analysis to cases of straight-forward inconsistencies. Violations of consistency are rare in the reasoning patterns of either normal subjects or subjects with delusions, but it is not necessary to report mutually contradictory beliefs in order to deserve a charge of bad integration. Think about the phenomenon of double-bookkeeping: bad integration is observed when beliefs are simply in tension with one another (without being straight-forwardly inconsistent), fail to be mutually supportive, or point in different directions.

My strategy against the application of the procedural rationality constraint on belief ascription to the case of delusions will be to argue that ordinary beliefs also fail to satisfy the demands of procedural rationality, and in a qualitatively similar way to delusions. We shall be reminded of beliefs that are not well-integrated in a system and give rise to pervasive and persistent dissonance. Many of the observed 'inconsistencies' in normal cognition are hard to explain within a framework where the relationship among beliefs are governed by rationality. The concession that norms of rationality can be 'suspended' if parts of a subject's mind are found to be fragmented needs further examination. Why are these exceptions to the norm of good integration allowed for belief states, but not for delusional states? Do beliefs really clash with one another only when they belong to different 'fragments' of a subject's mind? If the arguments and examples I offer are convincing, we will have to revisit our theory of the con-straints that apply to beliefs. As a result, considerations about bad integration will no longer be sufficient to deny that delusions are beliefs.

## 2.2 Bad integration in beliefs

In the literature on the nature of delusions, there is a marked tendency to ide-alise ordinary beliefs and to accentuate the contrast between their rationality and the irrationality of delusions. Beliefs are governed by norms of rationality, delusions aren't. Whether and to what extent ordinary beliefs are procedurally rational is of course controversial. The psychological literature on human rea-soning has shown that most (if not all) humans fall prey to systematic mistakes in deductive, statistical, and probabilistic reasoning (for a review, see Stein 1996; Samuels *et al.* 2002), and often exhibit dissonant attitudes (e.g. Thaler and Tversky 1990; Wilson and Hodges 1994). Although there are significant individual differences in reasoning performance (Stanovich 1999), and certain reasoning biases may be more pronounced in deluded and high risk samples, there is a concrete possibility that delusions and beliefs are continuous in their procedural irrationality and that, with respect to beliefs, the conditions for intentionality and those for rationality should be kept distinct.

As we saw in Chapter 1, some argue that it is impossible to ascribe to an individual a pair of inconsistent beliefs (Dennett 1981, p. 95), and other forms of procedural irrationality such as basic reasoning mistakes are also seen as a serious obstacle to the adoption of the intentional stance. If a subject does not behave rationally, then her behaviour cannot be predicted on the basis of the ascription of intentional states, such as beliefs.

> It is at least not obvious that there are any cases of systematically irrational behavior or thinking. The cases that have been proposed are all controversial, which is just what my view predicts: there is no such a thing as a cut-and-dried or obvious case of 'familiar irrationality'. This is not to say that we are always rational, but that when we are not, the cases defy descriptions in ordinary terms of belief and desire.
>
> (Dennett 1998d, p. 87)

Within Davidson's theory of belief ascription, the idea of a subject with inconsistent beliefs is not to be ruled out completely, but Davidson's background argument requires that no individual be ascribed an obvious inconsistency, that is, an inconsistency between beliefs that are simultaneously activated. For instance, the conjunction of two contradictory statements could not be ascribed to someone as a belief. Davidson concedes, though, that dissonant attitudes can be ascribed as beliefs if these are not simultaneously activated (maybe 'stored' in different mental compartments).

Independent of the specific formulation of theories of belief ascription relying on the rationality constraint, it is fair to say that friends of the rationality constraints see lack of coherence in a belief system as the arch enemy of belief ascription. I shall suggest that many ordinary, typical beliefs fail to satisfy the demands of procedural rationality, and in particular are badly integrated with one another. Although experience in everyday interpretation should leave us with no doubt that people's beliefs often lack coherence, having some experimental back-up is always desirable, and suggests that such deviations from procedural rationality are not the exception to the rule, but widespread and systematic.

We do not have copious evidence of subjects believing the conjunction of two contradictory statements, but we can find evidence of subjects believing the conjunction of a statement with another, where the latter undermines the former, or of subjects having beliefs that are not well-integrated with one another or consonant with other attitudes. Helen decides not to swim in the river because she believes that it is contaminated but the next day she regrets not having had that swim. In the departmental meeting Stephen sincerely reports that his new colleague is hard-working, competent and fully qualified, but he predicts that she will make a mess of the annual report. In the first example, dissonance is diachronic as the dissonant attitudes are entertained at different times, whereas in the second it is synchronic as the dissonant attitudes are entertained simultaneously. Obviously, changes of attitudes or nuanced attitudes can be rational and well-motivated. New evidence about the state of the water in the river can become available to Helen and cause her change of attitude. Some information about the specific challenges involved in the preparation of the annual report can be the reason why Stephen predicts his colleague's failure. But in absence of special considerations, dissonance constitutes a challenge to theoretical rationality.

### 2.2.1 Preference reversals

The evidence on preference reversals is still discussed in the psychology and economics literature as evidence of inconsistency. Violations of procedure invariance and description invariance are frequently observed in a variety of contexts. The principle of procedure invariance tells us that, given two options, if one prefers the A to B, then this preference should not be reversed when the method for eliciting the preference changes. Yet, subjects often state a preference for A over B (*choice*), but are prepared to pay more to obtain B rather than A (*pricing*).

Take two lotteries, a relatively safe one, where one has 10% chance of winning nothing and 90% of winning £10; and a relatively risky lottery, where one has 10% chance of winning £90 and 90% of winning nothing. If asked to choose, people usually prefer to buy a ticket for the safe lottery. If asked at what price they would sell their ticket, they set a higher selling price for the ticket of the risky lottery. This phenomenon is observed in different contexts of choice and matching too. If asked whether they prefer to live 20 years with migraine 5 days a week or 10 years with migraine 5 days a week, many research participants prefer the latter option. But then, when they are asked how many years of good health 20 and 10 years of frequent migraines would be worth, most participants match the former option (living 20 years with migraines) with a higher number of healthy life years than the latter option (living 10 years with migraines) (Stalmeier *et al.* 1997).

The classic example of violation of procedure invariance in the literature is the Traffic Problem (Tversky and Thaler 1990).

1) The Minister of Transportation is considering which of the following two programs would make the electorate happier:
   - Program A is expected to reduce the yearly number of casualties in traffic accidents to 570 and its annual cost is estimated at $12 million.

- Program B is expected to reduce the yearly number of casualties in traffic accidents to 500 and its annual cost is estimated at $55 million.

Which program would you like better?

2) The Minister of Transportation is considering which of the following two programs would make the electorate happier:
   - Program A is expected to reduce the yearly number of casualties in traffic accidents to 570 and its annual cost is estimated at $12 million.
   - Program B is expected to reduce the yearly number of casualties in traffic accidents to 500.

At what cost would program B be as attractive as program A?

Options 1 and 2 represent two different ways of eliciting people's preferences for one of the two life-saving programmes. In option 1, people are given all necessary information about the the two programmes: how many lives they would save and at which cost. When preferences are elicited in this way (*direct choice*), 2/3 of participants express a preference for programme B (which allows more lives to be saved, albeit at a higher cost). In option 2, people are told how many lives would be saved, and the cost of programme A, but they are not told the cost of programme B. Rather, they are asked at which cost programme B would become as attractive as programme A. When the preference is elicited this way (*price matching*), 90% of participants provide values smaller than $55 million for programme B, thereby indicating a preference for programme A.

If we take the evidence concerning people's responses to the Traffic Problem as ecologically valid and reliable, it tells us something interesting about dissonance of attitudes. It tells us that it is very likely that each of us would have two dissonant beliefs about what the Minister of Transportation should do if we were presented with the Traffic Problem. We believe that the Minister should implement programme B in order to save the lives of 70 more people a year, even if the programme costs $43 million more than programme A. We also believe that the Minister should implement programme A, which would save fewer lives, unless programme B costed considerably less than $55 million. Depending on the method of elicitation of the preference, we would attribute different monetary value to human lives.

Another common behavioural pattern in the expression of preferences is the violation of description invariance. Given two options, if a subject prefers A to B, then this preference should not be reversed when one or both of the options are described in a semantically different but logically equivalent way. The classic example of violation of the principle of description invariance in the literature is the Asian Disease Problem.

1) Imagine that the United States is preparing for the outbreak of an unusual Asian Disease, which is supposed to kill 600 people. Two alternative programs to combat

the disease have been proposed. Assume that the exact scientific estimates of the consequences of two programs are as follows:
- If program A is adopted, 200 people will be saved.
- If program B is adopted, there is a 1/3 probability that 600 people will be saved and a 2/3 probability that no people will be saved.
Which program should be adopted?

2) Imagine that the United States is preparing for the outbreak of an unusual Asian Disease, which is supposed to kill 600 people. Two alternative programs to combat the disease have been proposed. Assume that the exact scientific estimates of the consequences of two programs are as follows:
- If program A is adopted, 400 people will die.
- If program B is adopted, there is a 1/3 probability that nobody will die and a 2/3 probability that 600 people will die.
Which program should be adopted?

Tversky and Kahneman (1981) who originally devised this task found that the formulation of the problem had a significant effect on people's responses. When the problem was formulated as in (1), 72% of the research participants believed that programme A should be adopted. However, when the problem was formulated as in (2), only 22% believed that programme A should be adopted. Programmes A and B are equivalent in the two versions of the problem. Participants are risk-averse when the solutions are presented in terms of lives saved, but they are risk seeking when the solutions are presented in terms of lives lost. According to the authors, subjects violate the principle of descriptive invariance, according to which complementary re-descriptions of the same outcome should not affect choice. This phenomenon is especially common with respect to emotionally charged or ethically sensitive concepts, such as those of life and death (Bleichrodt and Pinto Prades 2009). Since this original study, different versions of the task have been designed, and the framing effect has remained substantial, even when the task was adapted contextually and given to professionals who do have to make risk-related decisions, such as physicians and businesspeople. New interpretations of the results have been offered which potentially reduce the extent to which problem formulation affects preference (e.g. Bless *et al.* 1998; Li and Xie 2006), but the effect has not been eliminated entirely. In a review article on the influence of framing on decisions where risk is involved, the existence of framing effects in confirmed in a number of experiments, although the size of the effects seems to depend on features of the experimental settings (Kühberger 1998).

These phenomena concern primarily preferences rather than beliefs, but it is not hard to see that they are relevant to claims about procedural rationality, and contribute to challenging the common assumption that ordinary beliefs are well-integrated with one another and belong to largely coherent systems.

Independent of whether we agree with Thaler and Tversky that preference reversals are evidence of inconsistency, they are most definitely evidence of poor integration. Beliefs about the best solution to a problem seem to be hostage to the way in which the available information is presented and processed.

## 2.2.2 Beliefs about the probability of events

Judgements of probability seem to be also very sensitive to how the case is described, highlighting possible elements of dissonance between attitudes towards the probability of certain events. In a classic study by Tversky and Kahneman (1983), research participants were first given the description of a person and then asked to assess the probability of some statements concerning that person.

> Description: Linda is 31 years old, outspoken and very bright. She majored in philosophy. As a student she was deeply concerned with issues of discrimination and social justice and also participated in anti-nuclear demonstrations.

Participants were asked to evaluate the probability of a number of statements, including the following:

i) Linda is a bank teller
ii) Linda is a bank teller and active in the feminist movement.

In the original study, 85% of the research participants judged (*i*) less probable than (*ii*), violating the conjunction rule, according to which the probability of both of two events occurring must be less than or equal to the probability of either event occurring individually. This is a basic rule of probability: the conjunction of two events cannot have greater probability than each of the conjuncts. The explanation offered by Tversky and Kahneman is that people are misled by the heuristic of *representativeness*. We organise information in the most economic way by associating a career, for instance, with the profile of a person whose description bears a relation of resemblance with interests or tendencies that are common to people who choose that career. Linda's profile is not representative of a bank teller. On the contrary, her interests in philosophy and social issues make her representative of a person which is active in the feminist movement. Considerations about representativeness should not influence the participants' response, since the conjunction rule is valid independently of the content expressed by the conjuncts. But Tversky and Kahneman (1982a) claim that participants who are not satisfied by (i) regard (ii) more probable, although (ii) is the conjunction of (i) and something else, and thus cannot be most probable than (i). Given that the description of Linda's personality *fits better* (is more representative of) a feminist than a bank teller, participants erroneously judge (ii) more probable than (i).

This experiment has been replicated many times, and extensively discussed. Some expressed doubts about the possibility of drawing general conclusions (such as 'Humans don't understand probability') from the results. In particular, Gigerenzer wanted to show that it would be too hasty to conclude on the basis of the Linda task that people are unable to recognise the conjunction principle and to conform to it. So he developed a different version of the experiment where participants are not asked to evaluate the probability of statements about a person's choice of career, but about the frequency of an event in a larger class of events. Gigerenzer argued that, given how probability is understood, the conjunction principle is more likely to be obeyed when problems are framed in a frequentist way. The new version of the Linda case was tested: participants read the same description of Linda and then they are told that 100 people fit that description. Next, they are asked to indicate how many of these 100 people are $i^*$) bank tellers, and $ii^*$) bank tellers and active in the feminist movement. The performance dramatically improves when the task is presented this way: Hertwig and Gigerenzer (1999) found that all participants answered that ($i^*$) was more probable than ($ii^*$). In Gigerenzer's later work (2008, p. 72), the explanation offered for this result is that people understand the problem in its original formulation as a problem about plausibility and apply contextually relevant considerations when they offer a solution. In the frequentist formulation, the problem appears as a problem about probability, not plausibility, and participants have no hesitation in applying the conjunction rule.

The case of differences in responses when probability judgements are elicited in different ways may speak in favour of a particular theory about human rationality and about our folk understanding of probability, but that is not the debate that interests us here. Rather, these significant differences in reasoning performance across versions of the task indicate that people are prone to forming and maintaining beliefs and making decisions that are not necessarily well-integrated and consistent with one another. Gigerenzer might be right that logical mistakes reveal intelligent and adaptive responses, but it is not at all clear why the same people who find it more plausible that Linda is a feminist bank teller rather than a bank teller and nothing else, also find it more likely that a greater number of people fitting Linda's description are bank teller rather than feminist bank tellers. It is not that the conjunction of these attitudes cannot be explained satisfactorily, but it reveals an underlying fragility in the grounding for our attitudes, and makes the possibility of bad integration within a belief system a very concrete danger.

### 2.2.3 **Dissonant beliefs**

Let me offer some other examples of dissonant beliefs that do not come from the psychological literature but can be observed in patterns of everyday reasoning. Richard Foley (1998) mentions an interesting case of dissonance among beliefs: this is when an individual has some strongly held belief in the efficacy of a certain method, but also acquires reliable information about the limitations of that method. The example is that of the use of personal interviewing. Interviews are widely used to assess job candidates, to examine prospective graduate students, and to grant parole to committed criminals. The purpose of such interviews is to allow the interviewer to predict whether the person being interviewed, respectively, will be successful at her job, will become a good student, or will avoid re-offending. Given their purpose in assisting such predictions, interviews have been proved to be a very poor method, mainly because the interviewer tends to be distracted by irrelevant features (personal appearance and mannerisms) rather than focusing on the features of the interviewee which would be relevant to making the prediction.

Believing that personal interviews are useful when one uses them is clearly at odds with trusting the psychological evidence on interviews being poor predictors of future performance, so entertaining these two beliefs causes dissonance that is rarely resolved either by revising one's beliefs about the utility of interviews or one's trust in the psychological evidence. Notice that this type of dissonance applies to other methods in other contexts, and is often characterised by the thought that one is immune from the mistakes made by other people in similar circumstances, such as being fooled by the pleasant mannerism of a job candidate when making an appointment. Analogously, people trust their own introspective reports, but may be suspicious about those of others, especially after being convinced by data about the limitations of introspection. People might be impressed by the results of the Milgram experiment (1974) on obedience to authority, but come to think that, in the experimental situation or in equivalent real-life situations, they would not obey authority figures at the expense of their most valued principles. There is nothing surprising in these observations, as we know that there are self-serving biases inviting us to form largely positive images of ourselves. But when positive attitudes about our own use of a certain method, or our own capacity to behave in a way that we consider morally acceptable are compared with our fairly pessimistic attitudes towards what other people do, an element of dissonance, and even deception, is present. When we think about subjects with delusions, and their protestations that, although the event they report to believe is really unusual, it has happened *to them*, the literature on self-serving biases and attribution biases comes to mind and provides solid basis for the thesis that there is significant continuity between delusional and non-delusional thought.

A case that often involves open conflict between a subject's beliefs is superstition. People maintain superstitious beliefs, beliefs about magic or beliefs about supernatural phenomena that are contrary to their own commitment to the principles of science. Vyse (1997) reports how college students have superstitious beliefs about how to pass exams (dressing down helps), gamblers perform rituals in order to bring good luck to themselves (dropping the dice is a bad omen), and people in show-business or in professional sport have their own superstitious beliefs and practices. Some superstitious beliefs are not specific to any subculture and are very widely shared: police officers, medics working in emergency rooms and mental health workers are reported to believe that more crimes, accidents, and psychological crises occur during nights of full moon (Vyse 1997, p. 36). Knowledge of the likely causes of crimes, accidents and psychological problems does not seem to prevent people who have daily experience of these events from reporting (and acting on) implausible beliefs that are also badly supported by the evidence available to them. Education, even scientific education involving critical thinking and an appreciation of empirical methods of investigation, is not consistently shown to reduce the occurrence of superstitious beliefs, which are common among academics. Also in this case, the similarities with the delusions literature spring to mind: people with delusions of thought insertion believe that it is not plausible that instruments for inserting thoughts into other people's minds are available to their neighbours, and people with Capgras know how unlikely it is that aliens have substituted their dear ones. But this does not prevent them from reporting and endorsing their delusional stories, which might affect their everyday behaviour as superstitious beliefs affect the behaviour of highly educated and sensible people.

It is not hard to see how the phenomena I described challenge the procedural rationality constraint on the ascription of beliefs and premise one of the bad integration objection which states that: In order for $p$ to be ascribed as a belief to a subject, $p$ needs to be well-integrated with the subject's beliefs. If ordinary beliefs, such as beliefs about which solution is more effective in limiting the damage of a disease outbreak, or beliefs about what causes one's poor performance in a exam, fail to be well-integrated with other beliefs, then it seems implausible to suggest that good integration is a constitutive feature of beliefs. The bad integration objection is guilty of double standards: it denies belief status to delusions because they are badly integrated with the subject's beliefs, but it does not deny belief status to judgements about the best possible solution to a problem or about the causes of personal failures, when these are in conflict with other things subjects are committed to. To escape the 'double standards' accusation, we should either deny that judgements such as those we make in the Asian Disease Problem or superstitions are belief-like, or lift the bad integration objection to the belief status of delusions. The best option is a straight-forward rejection of the procedural rationality constraint on the ascription of beliefs. But the friends of the constraint on the ascription of beliefs have a few more aces up their sleeves.

## 2.3 **Recovery after 'Socratic tutoring'**

The 'double standards' accusation can be rejected if significant difference can be found between failures of integration in ordinary beliefs and in delusions. Let me consider two influential accounts of such difference, based on (1) the capacity to restore procedural rationality and (2) the explicability of failures of integration.

First, one might argue that, even when beliefs appear to be badly integrated, people with dissonant beliefs or inconsistent preference sets are *disposed to restore* well-integration when they are made aware of their deviations from norms of procedural rationality. With a bit of 'Socratic tutoring', they see the light. People with delusions, instead, are resistant to cognitive probing, because their deviations from norms of rationality run deeper. Alternatively, or in addition to the previous argument, one might suggest that in ordinary subjects deviations from norms of procedural rationality can be explained by the phenomenon of compartmentalisation: subjects are not aware of having conflicting beliefs or inconsistent preferences. Poor integration in people with delusions, instead, cannot be excused, because it cannot be explained by reference to compartmentalisation. Behind both moves, there is one general idea: even if we concede that ordinary beliefs may violate norms of procedural rationality, delusions are significantly different, different *in kind*, from such irrational beliefs. Delusions, as opposed to procedurally irrational beliefs, cannot be 'corrected' and cannot be 'excused'.

### 2.3.1 **Restoring rationality**

Both attempts at rescuing the procedural rationality constraint on belief ascription are unconvincing. Let's start with the claim that the procedural rationality of subjects with delusions is of a more serious kind than the occasional, temporary and revocable procedural irrationality of ordinary subjects. According to the background argument, one can concede that delusions and mundane irrational beliefs can be both affected by bad integration—failures of procedural rationality are not a promising demarcation criterion between delusions and beliefs after all. However, one can argue that there is a substantial difference between subjects with ordinary beliefs, even irrational ones, and subjects with delusions. When they deviate from norms of procedural rationality, the former maintain the capacity to recover and are disposed to act in such a way as to reduce bad integration and eliminate dissonance between attitudes. The idea that people are disposed to reduce or eliminate dissonance among their attitudes is not new, and is at the basis of the theory of cognitive dissonance developed by Leon Festinger:

> If dissonance exists between two cognitive elements or between two clusters of cognitive elements, this dissonance may be reduced by adding new cognitive elements which produce new consonant relationships. One would then expect that in the presence of dissonance, one would observe the seeking out of information which might reduce the existing dissonance.

(Festinger 1957, p. 126)

What is new is the suggestion that procedural rationality does not consist in conforming to the norm of good integration (and other relevant norms), but in *being disposed to restore* good integration when violations of this norm are detected. Will this version of the constraint solve the issue of double standards? If subjects with delusions cannot recover from violations of norms of rationality, and other subjects can, then a relevant difference between them has been identified.

However, the claim that people with procedurally irrational beliefs are disposed to restore rationality is not compatible with the psychological evidence showing that research participants are extremely resistant to changing their answers to tasks such as the Asian Disease Problem after debriefing (Stalmeier *et al.* 1997; Lichtenstein and Slovic 1971). This is not an isolated finding, as similar resistance to cognitive probing has been observed with respect to tasks which involve other violations of norms of procedural rationality, such as the conjunction fallacy (Tversky and Kahneman 1983), and with respect to beliefs about the self, or superstitious beliefs, which persevere even when challenged on the basis of other beliefs that the subject endorses. Anecdotal evidence supports these findings: I often ask undergraduate students in their final year of a philosophy degree to take some of the reasoning tests studied by psychologists (such as the Asian Disease problem). Most of those who provide largely inconsistent answers are keen to find faults with the ecological validity of the reasoning tasks and refuse to concede that 'they made a mistake', even after debriefing. These are students who have passed a logic exam in their first year, and received extensive critical thinking training since then.

As we already mentioned, the claim that subjects with delusions are resistant to cognitive probing also needs to be qualified. There are strong indications that cognitive behavioural therapy is efficacious in reducing the rigidity of delusional states, and the preoccupation of the subject with the topic of the delusion (Coltheart 2005b; Kingdon *et al.* 2008). Although the evidence gathered so far does not suggest that cognitive behavioural therapy is effective in leading the subject to abandon a delusion altogether, cognitive probing does contribute to the subject adopting a more critical attitude towards the content of the delusion. This partial result is not surprising, as this is what we would expect if the delusion were a belief that one had powerful motivational reasons not to reject—the alternative to endorsing the delusional content often consists in conceding that one is or has been mentally unwell.

These considerations recommend caution in advocating a qualitative gap between delusions and beliefs on the basis on the subjects' capacity to restore conformity to the norm of good integration. The charge of double standards has not been satisfactorily addressed yet.

### 2.3.2 Excuses for bad integration

Here is the second argument for the view that there is a qualitative difference between delusions and procedurally irrational beliefs. If deviations from norms of procedural rationality affecting a subject's mental states can be made sense of and *excused*, then they do not compromise the belief status of those mental states.

It is understandable why people might have dissonant cognitions, if we advocate the notion of compartmentalisation (Davidson 1982, 1985b) or mental partitioning (Lewis 1982; Evnine 2008). In a version of compartmentalisation, limited resources in memory and attention force subjects to store beliefs in different compartments of their mind, and prevent subjects from attending to the conflicting beliefs all at once. In another version, the 'boundaries' dividing one compartment from the other are not simply due to feasibility issues, but to motivational factors, as in textbook cases of self deception. Boundaries of different nature can of course co-exist. As a result of compartmentalisation, subjects might forget their previous commitments when they form a judgement anew, or fail to realise existing cognitive conflicts. The view is that, although ordinary believers can be *diachronically* inconsistent on some occasions, and have conflicting beliefs in different compartments of their minds, they are never *synchronically* inconsistent.

> One might believe two things independently that, when one puts them together, one sees cannot both be true. If one is committed to the view that contradictions cannot be true (or rationally believed), one will take this fact as a reason for suspending belief

in one or both of the propositions involved. One might further specify this scenario in either of two ways. According to one of those ways, one comes to see that, whatever one's initial impressions were, belief in one or both of the propositions was, after all, not rational. According to the second way, one was rational in believing the conjuncts previously, but ceases to be so when one sees that they cannot both be true.

(Evnine 2008, p. 56)

The mere act of co-attending to mutually conflicting beliefs would alert subjects to the risk of inconsistency and lead them to restore procedural rationality. People with delusions, instead, can also be synchronically inconsistent, as in some of the examples we reviewed earlier in this chapter—so compartmentalisation cannot be advocated to explain their procedurally irrational behaviour.

In the context of the debate on the belief status of delusions, there are reasons to believe that the move from explicability is unhelpful. First, nothing prevents us from regarding poor integration in delusions as the result of compartmentalisation, and thus conclude that the procedural irrationality of delusional states is of the explicable kind. In delusions that are more likely to present obvious and explicit inconsistencies (monothematic delusions) the tension is often due to the delusion being heavily circumscribed, and one could well argue that circumscription is nothing but an extreme form of compartmentalisation, due to reasoning deficits, motivational factors, or a combination of the two. Polythematic delusions, such as the case of persecution previously reviewed, tend to present fewer obvious inconsistencies. But they still suffer from bad integration, because they are not in an epistemologically healthy relationship of mutual support with one another and with the subject's beliefs. To these delusions, considerations about circumscription pply to a lesser extent (Davies *et al.* 2001), as polythematic delusions tend to give rise to comprehensive narratives through which much of the subject's experience is interpreted. This suggests that the correlation between compartmentalisation and the presence of inconsistencies *supports* rather than *undermines* the continuity between delusions and beliefs. Delusions do not seem to behave in a qualitatively different manner from typical beliefs: as we would expect, in both cases bad integration is more of an issue when belief-like states are relatively insulated from the rest of the subject's cognitive life.

A more general worry is whether compartmentalisation is ever a *good* excuse for procedural irrationality. If we interpret compartmentalisation as a necessary evil, due to limited resources in human cognitive architecture or an inevitable mechanism of self-protection, then the excuse is an 'ought-implies-can' move. On some occasions, we have beliefs that are not well-integrated with one another because we cannot work out all the active relations between all the beliefs we have, or because a defence mechanism has been triggered, driven by the non-conscious desire not to have one's self confidence or emotional instability compromised. But these considerations apply only to a subset of cases of bad integration. Some cases of bad integration do not fall nicely in one of these two categories and still demand an explanation. People who endorse conflicting attitudes in reasoning tasks are fiercely resistant to reviewing their answers even after they have been explained the principles of reasoning relevant to the tasks. When the attention of the subjects is drawn to the conflict between the attitudes they have endorsed and they do not revise their attitudes even if they have no particular emotional or personal invest-ment in the tasks, neither of the ready 'excuses' for bad integration seem to justify their procedurally irrational behaviour.

### 2.3.3 Subscription to norms of rationality

Conceding the possibility that subjects might have badly integrated beliefs that are not simultaneously attended to has serious implications for the formulation of the rationality constraint on belief ascription (Davidson 1985a). One simple, maybe naïve, formulation of the constraint is that subjects can be ascribed beliefs if they conform to norms of procedural rationality. Accordingly, the first premise of the bad integration argument says that:

> i) In order for b to be ascribed as a belief to a subject, b needs to be well-integrated with the subject's beliefs.

In the light of the background argument and the thesis about subjects with beliefs being able to recover from violations of procedural rationality, the notion of conformity should be unpacked and given a disjunctive treatment. Either a subject has beliefs that are coherent with one another and well-integrated in a system, or she is disposed to revise those beliefs that do not cohere with one another and are not well-integrated in a system in order to conform to the norms of procedural rationality.

> i*) In order for $b$ to be ascribed as a belief to a subject, either $b$ needs to be well-inte-grated with the subject's beliefs, or its bad integration with the subject's beliefs needs to be amenable to revision (when the subject is made aware of there being a case of bad integration).

Adopting this disjunctive account of what it is to be rational is in the spirit of the background argument. It seems *prima facie* possible to reconcile the necessity of the rationality constraint on belief ascription with islands of bad integration in a largely coherent belief system. The interpreter might ascribe to the speaker a pair of conflicting beliefs if such doxastic conflicts can be remedied by the speaker when she becomes aware of them. In the light of the background argument and the thesis about subjects with beliefs being excusable from violations of procedural rationality, the notion of conformity should again be unpacked and given a disjunctive treatment:

> i**) In order for *b* to be ascribed as a belief to a subject, either *b* needs to be well-integrated with the subject's beliefs, or its bad integration with the subject's beliefs needs to be of the 'explicable' sort.

I have argued elsewhere (Bortolotti 2003) that, when we replace (i) with versions of (i*) and (i**), the rationality constraint on belief ascription loses some of its original appeal. What is distinctive and attractive about classical interpretationism is that the conditions that a mental state needs to satisfy to qualify as a belief can be straight-forwardly read off speakers' observable behaviour.

> What is distinctive about the interpretationist account is the attempt to characterise a creature's beliefs by reference to the creature's behavioural patterns. There is a clear sense in which attributions of belief and desire [...] are supervenient on behaviour more broadly described.

> (Davidson 1975, p. 159)

In (i*) and (i**), the conditions relevant to assessing whether a mental state can be ascribed to a subject as a genuine belief are not straight-forwardly apparent in behaviour because they make reference to further behavioural dispositions (what the speaker would do if challenged, etc.) or to the underlying mechanisms responsible for the apparent violation of rationality (whether it is a case of compartmentalisation). Formulations (i*) and (i**) prompt the following question: why do subjects with beliefs have this capacity for restoring conformity to norms of rationality? The answer is that they *subscribe* to norms of procedural rationality. With respect to classic formulations of the rationality constraint on belief ascription, the background argument brings the new notion of subscription to norms of rationality to the fore. If subjects with beliefs are never impervious to recovery from violations of norms of rationality, then, according to Davidson, the rationality constraint is undefeated. One can still hold true that there is some necessary connection between having beliefs and being rational, since subjects are disposed to restore conformity to norms of procedural rationality, once the conflicting beliefs are co-attended to. What makes subjects recover is their subscription to a principle according to which there ought to be coherence and good integration in belief systems. Subjects are not required to be able to formulate the fundamental principles of rationality, nor are they required to recognise such principles (and the violations of such principles) in all the relevant circumstances (Davidson 1985a, p. 352). However, they must have some non-explicit knowledge of the principles, and such competence is supposed to manifest in the general conformity to those principles. A useful analogy is with speakers who may not be able to make explicit the grammar rules of their native language, in spite of their general observance of those rules.

> For a person to 'accept' or have a principle like the requirement of total evidence mainly consists in that person's pattern of thoughts being in accordance with the principle without being aware of it or able to articulate it.
>
> (Davidson 1985b, p. 81)

One can fail to conform to norms of rationality without being irrational, because rationality is subscription (not conformity) to norms of rationality. What is not clear is whether Davidson thinks that a subject's subscription to norms of rationality implies that her patterns of behaviour largely conform to such norms. In other words, is conformity to norms necessary for subscription?

> I think everyone does subscribe to those principles [= principles of decision theory], whether he knows it or not. This does not imply, of course, that no one ever reasons, believes, chooses, or acts contrary to those principles, but only that if someone does go against those principles, he goes against his own principles. I would say the same about the basic principles of logic, the principle of total evidence for inductive reasoning, or the analogous principle of continence. These are principles shared by all creatures that have propositional attitudes or act intentionally.
>
> (Davidson 1985a, p. 351)

> The possibility of inconsistency depends on nothing more than this, that an agent, a creature with propositional attitudes, must show much consistency in his thought and action, and in this sense have the fundamental values of rationality; yet, he may depart from these, his own, norms.
>
> (Davidson 1985a, p. 353)

In the case of inconsistencies excused by compartmentalisation, conformity to norms of rationality does not seem to be a necessary condition for subscription. Subjects with beliefs can be found to endorse inconsistent beliefs and are expected to restore conformity to norms of rationality only if the deviation from norms of rationality is detected and made salient to them. Do we need these constraints on the ascription of beliefs?

### 2.3.4 Charity and explicability

On the basis of the background argument and the application of notions such as subscription, compartmentalisation and recovery, occasional and temporary violations of norms of rationality are treated as an exception to the rule or an occasional mistake that can be 'corrected'. One of the arguments for the qualitative difference between delusions and (irrational) beliefs is that the latter but not the former are amenable to this 'correction' due to their explicability.

> [...] when a mistake is agreed to have been made we will often look for, and find, a reason why it was made, not just in the sense of cause or regularity in its making but in the sense of some excuse which reconciles the mistake with the idea that, even in making it, the perpetrator was exercising his or her rationality.
>
> (Heal 1988, p. 99)

Consider the following examples.

- Whenever Nishad takes an exam, he wears the chain that his grandmother gave him, because he believes that the chain brings him luck and protects him from harm. He knows that, in general, objects have no special power on people or situations, but he makes an exception in this case.
- Bob believes that the person who lives in his house and looks identical to his mum is not his mum, but a cleverly disguised Martian, and develops a growing sense of hostility towards the impostor.

Suppose Bob and Nishad are otherwise perfectly rational subjects. Is there a sense in which judgments of rationality can discriminate between them? One main difference is that Nishad's belief in the powers of the chain is common and familiar, whereas Bob exhibits a very rare condition, as a result of which his report is unexpected and perplexing for all those who lack an insight into his medical history. Is it plausible that there is a qualitative gap between the irrationality of Nishad's and Bob's reports? For the background argument to be vindicated, it should be the case that Nishad is easily disposed to revise his belief about the powers of the chain, whereas Bob preserves his delusion in spite of challenges. In addition, the background argument would invite us to conceive of irrational beliefs as 'mistakes that can be corrected'. A suitably located interpreter could exercise charity and reinterpret the reports as saying something different, and more sensible, in the light of the other sensible beliefs that Nishad and Bob happen to have. But the background argument is at a loss with *both* familiar and exotic instances of irrationality. Nishad will not easily give up his belief that the chain brings him luck, and will explain away apparent counterevidence. Bob will be resistant to cognitive probing and continue to believe that his mother has been substituted notwithstanding the incredulity of his relatives and friends. This is not to say that the idea behind the background argument is totally misguided: there are some false beliefs that can be revised and crumble under the gentle pressure of charitable interpreters. But 'corrigibility' and the disposition to restore rationality where its norms have been infringed cannot be taken as a general feature of subjects with beliefs, and tend to work best in cases in which a belief is false or irrational because it contains a concept that has not been fully grasped.

- Jennie admires the beautiful tree in front of her, and says she would like to see more elms in the park. Her friend Tommy makes her notice that the tree she is looking at is a beech. Tommy can make sense of Jennie's false belief because it is a simple mistake she made as a result of misapplying a concept: she saw a tree and thought it was an elm. She rightly believes that elms are trees, and that there is a tree in front of her, but she does not realise that the tree in front of her is actually a beech.
- Bert goes to the doctor and claims he has arthritis in his thigh. The doctor fully understands him, even if Bert made a mistake. Arthritis is a condition of the joints only. The doctor realises that Bert must have a pain in his thigh and describes it that way because he does not completely master the concept 'arthritis'.
- Roxanne is helping her dad to fix the car. Roxanne's dad raises his head and asks her to pass him the sandals. She notices that there is a pair of sandals in the garage, but also realises that what her dad wants is the spanner. In fact, when Roxanne does pass him the spanner, her dad thanks her and goes on fixing the car. He had a slip of the tongue.

There are strong analogies between these three cases. The speaker makes a mistake that the interpreter can understand and 'correct' on the basis of clues about the speaker or the surrounding environment. It is open to the interpreter to apply the principle of charity and make sense of the fact that Jennie is referring to a beech, Bert is talking about a pain in the thigh and Roxanne's dad wanted the spanner. This is possible because we know that Jennie and Bert would not be resistant to revise their statements if an 'expert', or an otherwise suitably located interpreter, were to explain to them, respectively, the difference between elms and beeches and the exact meaning of arthritis. We also realise that Roxanne's dad would recognise his mistake if it were pointed out to him. These cases are the ones that the background argument is best suited to account for. The interpreter makes sense of what is going on by reference to the evidence that the speaker has for what she believes and to her behaviour in the context.

The same strategy cannot be easily applied to delusional states, or other procedurally irrational beliefs that are resistant to revision. Which true belief of Bob will help us rationalise his conviction that the person who looks identical to his mother is actually an alien? He knows how unlikely it is for Martians to replace Earthlings with identical replicas but this does not undermine his conviction in the content of his delusion. Which true belief of Nishad can explain his conviction that the chain has powers? He knows that what people wear is unrelated to what happens to them but does not give up his belief about the chain. As a charitable interpreter, I could take Jennie as saying: 'There is a beech in front of me', instead of 'There is an elm in front of me'. How could

I reinterpret Bob and Nishad? If I interpreted Bob as having the belief that he is suffering from the Capgras delusion, I could not make any sense of his behaviour, especially of his increasingly hostile behaviour towards his mum. My 'charitable' ascription would not be helpful in attempting to explain and predict Bob's behaviour in intentional terms. If the idea behind the background argument is plausible at all, it is plausible in those cases in which the believer makes a revocable mistake or is in partial ignorance. In other cases, the idea that we are better off when we take the believer to endorse something true and sensible seems not to be supported by our experience as everyday interpreters of others. We seem to ascribe beliefs to people who make reasoning mistakes and are inconsistent or delusional, just because we allow the same possibility that the procedural rationality constraint denies, that the person in front of us might not be rational and might not tell us something true.

I have argued that one common strategy to challenge the doxastic conception of delusions is to assume that conformity to norms of procedural rationality is a necessary condition for the ascription of beliefs. Given that delusions (mono- and polythematic ones) seem to be badly integrated with the subject's beliefs and often give rise to dissonance among attitudes, they fail to satisfy norms of procedural rationality and should be denied belief status. My reply has been two-fold. It is true that delusions can fail to integrate in the subject's belief system, and I have offered some examples in support of that claim. But I rejected the conceptual claim that the satisfaction of norms of procedural rationality is necessary for belief ascription. Scepticism towards the rationality constraint comes from the observation that ordinary beliefs also fail to satisfy norms of procedural rationality, and that dissonance among attitudes is a very common form of irrationality.

A friend of the rationality constraint could rebut that there is an important difference between delusions and beliefs: whereas subjects with delusions cannot restore conformity to norms of rationality, and their delusions are impervious to revision even after Socratic tutoring, subjects with procedurally irrational beliefs preserve the capacity to restore conformity to rationality. If they are invited to draw attention to dissonant beliefs, they are also behaviourally disposed to reduce or eliminate the existing dissonance. These behavioural dispositions show that they subscribe to norms of procedural rationality even if they do not always conform to them. Both the empirical and conceptual claims made in this reply raise concerns. Empirically there is no such a sharp divide: normal subjects are not always disposed to restore conformity to norms of procedural rationality, and subjects with delusions are not always impervious to counterargument. As a fix to the rationality constraint on belief ascription theory, the introduction of the notion of subscription creates more problems than it solves. The notion of subscription to norms of rationality is underspecified and no coherent and unitary account is given of the relationship between subscribing to a norm and conforming to it. If subscription to norms of rationality implies general conformity to such norms, then subscription is robustly linked to observable behaviour and can play a role in the practice of radical and everyday interpretation, but there is still a tension between the procedural rationality constraint and the observation that subjects have dissonant attitudes. If subscription does not imply conformity, as the appeal to the notion of recovery suggests, the idea that one can ascribe beliefs to a subject by reference to her observable behaviour, which is distinctive of the interpretationist picture, has to be qualified or even substantially revised.

## 2.4 **The indeterminacy argument**

The rationality constraint on belief ascription tells us that the interpretation of irrational behaviour is always problematic because our attempts to describe, explain, and predict behaviour in folk-psychological terms necessarily rest on an assumption of rationality. This view of folk psychology as tied to a general assumption of rationality is widely supported and different versions of this idea can be found in the philosophical literature:

> If we are intelligibly to attribute attitudes and beliefs, or usefully to describe motions as behavior, then we are committed to finding, in the pattern of behavior, belief, and desire, a large degree of rationality and consistency.
>
> (Davidson 1974b, p. 237)

> It is clear that the scope for indeterminacy diminishes when we require [...] that interpretation should meet various standards of plausibility, rationality and consistency.
>
> (Child 1994, p. 70)

> Propositional attitudes have their proper home in explanations of a special sort: explanations in which things are made intelligible by being revealed to be, or to approximate to being, as they rationally ought to be.
>
> (McDowell 1985, p. 389)

> When we are not [rational], the cases defy description in ordinary terms of belief and desire.
>
> (Dennett 1987, p. 87)

As we saw in Chapter 1, and in this chapter by reference to procedural rationality, the *strong* necessary claim would hold that behaviour that departs from norms of rationality to a significant extent *cannot* be intentionally characterised *at all*. An example of a strategy that stems from the endorsement of the strong necessary claim is the 'hard line' in Dennett's intentional system theory. According to Dennett, one cannot adopt the intentional stance in order to make sense of or predict the behaviour of a system that departs from norms of rationality. Depending on the aims of the interpreter and on the complexity of the system's behaviour, the physical or the design stance might be adopted instead. The rationality constraint can also be interpreted as the *weak* necessary claim that if the subject's behaviour is not rational then the subject *cannot* be ascribed belief states *with determinate content*. This claim concerns cases in which behaviour that departs significantly from norms of rationality eludes the interpreter's explanation or prediction, because it is not determinate which belief contents the subject is genuinely committed to. The indeterminacy argument can equally apply to constraints on belief ascription that start from assumptions of procedural, epistemic or agential rationality. Here, I primarily consider violations of procedural rationality.

   i) In order for *b* to be ascribed to a subject as a belief with determinate content, *b* needs to be well-integrated with the subject's beliefs.

   ii) Delusions are badly integrated with a subject's beliefs.

Thus, delusions cannot be ascribed as beliefs with determinate content. As a consequence, explanation and prediction of the subject's behaviour in intentional terms is compromised.

## 2.4.1 Delusions and interpretation

Consider the following cases. Someone says: 'There are flies in my head.' One might not be able to determine what this person is trying to say. Is he metaphorically alluding to a state of confusion or dizziness? Or does he (literally) believe that there are flies in his head? If further information about the speaker or the situation is not available to the interpreter, no determinate belief content will be ascribed to the subject. A subject with Cotard delusion reports that she is dead, and believes at the same time that dead people don't speak and don't move. Would an interpreter ascribe to her the belief that she is dead? A subject with Capgras claims that his wife has been replaced by an impostor but does not seem worried about his wife's safety. Would an interpreter ascribe to him the belief that the woman in his house is not his wife but an impostor? The indeterminacy objection concedes that circumscribed and monothematic delusions can be ascribed to a subject as beliefs, but argues that the content of the ascribed beliefs might not be sufficiently determinate to support explanation and prediction of behaviour in intentional terms. Indeterminacy might affect interpretation when reported attitudes are dissonant, when they are not reflected in behaviour, or when their content is so implausible that we cannot understand how the subject can commit herself to it. This strategy is an example of the 'soft line' in Dennett's intentional system theory.

> In cases of even the mildest and most familiar cognitive pathology – where people seem to hold contradictory beliefs, or to be deceiving themselves, for instance - the canons of interpretation of the intentional strategy fail to yield *clear, stable* verdicts about which beliefs and desires to attribute to a person.
>
> (Dennett 1998c, p. 28, my emphasis)

It is true that behaviour that deviates from norms of rationality can be more challenging to interpret. However, the nature of the relationship between rationality and intentionality is not at all clear. Is the subject's irrationality responsible for the challenges faced by the interpreter? Not necessarily, or so I shall maintain. Failures of rationality are neither necessary nor sufficient for interpretation to be compromised on the account of indeterminacy. Interpretation is often compromised when the interpreter has limited knowledge of the environment shared with the subject, or of the subject's relevant cognitive features. The difficulty in interpreting the behaviour of the man who says that there are flies in his head might not be due to his irrationality. It might very well be due to the interpreter's lack of familiarity with the speaker and with the specifics of the situation. Maybe the speaker's psychiatrist or one of his closest friends would be better placed than a stranger to understand the prima facie puzzling utterance, and ascribe to the speaker beliefs with determinate content. The speaker can genuinely believe that his head is being infested with flies. Some patients affected by schizophrenia or in the first stages of dementia report that they feel insects moving inside their heads, and some drug users suffer from the delusion that there are insects crawling under their skin— consequently, they engage in obsessive scratching. If the speaker is in one of these conditions, it does make sense to interpret the utterance 'There are flies in my head' literally, and although the content of that sentence remains implausible, the fact that the speaker is uttering it is not as perplexing as we might have thought at first, given that the speaker might be subject to abnormal experiences which would be somewhat explained by the presence of flies in his head.

What is doing the work in preventing the determinate ascription of belief contents is not a failure of rationality on behalf of the subject, but scarcity of relevant information on behalf of the interpreter. This phenomenon is a general one, and is not observed exclusively in cases in which subjects suffer from mental illness. It is as difficult to ascribe a belief with determinate content to a brain-damaged person suffering from delusions as it is to ascribe beliefs with determinate content to people from radically different cultures, human infants or non-human animals. The difficulty in ascribing beliefs with determinate content to these individuals is not necessarily due to their exhibiting behaviour that departs from norms of rationality. Important factors are the interpreter's lack of experience in recognising verbal and non-verbal behavioural responses that are different from her own, and the difficulty in projecting intentional states with content on subjects who have a different cultural background or psychological make-up. To some extent, the emphasis on the impact of differences between subjects and interpreters for the success of belief ascription is a trivial point. Isn't it easier for us to describe, explain, and predict in intentional terms the behaviour of a person who shares our interests, opinions, and desires than that of a person who doesn't? With time, we become more experienced at figuring out what individuals who are relevantly different from us might believe and desire, but the initial attempts at interpretation are characterised by a degree of uncertainty that compromises explanation and prediction of behaviour (e.g. 'Did he mean that? Or was it a joke?') Some of the differences between interpreters and subjects of interpretation have nothing to do with the satisfaction of normative standards of rationality, and yet have pervasive effects on the specificity of content of the beliefs we are able to ascribe to them.

### 2.4.2 Two notions of rationality

The apparent plausibility of the view that explanation and prediction of behaviour in intentional terms rest on the assumption that the subject behaves largely rationally is due to the equivocation between two notions of rationality—rationality as conformity or subscription to epistemic norms, and intelligibility of observed behaviour. The claim that rationality is a precondition for the ascription of beliefs is much more plausible if we have in mind the weaker notion of rationality that is met by any form of intentional behaviour; but the claim that rationality is precondition on the ascription of beliefs is interesting and non-trivial only if the notion of rationality is intended as conformity or subscription to epistemic norms.

There is a sense in which folk-psychological explanations of verbal reports and other types of behaviour are all rationalisations, that is, they are an attempt to establish meaningful connections between seemingly disconnected events in order to make them intelligible. Think about the case of Stewart, who puts on his hat and scarf before facing a cold wind. An interpreter acquainted with the circumstances in which Stewart acts in this way, might ascribe to Stewart the belief that it is cold and windy outside, the desire to be protected from the cold wind, and the belief that wearing the hat and the scarf will constitute effective protection. Stewart's action is rationalised because his behaviour can be made sense of by the ascription of intentional states that explain the action. But Stewart's behaviour does not necessarily meet the standards of rationality for thought and action. Wearing hat and scarf may not be an effective protection in the circumstances, and it may not be the best action available to Stewart. For instance, it may be better for Stewart not to step outside at all until the wind has gone—the hat will fly away in the wind and the scarf will not be warm enough to protect him from the cold. These considerations are relevant to whether Stewart's reported states and observable behaviour conform to norms of rationality, but not to whether they are intentional states and intentional behaviour. In the literature the relationship between the two notions of rationality has not been properly explored. Does the explanation of Stewart's behaviour in terms of his beliefs and desires (and possibly other intentional states) presuppose that Stewart meets standards of rationality? Do we need to assume that the beliefs and desires Stewart entertains are those he *ought to have*, or that his action conforms to what *he ought to do* (as Dennett's intentional stance requires)? The answer to both these questions is obviously no. For the purposes of establishing intelligibility and proceeding to explaining and predicting behaviour intentionally, all we need is that the subject has a reason for reporting her attitudes or acting as she does that can be cashed in intentional terms. Whether her attitudes or actions meet standards of rationality is beside the point.

In the attempt to identify the mark of intentional action, some philosophers have argued for the view that there cannot be intentionality without conformity or subscription to norms of rationality, but their best evidence only supports the claim that intentional behaviour must be intelligible or amenable to rationalisation. When Child (1994) characterises what the conditions for interpretation are for Davidson, he endorses the view that they involve a demanding notion of rationality as satisfaction of normative standards.

> Rationality includes everything relevant to saying what constitutes a *good* argument, a *valid* inference, a *rational* plan, or a *good* reason for acting, and everything relevant to the application of those notions to the particular case; it includes practical rationality, not just theoretical rationality; it involves inductive as well as deductive rationality; and considerations about rationality are relevant too, in assessing how a belief and desire must cause an action that they explain.
>
> (Child 1994, pp. 57–8, my emphasis)

Why should we endorse the view that rationality is a constraint on the ascription of intentional states? There can be arguments that are not good arguments, plans that are not rational, and inferences that are not valid. To claim that these arguments, plans, and inferences are not instances of intentional behaviour seems implausible. It might be much more appealing to claim that there is a limit to how irrational intentional behaviour can be. Is a very bad argument still an argument?

There is a reply to the contention that irrationality is not always responsible for failures of interpretation. Is it not the case that when the observed behaviour fails to satisfy norms of rationality, then it is also difficult or impossible to rationalise it? The most compelling examples are inconsistencies. Suppose that for some $p$ and some $q$, Mark reports that $p$ and that not-$p$, that $q$ and that not-$q$, and so on. If Mark reports both that the cherry tree in his back garden is dead, and that it is not dead, should we predict that he will wait for cherries next spring? It seems that one cannot predict or explain Mark's behaviour in intentional terms when his belief reports are just plainly inconsistent. Verbal reports are good evidence (not conclusive evidence) for what one believes and additional evidence for the interpreter comes from the observation of relevant behaviour. In the case at hand, the interpreter has conflicting evidence and very few indications of what may be going amiss. It is possible that Mark is particularly bad at reporting what his genuine mental states are like or that only further evidence will settle the issue—for instance, it would be evidence for Mark's belief that the cherry tree is still alive if he watered it regularly.

The example can also be used to challenge the distinction between intelligibility and rationality. I suggested that intelligibility is a plausible but trivial condition on the ascription of beliefs, whereas the rationality constraint would be interesting, but too demanding. A critic could suggest that the two notions turn out to be much closer than I described them, given that the failure to satisfy standards of procedural rationality (such as the inconsistency in Mark's reports) brings about a failure of intelligibility. A reply would be to argue that the project of treating people like Mark as subjects with beliefs is not necessarily doomed. Unless Mark reports badly integrated attitudes synchronically, at any one time Mark will endorse either $p$ or not-$p$ and the interpreter will make an attribution on the basis of Mark's reports and other observable behaviour which will constitute evidence for what Mark believes at that stage. Why did Mark look at the tree with tears in his eyes on Monday? Because he believed it was dead. Why was he so excited about picking cherries on Tuesday? Because at that time he believed that the tree was still alive. It is possible that Mark 'changed his mind' or that he had both attitudes from the start, but one was activated and operative on the Monday, and the other was activated and operative on the Tuesday. If Mark endorses the conjunction of two contradictory statements, the interpreter may just have to give up.

In our daily life we encounter people who declare that some issues are really important for them, and then do nothing to contribute to their understanding or resolution; people who at the same time fear and desire some life-changing outcome; people who are torn between what they would like to believe and what the evidence tells them to believe. Mark's behaviour is perplexing in a way in which these common behaviours aren't, because these behaviours are complex, whereas our example is straight-forward (in the underspecified way in which we presented it). Although it is true that we do not witness regularly the endorsement of open contradictions, the difference between Mark's surprising verbal behaviour and more familiar cases seems to be a difference in degree of integration. In this case it is right that a violation of a norm of rationality is present and a subject's behaviour results as unintelligible to interpreters, but the fact that on one occasion unintelligibility and irrationality co-occur is neither a reason to think that they should be collapsed, nor a reason to think that they play the same role in constraining belief ascription.

Where there is a failure of intelligibility, interpretation is compromised, for the very simple reason that to interpret behaviour is to make it intelligible, to rationalise it in the weak sense I proposed. But the reason for the failure of intelligibility may vary, and cannot always be found in cases of irrationality. Some instances of behaviour may not be intentional, or may be misunderstood due to relevant differences between the interpreter and the subject of interpretation, or due to the interpreter's limited knowledge of the shared environment or of the subject's cognitive situation. For instance, Mark's behaviour would become much less perplexing if we knew that he had a memory impairment or that he suffered from a dissociative disorder in the context of which bad integration among beliefs is not uncommon.

### 2.4.3 Interpreting in the real world

When difficulties in interpretation emerge and the interpreter cannot ascribe beliefs with determinate content, the problem does not necessarily lie in the subject's failure to behave rationally. So far, I have just hinted at some factors that might be relevant, but here I shall argue that most of the difficulties interpreters encounter when they fail to ascribe intentional states with determinate content are due to the subject's behaviour being outside of the scope of application of the heuristics that guide (as opposed to constrain) the interpretive exercise. Considerations about rationality might still have an important role to play at the level of heuristics, together with considerations about the plausibility of the subject's beliefs and their similarity to the interpreter's beliefs. However, considerations of rationality, plausibility, or similarity of behaviour are not necessary conditions for the intentional characterisation of behaviour.

It is a precondition for ascribing intentional states that the interpreter masters folk-psychological concepts. A theory of mind usually emerges between 2 and 3 years of age, allowing us to distinguish between external reality and representations of reality by ourselves and others. In the much cited and controversial false-belief task (see Leslie 1987; Wimmer and Perner 1983), children younger than 3 years of age fail to ascribe false beliefs to the character of an incomplete fictional story and, as a consequence, cannot predict accurately what the character will do in the rest of the story. There are doubts about the ecological validity and the implications of the test (Bloom and German 2000, Repacholi and Slaughter 2003), and multiple versions of the false-belief task have been designed since the original studies (Call and Tomasello 1999). Independent of one's stance on the false-belief task as a reliable indicator of a theory of mind, it is very likely that different skills are associated with different capacities and levels of development. For our purposes here, it is sufficient to agree that explanation and prediction of behaviour in intentional terms require some (implicit) grasp of the notion of belief. By reflecting on the data gathered in the false-belief task and other relevant psychological evidence, it is fair to conclude that humans are not born competent folk psychologists but acquire mind-reading capacities in the course of their normal development.

Although familiarity with the subject's cognitive and social context is not a precondition for successful interpretation, shared background knowledge between interpreter and subject, or at least good potential for communication between them, is likely to impact on interpretation and on the determinacy of the ascribed belief contents. It is a common experience among people who move to a new environment without being completely fluent in the local language, or without being accustomed to local conventions, that misunderstandings ensue in the way in which their verbal and non-verbal behaviours are interpreted. The importance of shared background and communicability is emphasised in those situations in which interpreter and subject are significantly different in their cognitive capacities and are also unable to communicate effectively, either verbally or non-verbally. These are the circumstances that justified the use of the term 'radical interpretation': you need to imagine that you are an anthropologist in a far-away land, meeting people who speak a language radically different from yours, and from other known languages, and trying to make sense of their utterances by relying exclusively on the causal relations between them, yourself and the shared environment (Quine 1960; Davidson 1973). There is no need to construct such a remote scenario, as we all have experience of radical interpretation at home: trying to understand whether a kitten is hungry, and guess which type of food he prefers, can prove challenging; figuring out why a baby cries is just as difficult. The environment is shared, and some assumptions are made, but the cognitive situations of interpreter and subject of interpretation are radically different, and communication is impeded by lack of a common language.

Significant factors in more and less radical instances of interpretation are the interpreter's assumptions about the behaviour of the subject. One such factor is the assumption that the subject's behaviour will be rational. Such assumption needs to be clearly distinguished from versions of the rationality constraint on belief ascription. As we saw earlier, there are weak and strong versions of the rationality constraint on belief ascription. According to the weak version, the interpreter will not ascribe beliefs with determinate content to the subject unless the subject is rational. According to the strong version, the interpreter will not be able to ascribe beliefs to the subject at all unless the subject is rational. The assumption of rationality should not be phrased in either of these ways, as it is a contingent claim, not a necessary one. The assumption the interpreter makes is that the subject of interpretation behaves in a way that is rational. But this assumption is revisable, and can be adapted according to the specifics of the situation. Rationality here is not *constitutive* of *all* minded beings but it is a *heuristic* for the interaction with *some* minded beings, those beings whose behaviour is likely to conform to certain standards of rationality, e.g. well-educated adult humans with no statistically abnormal reasoning impairment.

Let me offer a couple of examples. On Wednesday I visited my friend Dan at the hospital. He had just undergone some surgery and he was still under the influence of a general anaesthetic. I asked him how he was feeling and we talked for ten minutes. During our conversation he seemed fine and gave me a fairly detailed account of what the doctor had told him earlier. On Friday I go back to the hospital to check if he is still fine. He is, but he has no recollection whatsoever of the conversation we had on Wednesday. Actually, he seems not to realize I had been there at all. He tells me that he thought he saw me in a dream. I ascribe to him the belief that I didn't go to see him on Wednesday. How do I arrive at this accurate and successful ascription? I have no reason to think that Dan is being insincere; I know he usually has a very good memory; but I also know he was under an anaesthetic when he saw me. This helps me make sense of the fact that he cannot remember our conversation. There is no unique route to interpreting Dan's behaviour successfully in this case. I can either reflect on what I would have been like if I had been in Dan's shoes, and arrive at the conclusion that in the same conditions I would have behaved similarly to Dan. Alternatively, if I have never experienced disorientation after a general anaesthetic, I will appeal to the generalisation that people are not fully aware of what happens to them when they are under the influence of an anaesthetic. This background information derives from my previous experience: either experience of my own behaviour, or experience of interactions with other subjects in similar circumstances, or indirect experience due to things I have heard or read before. The information that allows me to interpret Dan's sincere assertion that he doesn't remember my earlier visit is independent of judgements of rationality.

One might object that I am surreptitiously reintroducing the rationality constraint. Maybe the interpreter does not rely on the subject being rational, but he relies on the subject *not* being *irrational*. In Davidsonian jargon, the fact that Dan was under anaesthetic is an *excuse* for the fact that he forgot something he would not have forgotten otherwise, and that it makes his false belief more *explicable*. In ascribing to him the belief that I didn't go to see him previously, I justify him for forgetting my visit given his condition at the time. This is a clever and appealing response. But we need a more convincing argument for the view that rationality always has a role to play in interpretation. In the case just described, I am not relying on Dan being more or less rational, in the sense of his behaviour satisfying norms of rationality. Instead, I rely on some notion of statistical normalcy or well-functioning. It is not normal for Dan to be forgetting previous salient events. But the fact that he had still been under the influence of a general anaesthetic can make his forgetting behaviour normal. It would be misleading to claim that rationality requires for us to remember significant experiences in our recent past: if our memory functions well, then this is what we do, we remember significant events when they are not too remote. Our ability to remember past events is a sign that some of our cognitive capacities, those related to memory, are functioning well, rather than a sign of rationality. In the example, Dan is excused because his memory was not functioning well under the influence of an anaesthetic, but this seems to have no relevant connection with an assessment of his behaviour in terms of rationality.

Let's consider another example. While walking in the city centre, I am stopped by a man who is really excited and tells me that the dog resting on the steps of a nearby Catholic church raised his paw in a gesture of salute towards him. The man is convinced that he has just received a revelation (this example is adapted from a real-life case reported by Leeser and O'Donohue, 1999). The man's behaviour is unusual. The fact that he seems to derive a conclusion that is completely unjustified given the evidence available to him might not prevent me from ascribing to him (successfully) the belief that something significant happened to him, even though it is mysterious to me why he thinks the event he reports is significant. However, if I knew that the man suffers from schizophrenia and that in the past he has had other 'significant experiences' involving dogs and divine revelations, I could ascribe to him a more definite set of beliefs and attitudes. My knowledge that certain *rational* explanations of his behaviour become *less likely* given his history would make it easier for me to offer a tentative interpretation of his behaviour. I could use what I know about the behaviour of subjects with schizophrenia, and what I know about this man in particular, to make sense of what he said and of the way in which his report affected his behaviour.

Interpretation remains difficult in this case, but the difficulty seems to depend on the lack of shared beliefs between interpreter and speaker, and the scarcity of background knowledge. Some of the difficulties are attenuated by greater knowledge, on behalf of the interpreter, about the cognitive situation and history of the subject whose behaviour requires interpretation. My critic, the friend of the rationality constraint on belief ascription, could of course insist that where difficulties are found, they can be explained by the subject behaving irrationally (in this case, there would be a failure to satisfy norms of epistemic rationality). Although this reading is certainly more plausible in this latter example than it was in the former, a similar reply to the one I offered earlier could also be attempted in this case. Statistical normalcy is doing all the job! If the revelation had involved the appearance of a sacred image rather than the gesture of a dog, the reported belief would have been less difficult to interpret, and to be given specific content to, even if arguably it would have also been irrational from a purely epistemic point of view.

My suggestion is that we should view the practice of interpretation as guided by fallible (but generally successful) heuristics. By reflecting on the practice of interpretation we can sketch a very simple framework. When we interpret others we use our background knowledge constituted by some folk-psychological generalizations and by what we know about the subject to be interpreted and the surrounding environment. In some contexts we also adopt heuristics of similarity and rationality. That is, we tend to assume that people who are in some respects similar to us behave as we do, and we also assume that the typical human adult is largely consistent, reasons competently, and so on. The heuristics won't apply to all the instances of behaviour that we might be interested in interpreting, and even when they do apply, they will be applied in different ways and to a different extent depending on the situation and on the background knowledge about the individual subject. For instance, we might realize that competent reasoning is unlikely in traumatic circumstances and that even people who are similar to us in their opinions and social behaviour might act very differently from us and from their usual selves when they are tired, stressed or heavily intoxicated.[10]

---

[10] See Cooper, R. (2007) for an application of these debates to mental illness.

### 2.4.4 Heuristics *versus* constraints

The interpreter's assumptions are flexible and revisable heuristics, not constraints. They are supposed to guide the interpreter and help her to ascribe
intentional states with determinate content to a variety of subjects in a variety
of situations, but they are not criteria for deciding whether a subject's utterance expresses a belief. The suggestion that some folk psychological generalisation, considerations of similarity and rationality, and experience guide
interpretation is not an original suggestion: in the traditional debate about
how we read other minds, where the theory-theorists are opposed to the sim-
ulation-theorists, these factors are acknowledged and discussed, and other
issues are also addressed, as for instance whether this body of knowledge relevant to interpretation is available at the personal or sub-personal level. But my
point here is that, once we have this simple framework in place, we don't need
to find preconditions for intentionality in the rationality of subject's behaviour, as we already have some resources to explain the connection between
rationality and intentionality, without committing ourselves to a necessary
claim that is refuted day by day by our experience as interpreters. Belief ascription in the last instance is grounded on the interpreter's background knowledge, which includes some folk-psychological generalizations, some
information about the subject (the kind of subject and the individual), and
some information about the environment. A folk-psychological generalization
is something like: 'People whose bodily tissue is damaged experience pain,'
'Creatures avoid what they are afraid of,' and so on. The information about the
system that might turn out to be relevant includes data about the subject's
psychological make-up and stage of development, her belonging to some
linguistic or cultural group or community, and her background beliefs and
opinions. Of course, this information won't always be available to the interpreter. The same applies to the information about the environment, which
might include information about other agents in that environment that are
not being the direct focus of interpretation, or contextual factors that have a
causal impact on the subject and her behaviour.

   Think about the classic scenario of radical interpretation. I see a man pointing at a hopping rabbit and uttering a sentence in a language unknown to me.
Given what I can observe about the man and the environment (that there is a
rabbit, that the man seems to want to refer to the rabbit with his utterance,
etc.) and given my assumption that the man is sensitive to events in his environment, my working hypothesis will be that the man is uttering something
like: 'Look, there is a rabbit,' 'What a beautiful rabbit!,' or 'Dinner!' Only a
better acquaintance with the language that the man is speaking, or a better
acquaintance with the man's intentions and beliefs about rabbits, could make

my ascription more determinate. Even though I do not know much at all about the man, just by observing him I can assume that he is a normal adult human being with a complex network of beliefs and desires. If I knew that the man found rabbits particularly cute, I would guess that he might have meant to say: 'What a beautiful rabbit!' If it had come to my attention, instead, that the man finds rabbits delicious to eat, I would ascribe him the belief that the rabbit would make a fine dinner and predict that he will try to catch the rabbit. In interpreting the man's behaviour I am not necessarily relying on any rationality assumption. The man who finds rabbits cute is likely to exclaim 'What a beautiful rabbit!' because his appreciation of rabbits gives him a reason (not necessarily a good reason) to do so.

I can also focus on the rabbit, and notice that it accelerates when the man points at it and he starts running after it. Though there is no utterance to which I can ascribe meaning in this case, I might wonder why the rabbit hops faster and hides in a bush. The reason might be that the rabbit identifies the excited man as a potential predator and wants to avoid being captured (or, more simply, runs away because it is scared). In this case I shall still appeal for my ascription to the knowledge of the environment and the assumption that there are causal relations among the actors within the same environment. I shall also appeal to what I know about rabbits. Rabbits are not likely to engage in sophisticated, abstract, or self-reflective thought, but they might be able to form simple beliefs about their surrounding environment, and potential prey and predators are likely to attract their attention. In this scenario we have two cases of radical interpretation, yet there is no need for the interpreter to assume a conceptual link between rationality and the intentionality of belief states.

Rather, the interpreter's expectations and assumptions could be seen as a set of inductive generalizations triggered by contextual features of the environment shared by the interpreter and the subject and by what the interpreter already knows about the subject. These generalizations might be of very heterogeneous nature and might partially concern the reasoning capacities of the subject, the similarity of her opinions to those of the interpreter, or even her capacity to follow certain norms for the formation, integration, and revision of beliefs. But in some contexts, as we have seen, it is the assumption that the subject will behave irrationally that leads to a more determinate and effortless attribution. We sometimes expect the speaker to be irrational: when we ask undergraduate students to solve the Wason selection task, we expect many of them to fail the task. When we discuss politics with an obstinate friend we might expect her to defend a view that we find implausible. Often, it is the assumption that subjects with beliefs will not meet some standards of rationality that allows us to ascribe beliefs with determinate content or predict the intentional behaviour of others.

Even those who are persuaded by the distinction between the notions of rationalisation and conformity or subscription to norms of rationality can resist the rejection of a necessary constraint on interpretation. Maybe I am right that our everyday practice of interpretation is guided by fallible heuristics rather than by a general constraint, but it is still possible that there is a kind of constitutive constraint on interpretation. Maybe the constitutive constraint is not that a subject's behaviour must satisfy certain standards of rationality, but that the correct interpretation of a subject's behaviour is the one that makes best possible sense of that subject's total life and conduct: an overall intelligibility constraint has greater plausibility than a rationality constraint. But we might not need either. An overall intelligibility constraint would not serve to guide the actual practice of interpretation because interpreters have to deal with temporally bounded instances of a subject's behaviour; they are in conditions of partial ignorance about the environment, the subject's past and the subject's future; and they lack a general overview of the subject's interactions with the given environment. If we were happy to acknowledge that a constitutive constraint on interpretation need not be reflected in the practice of interpretation, the overall intelligibility constraint could be rescued. However, as we observed earlier, interpretationism is appealing because it attempts to clarify difficult theoretical issues such as the nature of intentional states and the conditions for having beliefs by analysing the actual practice of interpretation. If we endorse the constitutive version of the overall intelligibility constraint, the powerful link between the theoretical issues and our task as interpreters is broken. The conditions for belief ascription are no longer in step with the evidential bases on which we actually ascribe beliefs in real time in the real world, but will depend on the constraints applicable to an idealization of our actual practice of interpretation that does not necessarily reflect what we do when we ascribe beliefs. This seems to undermine the basic motivation for the interpretationist view. Of course, it is open to the modern-day Davidsonian to have a double account. That is, one can insist that there is a constitutive constraint that operates at the level of ideal interpretation and at the same time allow that other considerations (e.g. the interpreter's background knowledge and the heuristics she might use) play a major role in practice.

## Summary of chapter 2

In this chapter the main purpose was to review and assess the following objection to the doxastic conception of delusions: delusions are not beliefs because they are procedurally irrational.

In Section 2.1, we described the notion of procedural irrationality and focused on one norm, that of good integration in a belief system. By offering examples of mono- and polythematic delusions with varying degrees of circumscription and elaboration, we gathered evidence for the claim that delusions are typically procedurally irrational, and in particular they suffer from bad integration with one another, and with the subject's beliefs. In the same section we sketched some arguments for the view that delusions are other than beliefs: delusions are imaginings that the subject ascribes to herself as beliefs (mistakenly); delusions are not simply doxastic states but alternative realities in which the subject operates. Both the former argument, developed by Currie and colleagues, and the latter, developed by Gallagher, are examples of how versions of the procedural rationality constraints underlie objections to the doxastic conception of delusions.

In Section 2.2, we described cases of non-pathological beliefs which can be seen as violations of the norm of good integration. In order to make a stronger case for general beliefs being vulnerable to procedural irrationality, we considered a variety of cases: 1) preference reversals, where equivalent outcomes are judged differently according to the way in which they are described, or the method on the basis of which subjects arrive at their judgements; 2) beliefs about the probability of events which sometimes but not always track judgements of representativeness; 3) superstitious beliefs which conflict with other beliefs and values subjects endorse.

In Section 2.3, we developed an objection to arguments against the doxastic conception of delusions and considered some plausible responses. The problem with any argument structured around the rationality constraint on the ascription of beliefs is that many typical beliefs fail to satisfy the norm of rationality that is taken to be a precondition for the ascription of beliefs. This gives rise to a 'double standards' accusation: why should delusions, but not badly integrated beliefs, lose their belief status on the basis of their procedural irrationality? To this question, proponents of non-doxastic accounts of delusions usually respond with an illustration of the qualitative or categorical difference between delusions and procedurally irrational beliefs. By examining the notions of recovery from a violation of a norm of rationality; excusability on the basis of compartmentalisation; and explicability and charitable 'correction', I challenged the view that delusions are procedurally irrational in a qualitatively different way from badly integrated beliefs.

In Section 2.4, I have discussed and challenged the following view about the relationship between rationality and the intentionality exhibited by subjects with beliefs: even though it is possible to ascribe beliefs to systems that behave irrationally, the belief states we ascribe to them might not turn out to be determinate in content, and this shows that there is some weak but necessary relation between intentionality and rationality. I have suggested that there are other ways to explain the difficulties that the interpreter sometimes encounters in ascribing beliefs with determinate content: for instance, the interpreter might have limited knowledge of the subject's background beliefs, of the subject's psychological make-up, or of causal relations in the environment. Rationality does not necessarily have a major role to play in the ascription of beliefs, although considerations about the rationality of a pattern of behaviour might be useful in some specific contexts, as heuristics guiding the interpretation of fully competent human adults.

In order to make this point, I distinguished between intelligibility or rationalization, and the satisfaction of norms of rationality (such as bad integration). If Alex asserts that pigs have wings, claims to have some evidence for it or no evidence against it, defends the claim when challenged, and is disposed to manifest his commitment to the claim, then he believes that pigs have wings—and an interpreter will ascribe to him that belief and will be able to explain and predict Alex's behaviour in the light of that belief. But we need not assume that it is rational for Alex to believe that pigs have wings. Alex might have other beliefs that conflict with his belief (bad integration), might not have good evidence for his belief (lack of evidential support), or might have discarded good evidence against it (unresponsiveness to evidence), and might behave in a way that is not consistent with or explicable by his belief (attitude-behaviour inconsistency). These considerations affect judgements of procedural, epistemic and agential rationality but do not constitute a reason for the interpreter to deny that Alex believes that pigs have wings. Alex's behaviour is intelligible—and yet it is unlikely to satisfy norms of rationality.

# Chapter 3

# Epistemic rationality and belief ascription

> Delusions by their very nature are beliefs that reality has failed to constrain.
>
> (McKay, Langdon and Coltheart, *Sleights of Mind*)

> It is a natural hypothesis that the positive symptoms of schizophrenia will be correlated with impairments of epistemic rationality. As we remarked earlier, the central positive symptom of delusion seems *prima facie* to contravene the basic principles of epistemic rationality in so far as the delusional patient is in the grip of a distorted perspective on the world.
>
> (Bermúdez, *Normativity and Rationality in Delusional Psychiatric Disorders*)

In this chapter I consider a set of arguments for the view that delusions are not beliefs because they fail to meet the epistemic rationality constraint on belief ascription. When we discussed procedural rationality in the previous chapter, we focused on one norm (that can have different applications): good integration of beliefs and other intentional states. Here I consider two norms of epistemic rationality (which cannot always be kept completely distinct in their applications): good evidential support and responsiveness to evidence.

The lack of support argument concludes that delusions are not beliefs because they are not sufficiently supported by the available evidence:

i) In order for *b* to be ascribed to a subject as a belief, *b* needs to be well-supported by the evidence available to the subject.
ii) Delusions are not well-supported by the evidence available to the subject.
  Thus, delusions cannot be ascribed to the subject as beliefs.

The unresponsiveness to evidence argument concludes that delusions are not beliefs because they are not sufficiently responsive to the available evidence.

For instance, they may be maintained even if counterevidence becomes available.

  i) In order for *b* to be ascribed to a subject as a belief, *b* needs to be responsive to the evidence available to the subject.
  ii) Delusions are not responsive to the evidence available to the subject.
  Thus, delusions cannot be ascribed to the subject as beliefs.

In Section 3.1, I describe the central role of the notion of epistemic rationality in accounts of delusions. Delusions are defined in terms of their defying norms of epistemic rationality, and the *rigidity* or *fixity* of delusions is also an important diagnostic element. The most influential arguments against the belief status of delusions come from epistemic considerations.

In Section 3.2, my purpose is to turn to the empirical literature in order to establish whether the second premise of the lack of support argument and of the unresponsiveness to evidence argument is justified. When delusions are formed, are they totally unsupported, or badly supported by evidence? When they are maintained, are they excessively resistant to counterevidence? According to the most prominent accounts of delusion formation, there is usually some experience that the delusional hypothesis is aimed at explaining and there is some evidential support to which the subject can appeal in order to defend the content of her delusion, although the route from the experience to the delusion may be characterised by a faulty or viciously circular reasoning process. The relationship between evidence and hypothesis re-assessment is a complex one, and examples will be used to illustrate the claim that delusions may be more impervious to counterargument or empirical disconfirmation than many typical beliefs.

In Section 3.3, I examine the plausibility of the epistemic rationality constraint, by considering whether non-pathological beliefs are well-supported by evidence.

In Section 3.4, I ask whether they are responsive to evidence. The aim is to assess the first premise of the lack of support argument and unresponsiveness to evidence argument. People often endorse beliefs that are not well-supported by the available evidence and maintain beliefs in the face of powerful counterevidence. Evidence of epistemically irrational beliefs undermines the motivation for theories of belief ascription that rely on the epistemic rationality constraint.

In the end, I don't deny that delusions are epistemically irrational, for their resistance to counterevidence if not for their lack of evidential support, and I also concede that, in the typical case, they are epistemically irrational to a higher degree than non-pathological beliefs. But I resist the suggestion that delusions and epistemically irrational beliefs are qualitatively different.

Beliefs come in different shapes, and for some belief contents the question whether they are well-supported by evidence or responsive to evidence does not apply or makes little sense. For other belief contents, the relationship with the available evidence is crucial to their rationality, but does not determine their status as beliefs.

Considerations about the epistemic pitfalls of non-pathological beliefs and the epistemic merit of some reasoning styles that are conducive to accepting delusional hypotheses offer powerful reasons to resist the suggestion that epistemic rationality should be a precondition for the ascription of beliefs.

## 3.1 **Delusions and epistemic rationality**

Epistemic rationality provides norms that govern the formation, the maintenance, and the revision of beliefs. Delusions are paradigmatically conceived as violations of epistemic rationality. It is sufficient to look back at the definitions of delusions we cited in Section 1.4.1 to find that the most common characterisation of delusions is that of a belief which is not well-supported by the available evidence and resists counterevidence. For example, the DSM-IV (2000, p. 765) says that a delusion is:

> A false belief based on incorrect inference about external reality **that is firmly sustained despite what almost everyone else believes** and **despite what constitutes incontrovertible and obvious proof or evidence to the contrary**.
>
> (my emphasis)

Other definitions highlight the epistemic faults of delusions but also take into account the possibility of revision:

> Usually a delusion is defined as a false belief that is also strongly held such that it exerts a strong influence on behaviour and **is not susceptible to counter-arguments or counter-evidence** (or, at least, the delusion is unshakeable over a short timescale and in the absence of systematic attempts at belief modification).
>
> (Charlton 2003, p. 315, my emphasis)

> A delusion is a belief (probably false) at the extreme end of the continuum of consensual agreement. It is not categorically different from overvalued ideas and normal beliefs. It is held in spite of evidence to the contrary **but it may be amenable to change when that evidence is collaboratively explored**. In that case the belief may come to approximate more closely to ideas in keeping with the person's social, cultural, educational and religious background.
>
> (Kingdon and Turkington 2004, p. 96, my emphasis)

These definitions suggest that delusions can be revised in some circumstances and that they are (to some extent) sensitive to cognitive probing.

### 3.1.1 Cognitive probing

Even philosophers who argue that delusions are not necessarily irrational from a procedural point of view, concede that they are epistemically faulty. Bermúdez (2001), for instance, suggests that the claim that delusions are no more irrational than other beliefs is plausible with respect to procedural rationality but implausible with respect to epistemic rationality. Traditionally, philosophers have identified a constitutive link between beliefs and evidence (e.g. Price 1967) which has been preserved in many of the later accounts of beliefs in psychology and psychiatry. The theory tells us that beliefs are formed on the basis of evidence, and that they are responsive to evidence once they are formed (e.g. they cannot be maintained if powerful evidence against them becomes available). As we shall see, in Berrios (1991), this link has been relied upon in the attempt to argue against the doxastic conception of delusions.

We saw that the fact that beliefs aim at being well-integrated in a system is a core assumption in cognitive behavioural therapy and guides interventions in the case of delusions. The fact that beliefs respond to evidence is just as important to cognitive probing as the fact that they hang in a system. We shall see that, in the context of epistemic considerations, the deviations from the standards of epistemic rationality in the behaviour of subjects with delusions are often more accentuated than the deviations in the behaviour of normal subjects, That said, normal subjects also present biases in the gathering and weighting of evidence, and in the way in which they insulate certain beliefs from potentially disconfirming evidence. For instance, we all tend to be too conservative when asked to re-assess strongly held beliefs, and we are unlikely to modify such beliefs, even if convincing evidence against them becomes available. Further, we tend to revise more easily beliefs that are undesirable (e.g. negative beliefs about ourselves) and to maintain more strenuously beliefs that are desirable (e.g. beliefs that contribute positively to our self-image). In general, we attribute significance to events that concern ourselves, our responsibilities, and our achievements, even if, from an objective point of view, these events are in no way special and would deserve the same attention as events about the responsibilities and achievements of others.

Resistance to counterevidence, and the different weighing of evidence in relation to self-referential beliefs are common in subjects with delusions too, and in cognitive behavioural therapy these phenomena are treated by therapeutic applications of 'critical thinking': for instance, the therapist can invite the subject to consider alternative explanations for her delusional experience, and can invite the subject to think about novel (that is, previously ignored) pieces of evidence that count against the delusional state. Here is an example. If a woman believes that she is a witch, her belief will be challenged by the therapist when she acknowledges that she does not have any supernatural powers, as her conception of witches is likely to include the notion that they are able to, say, affect other people's behaviour with a spell, or cause catastrophes (Nelson 2005, pp. 143–4).

Coltheart (2005b) argues that cognitive behavioural therapy could have an important role to play in the treatment of subjects with delusions on the basis of considerations relevant to epistemic rationality. He observes how some subjects with Capgras delusion 'go in and out of the Capgras state' (p. 156). According to the two-factor account of delusion formation, the second factor is a deficit at the level of the hypothesis evaluation system and cannot be undone by cognitive therapy. However, the subject with delusions still *has* a hypothesis evaluation system. Coltheart speculates that, when the evidence against the delusional state is presented in an effective way, as in cognitive behavioural therapy where persuasive reasons against the delusional hypothesis are provided non-confrontationally and with constancy and systematicity, the subject is more inclined to reassess the delusional hypothesis and ends up losing confidence in it. Presenting evidence against the belief can encourage a suspension of judgement and lead the subject to doubt the content of the delusion. In the most favourable circumstances, the subject can even come to accept a more plausible hypothesis, at least for some time. Notice that in these challenges to delusional reports it is not always easy to distinguish elements of procedural and epistemic rationality. If we think about how the belief that Sarah is a witch fits with the evidence that Sarah cannot make any spells, we think in terms of epistemic relations between the content of her delusional state and how things are. If we think about how the belief that Sarah is a witch fits with other beliefs she has about witches (e.g. that they are evil), we think in terms of how the delusional state is compatible with her relevant background knowledge.

The fact that cognitive behavioural therapy has a record of positive outcomes, combined with some promising reports of individual cases in which cognitive probing was effective, suggests that subjects with delusions have not lost the capacity to 'recover' from their irrationality and can be sensitive to evidence in some circumstances.[1] Yet, the characterisation of delusions as unfounded and very resistant to counterevidence has inspired a number of influential anti-doxastic arguments.

---

[1] Arguably, cognitive behavioural therapy can help in conjunction with medication by intervening on anxiety, excessive preoccupation, and social withdrawal.

## 3.1.2 **Anti-doxastic arguments: delusions aren't probable explanations**

Reality testing is widely regarded as an important factor in determining whether a mental state is a belief state. In many accounts of belief, the acceptance of a belief and its maintenance are described as hostage to evidence, to how reality is. The subject forms a belief if evidence supports it, and is prepared to give it up if evidence against it becomes available. Very influential versions of arguments against the doxastic conception of delusions are based on the claim that delusions are detached from reality. Louis Sass (1994) argues that a subject with delusions refers to the private world of her experience when she reports delusional states, and does not engage with the real world. Apparent evidence for this account is that the subject often recognises the absurdity of the content of her delusion, but she does not regard such implausibility as a sufficient reason for her to abandon the delusional state (see also Gallagher 2009 and Young 2000). Another apparent reason to regard delusions as concerning non-actual realities comes from the phenomenon of double-bookkeeping, caused by the tension between the behaviour of the subject and her acceptance of the content of her delusions as true.

German Berrios goes further. By arguing that the utterances by subjects with delusions are 'empty speech acts', he doesn't just deny that they are beliefs, he denies that they are states with intentional content. As Berrios's argument strongly relies on having a particular view of what beliefs are, I shall describe it in more detail. This is what Berrios says:

> We must now test the hypothesis that, from the structural point of view, delusions are, in fact, beliefs. Price (1934) distinguished four elements that comprise a belief (P):
> a) Entertaining P, together with one or more alternative propositions Q and R;
> b) Knowing a fact or set of facts (F), which is relevant to P, Q or R;
> c) Knowing that F makes P more likely than Q or R;
> d) Assenting to P; which in turn includes (i) the preferring of P to Q and R; (ii) the feeling a certain degree of confidence with regard to P.
> Price's criteria are clear and elegant enough, but it is clear that no current textbook or empirical definition of delusion can be set in terms of these four criteria.
>
> (Berrios 1991, p. 8)

Berrios observes that delusions do not meet Price's criteria (a)–(d) for beliefs and concludes that we should not regard them as beliefs. He offers two main reasons for this anti-doxastic conclusion. First, rarely would there be a fact, or a set of facts, that is relevant to the content of the delusion (see point b). Here Berrios seems to dismiss the possibility that a delusional hypothesis is formulated *in order to explain* a certain event or experience, or that the subject's experience can lend evidential support to the content of the delusion.

Second, even if there were a fact, or set of facts, relevant to the content of the delusion, and in need of explanation, subjects would not themselves assign higher probability to the content of the delusional hypothesis than to that of alternative hypotheses (see points c and d). Independent of the plausibility of Price's criteria, which in my view offer an excessively narrow account of what beliefs are, Berrios' concerns can be turned into powerful arguments against the view that delusions are beliefs and have been very influential in the psychiatric literature. Thus, they deserve our attention.

Berrios seems to think that, when a subject S believes that P, part of what it is for S to have that belief is to take P to explain some fact of interest, and to regard P as more probable than some relevant alternatives Q and R that are also potential explanations for the fact of interest. Even if these conditions do not apply to all cases of belief (e.g. arguably perceptual beliefs do not *explain* anything), let's assume that they do apply to some type of beliefs, and that, if delusions were beliefs at all, they would belong to that type of beliefs. If the content of the delusion is not an explanation of some fact of interest, and is not regarded as more probable than relevant alternatives by the subject, it cannot be said to be *believed* by the subject. It could be the content of another intentional state, such as an act of imagination which does not need to be relevant to any specific fact, or does not even need to have a probable content. (A different argument would be necessary to support the claim that delusions are not intentional states at all, but empty speech acts. As we focus on arguments against the doxastic conception of delusions here, we shall not examine Berrios' further claims in this context. Let me just add that, although there are good reasons to challenge the belief status of delusions, it is very implausible to claim that delusional reports are entirely devoid of intentional content).

Here is an example of the standard process of belief formation according to Berrios. I went shopping and got some cookies. When I get home, I find no cookies in my bag. Why are there no cookies? Different potential explanations come to mind. I intended to get cookies, but then I forgot. Another possibility is that I got the cookies and paid for them at the cashier, but forgot to pack them with the rest of the shopping. A third possibility is that my evil neighbour made the cookies disappear with a spell. The fact that there are no cookies in my bag has many potential explanations which can be more or less plausible in context. Berrios assumes that if I seem to endorse an explanation that I do not regard as the most probable, then I cannot genuinely *believe* that explanation. The subject with delusions seems to endorse an explanation for a fact of interest that is less probable (in her own assessment) than alternative explanations. This account of delusional reports, according to which believing an explanation depends on assessing the probability of the believed event and finding it greater than the probability of competing explanations, leaves some questions unanswered. If subjects with delusions do not believe the content of their delusions, why do they behave as if they believed something they do not believe? Are they deceiving others or themselves? (In the metarepresentational account we previously discussed, subjects with delusions mistakenly believe that they believe the content of their delusions, but Berrios does not explicitly endorse a metarepresentational account, as he seems to think that an explanation of delusions involves neither first-order nor second-order beliefs).

Leaving further questions aside for the time being, is it plausible to make the claim that delusions lack evidential support and that there are no facts that they can be taken to explain? We can certainly tell a story according to which subjects develop their delusional hypotheses as a consequence of having an experience that they cannot explain otherwise. For instance, subjects with the Capgras delusion come to believe that their spouses have been replaced by impostors, because there is a fact that they experience and that is relevant to the content of their delusions, i.e. the fact that, all of a sudden, their spouses appear different to them. If there is a fact in need of explanation, and the substitution hypothesis can explain that fact, subjects have *some reason* to claim that their spouses have been replaced. Their reason for endorsing the substitution hypothesis might not be a *good* reason: subjects ignore alternative hypotheses (e.g. that something is wrong with their face recognition process) and do not take sufficiently into account the testimony of people they have no special reason to mistrust (e.g. relatives and doctors). But not having a good reason is different from not having a reason at all. It is true that the endorsement of the delusional hypothesis is not *well*-supported by evidence, but it is not completely ungrounded either. For those delusions that can be explained by reference to a powerful abnormal experience, the claim that the delusion is unsupported by evidence, or that there are no facts of interest that the delusion can be said to explain, seems implausible.

However, the doxastic account of delusions needs to account for the apparent disanalogy between delusions and beliefs in their relationship with evidence. The anti-doxastic argument by Berrios tells us that delusions do not behave like beliefs, because the subject does not come to doubt the content of the delusion on the basis of the available evidence as she would do in a typical case of believing. One could argue that, even if Price's criterion (b) were met by delusions, delusions would still fail to behave as if they were beliefs. My answer is that delusions do not behave like *rational* beliefs, but most beliefs do not behave like rational beliefs either. Subjects with delusions prefer a hypothesis with low initial probability, maybe involving the presence of aliens or clones, or an evil conspiracy against them, to a hypothesis that appears much more plausible given their other beliefs. It is true that this preference speaks against the subjects' epistemic rationality, but should it also speak against their having beliefs? It is fair to speculate that subjects with delusions do not regard the content of their delusions as more probable than relevant alternatives. The man who reports that his wife has been replaced by aliens and doesn't go to the police for fear that they would not believe him, knows that the content of his delusional state is not very probable. He knows that it is not going to be easily believed by other people. Endorsing a hypothesis with low probability may be a sign of epistemic irrationality, but does not necessarily constitute a knock-down argument against the view that the content of the delusion is genuinely believed. We can imagine other situations in which people believe things that they do not regard as more probable than relevant alternatives. Religious beliefs or beliefs in supernatural phenomena are a good example. Any Christian would agree that, in general, if the body of a dead man is not found in the tomb, it is more probable that the body were stolen than that the man resurrected from the dead. But this does not prevent Christians from endorsing the belief that Jesus resurrected from the dead and that his body was not stolen.[2]

### 3.1.3 Anti-doxastic arguments: delusions aren't responsive to evidence

The problematic relationship between delusions and evidence has also been emphasised in the philosophical literature by Currie and colleagues (Currie, 2000; Currie and Jureidini, 2001; Currie and Ravenscroft, 2002). They highlight the discrepancy between the content of the delusion and the content of the belief that would be warranted given the evidence available to the subject. On the basis of such discrepancy, they argue that delusions are more likely to be imaginings than beliefs.

Here is an anti-doxastic argument that can be developed on the basis of views about the appropriate source of belief states in belief formation and their sensitivity to evidence once they are formed. Currie and colleagues argue that perception offers material *more directly* to imaginings than to beliefs: in imagination we are happy to take the content of our experiences at face value (as subjects with delusions often seem to do). But when we form beliefs on the

---

[2] One might object that religious beliefs are not really beliefs, or are beliefs of a special kind, an exception to the rule rather than a core case. I shall come back to this point later in the chapter.

basis of perceptual experience, we seem to go through a *screening* or *filtering* stage where we assess hypotheses for plausibility before endorsing them.

> We might be readily *imagine* that a stranger's gaunt appearance signals that he has AIDS but be rightly very resistant to *believing* it without further evidence.
>
> (Currie and Jureidini 2001, pp. 159–60, my emphasis)

Let's flesh out this view by reference to a classic case of erotomania[3]:

> She realized he was empty without her and was pursuing her, but enemies were preventing them from uniting. The enemies included a number of people: people in her family, her classmates, neighbours and many other persons who were plotting to keep them apart. She knew that her conclusions were accurate because he would send messages to her proving his love. These messages would often present themselves as the license plates on cars of a certain state, the color purple and other indications that she received from the environment that proved to her that he loved her.
>
> (Jordan *et al.* 2006, p. 787)

The subject offers reasons to prove that the man she loves is in turn in love with her, but the 'evidence' she mentions (e.g. messages he sends her by means of licence plates) is not only insufficient to support her belief, but also seems to have no obvious connection to the content of the belief. The model defended by Currie and his colleagues could be made to work for the this example of erotomania and other similar cases: the delusional hypothesis is put forward in spite of its implausibility. A person in love could easily *imagine* that a certain licence plate is a 'sign' that her love is corresponded but she doesn't *believe* that there is any genuine evidential connection between the plate and the feelings that another person can have for her. The problem with the account, though, is that delusions of erotomania lead to action that is consistent with the content of the delusions, and they have inferential connections with the subject's beliefs (e.g. with beliefs about potential obstacles to the enjoyment of the alleged romantic relationship). These features are more likely to be features of beliefs than imaginings.

Good evidence in support of the belief that Karl is in love with Myra should be acknowledged by Myra and contribute to her coming to believe that Karl is in love with her. But if there is no good evidence to start with, or evidence against the belief becomes available at a later stage, then Myra should come to doubt the hypothesis, suspend judgement or even abandon the hypothesis altogether. In so far as they lack evidential support and resist counterevidence, delusions *are* epistemically irrational. Maybe the subject is not always epistemically

---

[3] Subjects having this delusion believe that another (usually of higher status) is in love with them.

blameworthy for entertaining the delusional hypothesis, but why is the hypothesis endorsed when more plausible hypotheses are available? More important still, why isn't the initially preferred hypothesis discounted later, when reasons against it pile up? One possible answer to these questions is that the content of the delusion is somehow encapsulated[4] as the content of some visual illusions.

The analogy between *perceptual* and *cognitive* illusions is difficult to resist:

> If certain stimuli trick your visual system into constructing an illusion, knowing that you have been tricked does not mean that the illusion disappears. The part of the visual system that produces the illusion is impervious to correction based on such knowledge.

> (Roser and Gazzaniga 2004, p. 56)

> [A delusion] can simply take over the content of the experience, as when a hallucinating subject has an experience of a pink rat and comes to believe that the pink rat is in front of him.

> (Currie and Jureidini 2001, p. 159)

We see the straw in a glass of water as bent or broken. We might even come to believe— for instance the first time that we are subject to the illusion— that the straw is bent. But then we revise our belief when we realise that our visual experience was misleading. Capgras patients have many good reasons to doubt that the content of their experience can be satisfactorily explained by their delusional state, including the authority of their doctors and the testimony of their families. The experience of recognising the voice of the spouse on the phone, but not recognising it when the spouse is in front of them, should have an effect on the Capgras patient that is similar to the effect of viewing the straw out of the glass after having been subject to the perceptual illusion that the straw was bent or broken. In the case of illusions, after seeing that the straw is not bent, we realise that experience had misled us to believe that the straw was bent and we give up the belief that it is. But subjects with Capgras fail to register the opportunity for a reality-check. They hear the same voice both when they talk on the phone with their spouse and when they talk to them in person, but recognise it in the former case and do not recognise it in the latter. They do not easily give up the content of their delusion in the face of other challenges made by relatives and therapists—'How can the impostor have this information?'; 'Why does she wear your wife's ring?', and so on.

---

[4] By that I mean that the endorsement of the content of the delusion is not amenable to change on the basis of the information available to the subject.

Considerations about encapsulation are compatible with the hypothesis that delusions are imaginings. Imaginings are not necessarily revised on the basis of new experiences, because they are not subject to reality testing.

> Imaginings are not apt to be revised in the light of evidence; the whole point of imagining is to be able to engage with scenarios that we know to be nonactual.
>
> (Currie and Jureidini, 2001, p. 160)

Rational beliefs are formed on the basis of robust evidence and are open to revision when emerging evidence makes them less likely to be true. If delusions cannot be rational beliefs, then they are not beliefs at all (Currie and Jureidini, 2001, p. 161). There is nothing wrong in the strategy pursued by the authors, once the rationality constraint on belief ascription is accepted. But there are beliefs that are extremely resistant to counterevidence and counterargument (such as prejudiced beliefs) which cannot be comfortably relabelled as imaginings given their role in inference and in action guiding. People sometimes behave as if they believed in horoscopes and assigned special significance to apparently random coincidences: rather than baptise all of these attitudes as imaginings by virtue of their having poor evidential support we could just acknowledge that there are epistemically irrational beliefs.

Tavris and Aronson (2008, pp. 60–61) report a fictional (but perfectly realistic) dialogue adapted from Gordon Allport's illustration of the reasoning of prejudiced people in his 1954 book, *The Nature of Prejudice*:

> Mr X: [Jewish people] think of nothing but money; that is why there are so many Jewish bankers.
>
> Mr Y: But a recent study shows that the percentage of Jewish people in the banking business is negligible, far smaller than the percentage of non-Jewish people.
>
> Mr X: That's just it; they don't go in for respectable business; they are only in the movie business or run nightclubs.

Here you have a non-pathological example of beliefs that are both badly supported by the evidence and maintained in the face of counterevidence. Tavris and Aronson comment that 'once people have a prejudice, they do not easily drop it, even if the evidence indisputably contradicts a core justification for it' (2008, p. 61). People who are in the grip of prejudice, just like Mr X, come up with reasons for their dislike of a certain group, and when a reason is challenged another takes its place, although such reasons are usually unfounded generalisations that often conflict not only with reliable data, but also with other beliefs about that group. One might of course argue that prejudiced beliefs are not typical beliefs, but their role in our mental economy certainly resembles the role of beliefs far more than it does that of imaginings. Moreover, additional cases of epistemically irrational beliefs are not hard to find.

## 3.2 **Delusions and faulty reasoning**

In this section, I review and discuss some evidence suggesting that people with delusions have faulty or biased reasoning. Reasoning biases often exhibited by subjects with delusions are continuous with the biases present in normal cognition. But as we did in the previous chapter, we consider one further argument for the categorical difference between delusions and beliefs. Maybe beliefs and delusions can both violate norms of epistemic rationality, but the epistemic irrationality of delusions is different from (more severe than) that of ordinary beliefs. The (ultimately unsatisfactory) argument attempting to show that delusions are irrational in a qualitatively different way says that delusions are not fleeting and excusable deviations from norms of epistemic rationality, because only a competence failure can explain the deviations from rationality attributed to subjects with delusions, whereas in normal cognition we can attribute temporary irrationalities to mere performance errors.

An enlightened rationality constraint theorist may suggest that, if reasoning is faulty in a non-permanent or non-systematic way in subjects with delusions, then delusions may be excused for their irrationality and receive intentional characterisation after all. The proponent of the anti-doxastic conception of delusions may insist, instead, that the reasoning 'mistakes' responsible for the maintenance (if not the formation) of delusional reports are a sign of competence failure. I shall make an apparent digression and present different positions about the nature of the cognitive failure responsible for the epistemic irrationality of delusions. Is it a performance or a competence failure? A clear verdict cannot be offered, because there is no reliable way to tell whether a reasoning mistake is due to performance or competence failure on the basis of the mere observation of systematic errors. But, as we saw in the previous chapter by reference to procedural rationality, delusions (as many irrational beliefs) cannot be easily re-described as errors to be explained on a background of rational beliefs.

It often proves difficult to argue that subjects with delusions exhibit normatively deviant reasoning. On the basis of some empirical studies on the relationship between evidence and hypothesis formation in subjects with delusions, the conclusion would be that their performance is not worse than, but different from the performance of normal subjects. One suggestion is that, in order to account for the difference between subjects with or without delusions, we cannot rely on the normative notion of epistemic rationality but we need to fall back on the notion of statistical normalcy. This means that, although some reasoning styles are more likely to contribute to the formation of delusions in certain circumstances (e.g. when there is a neuropsychological impairment), they are not necessarily marks of epistemic irrationality. The epistemic irrationality of delusions might be difficult to prove on the basis of performance in decontextualised reasoning tasks, but it becomes obvious and salient in conversations with subjects with delusions when they report, defend and cling onto their delusions. We expect the behavioural manifestations of delusions to be (at least in part) caused and explained by more basic reasoning tendencies—but the reasoning tendencies need not be always misleading in order to give rise to behavioural manifestations that are epistemically irrational.

Our purpose is not to arrive at an understanding of the causal mechanisms underlying the behavioural manifestations of delusions, but some views about the aetiology of delusions will be addressed, when they have implications for the nature of the epistemic features observed in the behaviour of subjects with delusions.

### 3.2.1 Empiricism and evidential support

Brendan Maher (1974, 1988, 1999, 2003) has famously argued that delusions are not ill-formed beliefs, and that there is nothing irrational in the relationship between the evidence supporting the delusional hypothesis and the formation of such a hypothesis. According to Maher, the abnormality of the delusion is entirely due to the abnormality of the experiences on the basis of which the delusion is formed. By reference to Maher's model, Blaney (1999) describes delusions for Maher as 'false but reasonable':

> Maher's central claim is that paranoid mentation can flourish even in the absence of a noteworthy thought disorder. Delusions are seen as 'normal theories'. Thus, delusional thinking is not inherently aberrant but results from the same kind of processes that people, including scientists, use to account for the data of observation. [...] An explanation is more likely to be judged delusional by others when the person holding it has access to unusual information, when his sensory experience is unusual, or his processes of selective attention are aberrant, causing him to focus on- or be puzzled by – information that other persons ignore.
>
> (Blaney 1999, p. 350)

Maher argues that deluded subjects do not violate normative standards of belief formation more often than subjects with beliefs do. The only significant difference between subjects with beliefs and subjects with delusions is that the latter have to account for abnormal experiences (often caused by brain damage). In the case of the Capgras delusion, the abnormal experience is the perception that the face of the spouse or relative is different, and it is due to the fact that there is no affective response to the face. The content of the delusional state is implausible because the content of the delusional experience is. Maher's position on the formation of delusions, labelled 'empiricism', has greatly influenced subsequent contributions to the debate about how delusions are formed, and about whether they should be regarded as rational. The most prominent accounts of delusion formation today embrace the empiricist position developed by Maher, but depart from the claim that delusions are just rational responses to, or plausible explanations of, abnormal experiences. The abnormality of the subject's experience is not sufficient by itself to explain the implausibility of the delusional state reported by the subject.

> According to Maher, delusions reflect perceptual abnormalities, that through normal reasoning lead to a mistaken conclusion. However, the fact that hallucinatory experiences do not necessarily evoke delusional interpretation suggests involvement of other factors as well. One of these factors may be information processing. Empirical studies have yielded evidence for cognitive abnormalities in deluded patients, particularly, a probabilistic reasoning bias or a 'jumping to conclusions' data gathering style, a selective information processing bias focused at threat-related information, an abnormal attributional style, i.e. strong externalizing and personalizing bias, and poor ability to understand and conceptualize the mental processes of other people (theory of mind).

> (Krabbendam *et al.* 2005, pp. 184–185. References omitted.)

A first difficulty with Maher's account is that there seem to be subjects who suffer from the same type of brain damage, and plausibly have the same experience, as the subjects who develop the delusion, but do not accept any delusional hypotheses.

> On Maher's view, […] [i]t follows that anyone who has suffered neuropsychological damage that reduces the affective response to faces should exhibit the Capgras delusion; anyone with a right hemisphere lesion that paralyzes the left limbs and leaves the subject with a sense that the limbs are alien should deny ownership of the limbs; anyone with a loss of the ability to interact fluently with mirrors should exhibit mirrored-self misidentification, and so on. However, these predictions from Maher's theory are clearly falsified by examples from the neuropsychological literature.

> (Davies *et al.* 2001, p.144)

This prediction from Maher's theory that appears to be falsified by available data on monothematic delusions is taken by Davies and colleagues to show that something else is required in order to explain the endorsement of the delusional hypothesis, apart from an abnormal experience (see also Young and de Pauw, 2002). Two-factor theorists may argue that a cognitive impairment at the level of reasoning competence is also necessary—the hypothesis evaluation system works below its optimal standards and does not veto the acceptance of the delusional hypothesis, even if the hypothesis is far from plausible and clashes with other things the subjects believes. Other theorists (e.g. Garety and Freeman, 1999) prefer to explain the cognitive failure in terms of a number of reasoning biases without identifying a specific cognitive deficit. A third option is to deny that there is any reasoning competence failure in subjects with delusions and characterise the potential failures at the level of reasoning performance. Although no permanent deficit in the hypothesis evaluation system is postulated, temporary and local reality-testing failures or motivational factors can be said to facilitate the acceptance of the delusional hypothesis.

Another difficulty with Maher's original account of delusions as 'false but reasonable' is that, even if the abnormality of the experience were to satisfactorily explain the acceptance of the delusional hypothesis and the formation of the delusion, this would not be sufficient to guarantee the overall epistemic rationality of delusions. We would still have to explain why delusions are maintained in the face of counterevidence. Gerrans (2002a) wants to resist the thought that monothematic delusions such as Capgras and Cotard involve necessarily a reasoning deficit, but distances his position from Maher's as he concedes that delusions violate norms of epistemic rationality. He argues that being a one-factor theorist, and thus denying that a permanent cognitive deficit is necessary for the formation of delusion, does not commit one to the claim that delusions are rational.

> Thus, one-stage accounts should not be thought of as claiming that a delusional subject is rational, where rationality is understood as revising ones belief according to idealized norms of deductive or probabilistic reasoning. Clearly, it is irrational, measured against canons of inferential consistency, to believe a proposition for which you have conclusive falsifying evidence (for example, to believe that you are dead, as the Cotard subject claims). Rather, the one-stage theorist should be understood as claiming that the actual psychology of belief formation, which departs considerably from ideal rationality, functions in the same way in normal and delusional subjects.
>
> (Gerrans 2002a, p. 48. References omitted.)

### 3.2.2 Competence *versus* performance

Given the purpose of our investigation into the status of delusions, it would be helpful to establish whether delusions are genuinely epistemically irrational in order to assess the second premise of the two arguments against the belief status of delusions. On the surface, the case seems settled. Not only do delusions appear as epistemically irrational to those who witness delusional reports, but, as we previously remarked, they are also routinely defined in terms of their faulty epistemic features in many influential accounts. The problem is that definitions of mental disorders are always controversial, and much of the resistance in accepting the DSM-IV definition of delusions is due to the suspicion that delusions are not as epistemically irrational as the DSM-IV would have them. The question whether delusions are genuinely irrational matters to the assessment of a number of influential positions in the debate about the doxastic nature of delusions. Whether the failure is described in terms of a cognitive deficit or a performance error might also have implications for the application of the rationality constraint on belief ascription to the case of delusions, and that is why we turn to the issue here.

In the context of familiar irrationality (e.g. common logical mistakes due to lack of attention), the background argument discussed in the previous chapter tells us that something can be a belief even if it does not conform to a norm of rationality, as long as the deviation from the norm is temporary, local or explicable in ways that do not threaten the conceptual link between rationality and intentionality. If delusions turned out to be the outcome of performance errors, then maybe we could just add them to the list of those apparent exceptions to the rationality constraint on belief ascription that do not constitute an insurmountable problem for the interpretationist. The irrationality of delusions would not be a threat to claims about the nature of belief-intentionality, because it would not stem from a systematic rejection of a fundamental norm of rationality, but from some mishap. As such, it could be 'excused'. As well as including delusions in the class of non-rational beliefs, this move would have the effect of defusing the special status of delusions as inherently puzzling: they would be on par with slips of the tongue and other cases in which a concept is used without being fully mastered by the speaker.

> Suppose someone says to you, 'The Statue of Liberty has a rather crowded location in the middle of Trafalgar Square in London, but anyone would have to admire the lions at its base; such a statue could only be English.' And so on. You might suppose that this is someone with wildly irrational beliefs about the Statue of Liberty. But the compelling diagnosis is that she does not attach the same meaning to the phrase 'the Statue of Liberty' as you do. When she says, 'the Statue of Liberty,' she means, 'Nelson's Column.' Then it all falls into place.

> (Campbell, 2001; p. 90)

Are delusional reports like the claim that the Statue of Liberty is in Trafalgar Square? Are they *mere* performance errors? As we shall see, the two questions are not equivalent, and furthermore it is not clear to what the competence/performance distinction refers to when applied to the cognitive failures that characterise delusions, because it is not clear what type of evidence would be sufficient to claim that competence, and not just performance, is compromised. As we anticipated, the two-factor theory says that delusions involve a cognitive deficit, and this deficit affects the hypothesis evaluation system. According to the view, the mechanism by which hypotheses are checked for plausibility before they are endorsed by the subject and gain the status of beliefs is present and is operative, but does not function well. The presence of a deficit is not the only possible explanation of the fact that subjects seem to endorse hypotheses that are implausible and not well-supported by the available evidence. The friends of the reasoning deficit account have been challenged to explain why delusions tend to cluster around the same topic and not all of the hypotheses accepted and endorsed by subjects with delusions are implausible and poorly supported by the evidence.

As we briefly saw in Chapter 1, two-factor theorists argue that the content-specificity of the delusion is not accounted for by the second, but the first factor. The neuropsychological impairment that causes a false pre-conscious prediction (e.g. in Capgras, the absence of an autonomic response when seeing one's spouse) is what determines the content of the delusional state. As Coltheart (2005, p.156) suggests, potential beliefs that are examined by the hypothesis evaluation system are usually rejected as implausible if they clash with other things that the subject believes or with the available data. But when a false prediction is caused by a neuropsychological impairment, the experience that constitutes evidence for the implausible hypothesis ('it's not my wife, it's a stranger') is too strong and too persistent to be dismissed, and generates a prepotent doxastic response that cannot be inhibited.

> Normal subjects usually assume perception to be veridical; they believe what they perceive. We might describe this transition from experience to belief as a *pre-potent doxastic response*. However, normal subjects are also able to suspend their unreflective acceptance of veridicality and make a more detached and critical assessment of the credentials of their perceptual experiences.
>
> (Davies *et al.* 2001, p. 153)

Alternative models of delusion formation prefer to describe the cognitive failure as a performance error (Hohwy and Rosenberg, 2005; Hohwy, 2007; Gerrans, 2001a). These authors agree with Coltheart and other two-factor theorists that delusion formation requires a cognitive failure, but prefer not to describe it as a deficit. Garety and Freeman, for instance, seem to explain the cognitive failure purely in terms of attributional biases and reasoning styles that do not constitute a deficit:

> [The results of the jumping to conclusion literature] should not be interpreted as evidence of a deficit, an inability to reason probabilistically or to test hypotheses, but rather of a tendency or bias to the early acceptance and, to a lesser extent, the early rejection of hypotheses.
>
> (Garety and Freeman 1999, p. 127)

It is not clear what hangs on something being a *deficit*. Garety and Freeman do not want to deny that the biases observed in people with delusions are persistent and affect a substantial portion of their reasoning, but probably refrain from talking about deficits because they want to emphasise the continuity between the reasoning styles that give rise to the formation of delusional and non-delusional hypotheses. Coltheart's position is pressed to specify what it is exactly that does not work in the hypothesis evaluation system: isn't there some tension in claiming that delusions are caused (among the other things) by a cognitive deficit and then insisting that they are continuous with other beliefs by virtue of they being formed by the same mechanisms that are responsible for belief formation? Hohwy (2007) converges with Coltheart on many aspects of the aetiology of delusions: it all starts with a falsified prediction that leaves the subject in need of an explanation for an unusual event. But Hohwy thinks that the failure of reality testing observed in many cases of schizophrenia, when something internal to the subject, for instance, is attributed to external causes, or vice versa, can be characterised as a performance failure. In the normal case, and in psychopathology, perception is predictive: the hypothesis with the highest posterior probability gives content to the subject's perception ('winner takes all'). The subject perceives what is suggested by her best prediction, the prediction 'with the lowest error signal'. In the successful cases, the subject's prediction can identify the real causes of her sensory data. However, this process can lead to delusions and hallucinations when the prediction fails.

> I therefore suggest that psychotic patients can have normal reality testing competence but that reality-testing performance is compromised. That is, they perceive what they best predict—what is associated with the globally smallest error signal. This is what gives them reality-testing competence. But since they may have some kind of trouble with predictive coding (with the detection of error signals and/or the formation and updating of generative models), the hypotheses that create the globally smallest error signal are in fact very bad hypotheses polluted with much internally generated noise. For healthy subjects they would be accompanied by relatively large error signals. However, since the globally best hypothesis is always favoured, patients cannot but believe that they represent real causes in the external world. They therefore develop, e.g. visual hallucinations or delusions.

(Hohwy 2007, p. 14)

In Hohwy's explanation the 'reasoning module' is intact, but when a 'pathological' perceptual input is to be processed, the reasoning outputs end up being irrational. In delusions, the perceptual input is pathological because the relevant experience is not available to further perceptual reality testing, and this makes it the case that the delusional hypothesis is not accompanied by the appropriate error signal. In this context, the performance/competence distinction is simply a distinction between a mechanism and its input. If the mechanism is faulty, there is a competence failure. If the mechanism is intact but the reasoning output is irrational, then there is a performance failure. Of course this way of characterising the distinction is useful if we have a good account of what causes irrational reasoning outputs when the mechanism is intact.

Coltheart speaks of deficit, and Hohwy of performance error, but the similarities in the description of what goes amiss in the formation of delusions greatly outweigh the differences, especially because both authors are keen to present the delusions as the output of the system that delivers ordinary beliefs. In order to adjudicate whether the problem is at the level of competence or performance, one would need to know more about the causes of the generation of error signals (for Hohwy) or about the causes of the impaired hypothesis evaluation process (for Coltheart). If the causes can be described as a permanent deficit that deviates from normal functioning, as opposed to a temporary mishap, then one might prefer to talk about competence failure rather than performance error, but the line can be blurred in more than one way.[5] For our present purposes we do not need to decide between these two accounts. Independent of the type of account we settle on, delusions resist characterisation in terms of mere exceptions to the rationality constraint on belief ascription or in terms of explicable errors— they are most certainly *not* on a par with slips of the tongue or cases of concept misapplication. The subject with delusions is guilty of the following (Davies and Davies, 2009): a) she accepts a hypothesis which does not have high probability given what she already knows; b) she underestimates the probability that the evidence would occur even if the hypothesis were false; and c) she ignores alternative explanations for the evidence. Now, (a) is a challenge for the subject's procedural rationality, as the subject should consider how the new hypothesis would fit with her other beliefs, before accepting it as a good explanation of the experience. But (b) and (c) are serious and systematic violations of epistemic rationality, and concern the relation between the evidence, the hypothesis chosen to make sense of the evidence, and the availability of other explanatory hypotheses. Even if we go along with Hohwy's model of predictive coding, and describe bad reality testing in delusions as a performance failure, we are faced with an error that cannot be excused in the light of the background argument.

Apart from differences in the terminology and in the emphasis on either the distinction or the continuity between factor one and factor two, current accounts of delusion formation would agree that delusions involve intentional states that are likely to violate norms of epistemic rationality. This leaves the

---

5 For the general difficulties in the project of pulling apart competence and performance when it comes to cognitive failures, see Stanovich (1999). Some of Stanovich's points are echoed in my brief discussion of Davidson's distinction between subscription and conformity to norms of rationality in chapter 2.

interpretationist in the usual, uncomfortable position of having to deny belief status to delusions that may be reported with conviction, argued for, and even acted upon.

### 3.2.3 Jumping to conclusions

In the previous sections we attempted to show that there is some consensus among modern-day empiricists that delusions involve a cognitive failure which has implications for the assessment of epistemic rationality. Delusions deviate from norms of epistemic rationality, and cannot be easily excused (by appealing to the abnormal nature of the subject's experience or mere interfering factors) when they do so. However, it has been suggested that subjects with delusions are no worse, and on some occasions even better, at responding to evidence than controls. Some studies show that normal subjects tend to arrive at decisions and formulate explanatory hypotheses in a very conservative way, requiring more evidence than is necessary with respect to the normative standards provided by, say, the application of Bayes's theorem. Subjects with delusions are more confident in arriving at a decision or in formulating an explanatory hypothesis on the basis of limited evidence than controls, therefore coming closer to meeting Bayesian normative standards (see Edwards, 1982; Huq *et al.* 1988; Garety and Freeman, 1999, p. 123). Huq and colleagues (1988) find that subjects with delusions perform tasks that involve epistemic rationality more accurately than controls. But focusing on the reasoning output alone might be misleading. First, the reasoning outputs provided by subjects with delusions tend to conform to the standards if we take Bayesianism as a source of standards of correctness for probabilistic reasoning. There is much controversy as to whether Bayesianism should play this role, and it is not obvious whether norms of epistemic rationality apply across the board, or only in specific contexts. That is why it is important to evaluate the reasoning process in its entirety, and in its relation to the subject's environment, rather than consider the single reasoning outputs in isolation. The maxim 'be conservative' can be a rule to apply or a bias to control for, depending on the structure of the environment in which a decision needs to be made.

> Although the deluded sample's response on two of the measures appears more 'Bayesian', being less subject to the 'conservatism' bias than normals, it is not possible to conclude that deluded people are better reasoners. One could argue here that an abnormal bias – a tendency to draw on little evidence and to be over-confident – is cancelling out a normal bias –towards conservatism in this type of (easy) probabilistic reasoning task. Conservatism of this type may, in certain circumstances, be ecologically valid, serving as a useful general strategy under conditions of uncertainty.
>
> (Huq *et al.* 1988, p. 811)

The empirical literature suggests that the reasoning performance of subjects with delusions reflects a data-gathering bias. More precisely, it has been argued that subjects with delusions 'jump to conclusions'; they need less evidence to be convinced that a hypothesis is true (Garety, 1991; Huq *et al.* 1988; Garety and Freeman, 1999), and are 'more hasty in their decision' (Moritz and Woodward, 2005, p. 203). In a recent meta-analysis of the jumping to conclusion literature, Fine and colleagues (2007) distinguish between different claims that have been previously conflated. When we describe subjects with delusions as jumping to conclusion, we might mean that 1) they require significantly less evidence than controls to decide whether a hypothesis is confirmed, or that 2) they seem much more confident than controls about the correctness of their hypothesis. These two phenomena are tested with different methodologies. In the classic task, there are two jars with beads. One jar contains 85% red beads and 15% green beads. The other jar contains 85% green beads and 15% red beads. The participants are shown beads that are supposed to come from one of the two jars and they have to guess from which jar they were drawn. In test one, which measures *hastiness of decision*, participants can request as many beads as they deem necessary to make a decision. In test two, which measures *confidence*, participants are shown a fixed number of beads and are asked how confident they are that the beads come from a certain jar. The conclusion drawn from the meta-analysis is that subjects with delusions are more hasty in their decision than normal and psychiatric controls in that they are likely to confirm a hypothesis on the basis of less evidence than controls. However, the data about confidence in the chosen hypothesis do not support the claim that subjects with delusions are more confident than controls.

> The critical feature of patients with delusion thus appears to be specific to a tendency to make a decision on the basis of less evidence than comparison groups.
>
> (Fine *et al.* 2007, p. 59)

It has not been conclusively established whether hastiness in decision-making is characteristic of subjects with delusions in particular, or subjects with schizophrenia in general. This issue matters to the role that the jumping to conclusions style has in the formation of the delusion: does it have a causal or a purely epiphenomenal role? In the review article, Fine and colleagues argue that jumping to conclusions is a characteristic of subjects with delusions in particular (both subjects with schizophrenic delusions and subjects with delusional disorders), although they do not exclude the possibility that it characterises a more general symptom or a family of symptoms of schizophrenia. One suggestion is that that jumping to conclusions is causally efficacious in the formation of delusions. In studies on samples at-risk-of psychosis, Broome and colleagues (2007) investigated whether the people who went on to develop the delusion were those who showed jumping to conclusions biases in previous reasoning tasks, but did not find convincing evidence in favour of a causal role of the biases in the formation of delusions – further studies are being planned in this area. Following previous theoretical accounts of the jumping to conclusions phenomenon (Young and Bentall, 1997; Dudley and Over, 2003; Garety *et al.* 2005), Fine and colleagues (2007) suggest that the phenomenon does not affect the *generation* of the delusional hypothesis, but its *acceptance*.

> The role of JTC in this account appears to be one of facilitating the precipitous acceptance of the delusional hypothesis.
>
> (Fine *et al.* 2007, p. 71)

It is not always possible to witness the moment in which a delusional hypothesis is first evaluated and accepted, and measure the extent to which the evidence available to the subject is sufficient to give rise to a hypothesis with delusional content. This difficulty is even more serious when the best 'evidence' for the delusion is an experience that cannot be shared with the subject. That is why the jumping to conclusions literature gives us some clues as to whether lack of evidential support can be a generalised feature of delusions. It is suggested that there is a reasoning style that affects the acceptance and maybe the formation of the delusion, and has potential consequences for the relationship between the content of the delusional hypothesis and the available evidence. Whereas a subject without a jumping to conclusions bias might think that evidence E is not sufficient to justify the acceptance of hypothesis H, a subject with the bias is disposed to make riskier decisions and to endorse H on the basis of E. Some hypotheses are accepted in spite of not being well-supported by the available evidence overall because subjects have a tendency to be less conservative in their predictions and explanations.

### 3.2.4 Attributional biases: me and others

Other behavioural dispositions might lead subjects to endorse hypotheses or maintain beliefs that defy epistemic rationality, although we do not know whether these tendencies are contributors to the formation or acceptance of their delusional state, or consequences of a general hypothesis evaluation deficit. An event may be taken to support a delusional hypothesis when in fact it does not constitute evidence for it. Not finding her house keys in her office can 'confirm' Lucy's belief that her evil colleagues have hidden or stolen her keys to upset her, when she has simply forgotten that she left her keys in the car. Thinking about the rejection rate of his papers in peer-reviewed journals, Alouk comes to believe that unsympathetic reviewers are trying to damage his academic career, instead of considering the possibility that the poor quality of his arguments was responsible for the unhappy outcome of his submissions.

Attributional biases are observer effects in judgements about the responsibility for a certain action or event. They comprise basic statistical errors and distorted memories that negatively affect the reliability of evidence. Typical attributional biases reveal an asymmetry between the first person ('me') and third parties ('others'). The fundamental attribution error is the tendency for observers to exaggerate the importance of dispositional, or personality-based, explanations for other people's behaviours and minimise the role of contextual information and external pressures. For instance, if we have a car accident involving another driver, we are likely to blame the other driver for the accident—they were driving too fast—and to excuse ourselves by reference to external or situational factors—the road was icy. In the context of criminal actions, this tendency is even more marked. Rapists tend to justify themselves by depicting their victims as seductresses or by attributing responsibility for their violent acts to alcohol or drug intoxication. (These examples are from Putwain and Sammons, 2002, p. 103).

Some subjects with delusions seem to have stronger attributional biases (Bentall and Kaney, 1996; Kinderman and Bentall, 1997) than subjects without, but the dominant bias varies according to the type of delusion. In delusions of persecution there seems to be a tendency to attribute self-referential negative events to external factors (*externalisation*) rather than to oneself. In particular, subjects with delusions of persecution attribute the responsibility for negative events to other people (*personalisation*). For instance, a man with persecutory delusions may attribute money problems not to external circumstances (a financial crisis), or to his own previous conduct (bad management), but to a conspiracy against him. In recent studies (Langdon *et al.* 2006; McKay *et al.* 2005b), personalising biases present in the normal population correlate with paranoid ideation, whereas externalising biases don't. Diez-Alegria and colleagues (2006) found that, although externalising biases may be found in normal and depressed populations as well as in subjects with delusions, the personalising bias characterises subjects with delusions in particular, and it is more pronounced in psychopathologies of greater severity. In contrast with what has been observed in delusions of persecution, in the Cotard delusion (the delusion that one is dead) there seems to be a tendency to attribute the responsibility for negative events to oneself (*internalisation*). This bias has been observed by Young and Leafhead (1996), reviewed by Gerrans (2000), and recently illustrated and tested by McKay and Cipolotti (2007).

> At neuropsychological assessment LU presented with the Cotard delusion. She repeatedly stated that she was dead and was adamant that she had died two weeks

prior to the assessment (i.e. around the time of her admission on 19/11/2004). She was extremely distressed and tearful as she related these beliefs, and was very anxious to learn whether or not the hospital she was in, was 'heaven'. When asked how she thought she had died, LU replied 'I don't know how. Now I know that I had a flu and came here on 19th November. Maybe I died of the flu.' Interestingly, LU also reported that she felt 'a bit strange towards my boyfriend. I cannot kiss him, it feels strange—although I know that he loves me.' Other presenting symptoms included reported sensations of dizziness, as well as musical hallucinosis (hallucinations of disco music), tactile hallucinations (a feeling of running water on her left forearm) and visual hallucinations (moving walls).

(McKay and Cipolotti 2007, p. 353)

People reporting Cotard often comment on their experiences feeling distant and less intense, as if they were detached observers of what happens to them rather than actors. Some say that their bodies have lost physical substance, that they no longer feel any emotion, or that even potentially distressing events leave them indifferent (see Gerrans, 2002a, p. 50). Instead of blaming the external reality or other people for this apparent change in perception or emotion, they seem to find these impressions consistent with, and possibly explained by, their own death. In the description of LU, McKay and Cipolotti remark how it was interesting that certain feelings or experiences that could have been explained otherwise (such as relating differently to her boyfriend) were instead explained by LU with her death 2 weeks earlier. With respect to the control group, when asked to report the most likely cause of certain events, LU was found to be more prone to internalising attributions both for neutral and negative events.

The unjustified asymmetry between 'me' and 'others' we observed in the attributional biases described earlier gives rise to fascinating dialogues with patients who claim to firmly believe their delusion, but have an insight into its implausibility. For instance, a man developed delusions about being able to see into the future and predict catastrophes after a head injury. When the experimenter asked him about how he would react if someone else was to tell him that they had the same powers, he recognised that he would have problems believing them unless they had the same accident as he did.

E: If you heard someone describing these visions, what would you think about them?

J: Well... if they were speaking to me I would think 'there's something wrong with your head'... I would think... 'why can you see things and I can't'.

[...]

E: What would you think if I said to you, before your accident, that I could foretell the future?

J: I would think it was a load of nonsense!

(Halligan and Marshall 1996, p. 248 and p. 258)

It is as if the subject had two epistemic standards: if others report the belief that they can see into the future, the implausibility of their belief content and the absence of independent evidential support for the belief would convince him that they were talking nonsense. But if the subject himself reports such a belief, then the implausibility of its content and its being badly supported by the evidence are no longer sufficient reasons to doubt or reject the belief. This vignette (which is not a-typical) seems to support a view of continuity between delusions and other beliefs, with respect to epistemic irrationality, as these asymmetries between 'me' and 'others', and the use of double standards or self-serving biases, are common in normal cognition. This approach seems to be the same as to all investigations of attributional biases and reasoning styles: there is no huge gap between the cognitive failures exhibited by subjects with and without delusions, but there is a sense that subjects with delusions may be in the grip of certain biases to a greater extent than relevant controls, where the bias in question varies according to the type of delusion and might lead to the endorsement of bizarre delusional hypotheses due to the presence of neuropsychological impairments.

Apart from jumping to conclusions and personalising biases, other anomalies have been found in subjects with delusions when they engage in probabilistic reasoning and theory of mind tasks. There are further studies suggesting that subjects with delusions are worse than controls at inhibiting the evidence of their senses when it conflicts with other things they know (Langdon *et al.* 2008b), that they have an accentuated need for closure which comprises a desire for clarity and structure (see Kruglanski, 1989, p. 14), and that they tend to give quick, decisive answers to complex questions (Colbert *et al.* 2006; Freeman *et al.* 2006). There might be an underlying cause for all these reasoning anomalies which contributes both to the adoption of hypotheses with little evidential support and to the perseverance with which subjects with delusions endorse such hypotheses, even in the face of counterevidence. Alternatively, the cause of the epistemic faults in hypothesis formation and assessment could be different for different delusions. Any conclusion should take into account the individual variation in the way biases affect reasoning, and the variation in individual performance that can be observed at different stages of the pathology.

### 3.2.5 Resisting counterevidence

Delusional reports manifest epistemic irrationality— subjects with delusions ignore relevant evidence or attempt to defend their beliefs from apparent objections with obvious confabulations. Good examples of resistance to counterevidence come from monothematic delusions, such as Capgras and Cotard.

> If in the course of people's lives they have learned that the faces of strangers generate weak or absent autonomic responses, and that such responses are strong when seeing the face of a loved one, what is a person to conclude when the face of someone who looks just like that person's spouse generates a weak or no autonomic response, rather than the expected strong response? Surely this must be the 'source' of the belief that the person being seen is a stranger rather than the spouse?
>
> (Coltheart *et al.* 2007, p. 643)

> We wanted to know whether the fact that JK had thoughts and feelings (however abnormal) struck her as being inconsistent with her belief that she was dead. We therefore asked her, during the period when she claimed to be dead, whether she could feel her heart beat, whether she could feel hot or cold [...]. She said she could. We suggested that such feelings surely represented evidence that she was not dead, but alive. JK said that since she had such feelings even though she was dead, they clearly did not represent evidence she was alive.
>
> (Young and Leafhead 1996, pp. 157–158)

Although resistance to counterevidence is the single most representative feature of delusions, the content of some delusional states makes it really hard to identify convincing *evidence* for their being false, and thus insulates them from rejection. Consider the previously considered case of Cotard delusion: it suggests that the relationship between data and belief is sometimes complex and circular. First, I interpret my experience (of detachment) in the light of a belief (that I'm dead) and then I regard the experiential data as supporting the belief, even if there are reasons to think that it does not—would I be feeling *anything* if I were dead? Similarly, Leeser and O'Donohue (1999) have argued that no argument or sensory data can count as 'powerful counterevidence' to the claim that an impostor has replaced a dear one. The delusional state becomes almost unfalsifiable. What would count as good evidence that a person physically identical to my mother is an impostor rather than my mother? It is only against some general background information (that impostors are relatively rare[6]) that the belief that the person I am seeing is an impostor rather than my mother loses plausibility. May it be, then, that resistance to counterevidence is epistemically *innocent*, at least in the case of some

---

[6] Stories of impostors are not so rare in fiction: see *The Talented Mr Ripley* (directed by A. Minghella, 1999, and adapted from a novel by P. Highsmith) or *Sommersby* (directed by J. Amiel, 1993 as a remake of a French movie).

bizarre delusions? Gary Young explains this in terms of a 'lucky match' between experience and explanatory hypothesis:

> The patient looks to the belief, 'That woman is not my wife; she is an impostor', to give some semblance of meaning to his sense of estrangement. Forming and accepting this belief then structures what he see when he looks at this woman—namely, an impostor. Why would he look to revise such a match up? From the patient's perspective, the validity of the belief and the authenticity of the experience are inextricably linked in so far as the congruence between belief and experience provides strong evidence for the validity of the former and the authenticity of the latter.
>
> (Young 2008, p. 872)

This viciously circular relationship between evidence and delusional content has been observed by others too: Gilleen and David (2005), Kapur (2003), Gerrans (2009), and Mele (2008) notice how selective attention to material that is relevant to the topic of the delusion reinforces the delusional interpretation of objectively neutral events and makes revision less likely.

In what conditions the content of a delusional report is first doubted and then revised is important in order to assess the claim that delusions are resistant to counterevidence in an epistemically suspicious way (and it is very important for decisions about the most suitable therapy). There is some evidence that, when faced with evidence that contradicts the delusion repeatedly, subjects lose conviction in the delusion and can also renounce the delusion (Brett-Jones *et al.* 1987; Chadwick and Lowe, 1990). When subjects are not probed, they tend to maintain their delusions, whereas when they are invited to think about alternative readings of the available evidence, their attitude towards the delusions becomes more flexible and the rigidity of the delusional states can be reduced. On the basis of these studies, Garety and Hemsley (1997, p. 53) conclude that delusions 'are in many respects like normal beliefs, in that they are multidimensional and potentially responsive to evidence and experience'.

## 3.3 Badly supported beliefs

Let's s see whether Garety and Hemsley are right that delusions are in many respects like normal beliefs. Are they alike with respect to their epistemic irrationality?

### 3.3.1 Beliefs about causes

Although people's beliefs about causation are largely in agreement with relevant normative standards, some systematic errors occur in causal reasoning (see Sloman and Fernbach 2008). Here are some common 'mistakes' in causal reasoning: giving excessive weight to temporal order of events; being subject to a conservative bias in the assessment of scientific theories; and making inaccurate judgements about the voluntariness of actions. The studies on causal, probabilistic and inductive reasoning suggest that non-delusional beliefs can be badly supported by the available evidence, and that there are systematic violations of epistemic rationality in ordinary cognition.

One body of evidence indicates that people are too sensitive to the temporal order of events when they establish causal relations. Although the observation of causes generally precedes the observation of its effects, temporality alone is not a reliable strategy for the identification of causal relations: as Lagnado and Sloman (2006) observe, the petrol gauge showing empty does not cause the car to stop, even if the former precedes the latter, and the fact that your computer crashes before mine due to an email virus does not mean that the your computer transmitted the virus to mine. Time order can be misleading in two ways: it can make us correctly infer that there is a causal connection between two events, but then it leads us to misattribute the direction of causality; or it may make us infer incorrectly that there is a causal connection between two events, whereas the events may be unrelated or caused by a third event. Lagnado and Sloman (2006) experimentally confirm the hypothesis that temporal order of events overrides information about covariation of the same events in judgments about causal relations, generating numerous errors in causal reasoning. Although temporal order is a useful heuristic in the identification of causal relation, it is not always to be trusted.

Another problem found in causal reasoning is the tendency to evaluate data on the basis of a preferred theory. This phenomenon has been observed generally in the formation of probability judgements, and in the acceptance or rejection of scientific hypotheses on the basis of reported data. Chinn and Brewer (2001) are interested in models-of-data theory, that is, how people represent and evaluate data. They make the following proposal:

> [W]hen people evaluate data, they construct a cognitive model of the data according to the perspective of the person who is reporting the data. This mental model consists of causal links, impossible causal links, inductive links, analogical links, and contrastive links. The individual seeks to undermine one or more of the links in the model, often by seeking alternative causes that invalidate particular links. If the individual succeeds in identifying a plausible alternative cause for an event, the data can be discounted. If the individual cannot identify any plausible alternative causes for any event in the model, then the entire model may be accepted.

> (Chinn and Brewer 2001, p. 337)

In the study they devised to test their proposal, Chinn and Brewer presented undergraduate students with reports of data relevant to the following two issues, whether the extinction of dinosaurs was due to volcanic eruptions, and whether dinosaurs were cold-blooded or warm-blooded. Subjects read about the initial theory on one of the two issues: the presented theory was well-argued for and contained many relevant pieces of evidence. Subjects were asked to rate their belief in the theory, and most of them became very confident that the theory was correct. Next, subjects were divided into two groups. In group one, subjects read about additional evidence *contradicting* the initial theory (e.g. Dinosaurs did not go extinct because of volcanic explosions, because eruptions were frequent but gentle) and then provided ratings and reasons for their ratings. In group two, they read about additional data *supporting* the initial theory (e.g. Dinosaurs went extinct because of volcanic explosions, because eruptions were frequent and violent), and also provided ratings and reasons for ratings. Finally, both groups were asked to what extent the additional data were inconsistent with the initial theory, and they provided both ratings and reasons for ratings. The assessment of the data was significantly influenced by the initial theory (as predicted on the basis of previous studies), but participants did not realise that. When the data were consistent with the initial theory, participants found the data convincing. When the data were inconsistent with the initial theory, they found the data unconvincing. But the reasons for the assessment of the data were not transparent to them and were not reflected in the reasons they provided for their ratings.

> Similar to many other researchers, we found that the undergraduates were more likely to discount data that contradicted their beliefs than to discount data that supported their beliefs.
>
> (Chinn and Brewer 2001, p. 375)

Overall, in this series of experiments, subjects showed a number of 'epistemic weaknesses': they almost never suggested counterexamples for theoretical claims based on data, but preferred to propose alternative causal explanations even if these were clearly underdeveloped due to the lack of elaboration; they used underspecified reasons to deny the impact of data on theories (e.g. 'There might be another reason why the experiment showed this'); they were not always 'fair-minded' and tended to deny evidence that conflicted with their preferred theory even if they did not have good grounds to do so (*confirmation bias*). In addition to suggesting that certain judgements people form ('Theory T is supported by the data and thus it is the best available explanation of phenomenon P') are not well-supported by the evidence, the results of the analysis by Chinn and Brewer show that there might be a tendency not to revise an accepted theory even when counterevidence becomes available.

The observation that people are not very good at establishing whether a theory is supported by the evidence may not be a clear indication of widespread epistemic irrationality: one might argue that expertise and critical thinking training are required to assess pieces of evidence and evaluate theories on the basis of their fit with the facts. Moreover, some background knowledge might be required to tell apart plausible from implausible explanatory models. But further evidence is available to suggest that people draw conclusions that are not always well-supported by the evidence—and that they ought to know better.

### 3.3.2 Beliefs about intentions

According to Wegner and Wheatley (1999), people tend to experience voluntariness with respect to actions that are in no causal relation with their thoughts, if the thoughts are prior to the actions (temporal priority), they are consistent with them (semantic consistency or compatibility), or they are the only apparent causes of those actions (exclusivity). They also experience involuntariness in situations in which external observers would attribute voluntariness, as in table-turning and hypnosis. The claim Wegner (2002; 2004) makes on the basis of these observations is that the *experience of conscious will* does not necessarily map onto the causal relations between intentions and actions: no matter what we think about his general thesis, the results of the experiments he describes strongly suggest that people make judgements (e.g. about the voluntariness of their own actions) that are not well-supported by the available evidence. The experiences of voluntariness and involuntariness Wegner describes in normal cognition or in psychopathology often do not reflect causal relations between intentions and actions, even if the pathological cases are much more likely to give rise to the formation of delusions. For instance, in alien hand syndrome, people feel that one of their hands is moving independently of their will, and either attribute such movements to an external source or claim that the 'alien' hand has a mind of its own.

Studies in social perception also confirm the tendency to infer causal relations between intentions and actions in other people when an action with a certain outcome is described. The problem is that the causal relations are not justified by the description of the action. In a recent experiment, subjects were asked to judge the moral responsibility of a man who shot another man under conditions of extreme duress (e.g. he had been given a drug which made him obey other people's orders). Predictably, subjects judged that these circumstances reduced the man's responsibility for the killing. But subjects who were told that the man wanted to kill the other man because he had done him harm in the past, attributed to the shooter far greater moral responsibility and did not discount the effects of the drug (Woolfolk *et al.* 2006).

Another related area of potential epistemic weakness is the judgement of the intentionality of actions: many recent studies have reported that people have a marked tendency to regard neutral descriptions of actions as intentional descriptions. Rosset (2008) argues that if the description of an event includes an agent, then the event is interpreted as willed, as if everything that anyone does is done intentionally. Rosset (2008) supports the claim that our judgements are affected by an *intentionality bias* with the results of some studies in which he asks subjects to decide whether some actions (which could have been done on purpose or by accident) are intentional. In particular, he notices that people are more likely to judge neutral sentences as intentional when they have limited time to make a choice. From this, he concludes that the *default* option is to take actions to be intentional, and only after explicit reasoning can actions be regarded as accidental. This seems to happen even for those situations in which, according to the subject's own judgement, actions are more likely to be accidental, such as 'He broke the window'. Even for more obvious accidental actions, such as 'She bumped into an old friend' or 'She found a penny', Rosset argues that additional processing is required to judge the action as unintentional. The intentionality bias has important implications for judgements of moral and legal responsibility, which are often connected with judgements of intentionality (see Broome et al. forthcoming). Rosset observes a potentially worrying asymmetry: we need to be constantly reminded that actions can be caused unintentionally, but we do not need any reminder that they can be caused intentionally, because the intentionality bias is at work. In a very influential series of studies, Knobe (2003; 2005) found that people are more likely to attribute intentionality to actions that are perceived as morally objectionable, suggesting that judgements of intentionality are not simply determined by facts about a person's attitudes and intentions, but are also sensitive to moral considerations. Knobe presented subjects with vignettes in which the same type of action was portrayed as having good or bad moral consequences. In the following (negative) version, 85% of subjects said that the chairman intentionally harmed the environment.

> The vice-president of a company went to the chairman of the board and said, 'We are thinking of starting a new program. It will help us increase profits, but it will also harm the environment.' The chairman of the board answered, 'I don't care at all about harming the environment. I just want to make as much profit as I can. Let's start the new program.' They started the new program. Sure enough, the environment was harmed.

But in the following (positive) version, only 23% of subjects said that the chairman intentionally helped the environment.

> The vice-president of a company went to the chairman of the board and said, 'We are thinking of starting a new program. It will help us increase profits, and it will also help

the environment.' The chairman of the board answered, 'I don't care at all about helping the environment. I just want to make as much profit as I can. Let's start the new program.' They started the new program. Sure enough, the environment was helped.

Knobe's results have been replicated, but there is no consensus on what general conclusion should be drawn from them. Some have suggested that it is too crude to ask subjects to answer yes-or-no to a question about attributions of intentionality in vignettes whose context is underspecified— maybe people are less prone to infer intentionality from moral relevance if the options are better articulated. Bertram Malle has argued that there is no significant bias when questions are presented to subjects in an unambiguous way: moral evaluations of behaviour do not necessarily cloud judgements of intentionality (see Malle, 2006). But even taking into account this critique of Knobe's studies, it is fair to suppose that there is a presumption in favour of ascribing intentionality in circumstances in which the agent's intentions are not fully explicit. This can be easily characterised as a case in which one forms beliefs (about whether an action was performed intentionally) which are not fully supported by the available evidence.

Can we identify elements of continuity between the epistemic irrationality of delusional reports and that of ordinary beliefs? Although differences remain, the weaknesses of causal reasoning that lead subjects to accept theories with little evidential support, and the inaccurate attributions of blame and responsibility due to the intentionality bias are observed in subjects with schizophrenia too. The subject's interpretation of the desires and intentions of others are at the origin of persecutory delusions (Charlton 2003), and the formation or justification of a delusional state often depends on attributions of meaning to physical and mental events relevant to the subject.

> An important component of patients' explanations for their experiences is their focus on the presumed positive or negative intentions of the putative agent: the *intentionalizing bias*. With their profound egocentric orientation, patients not only attach personal meaning to irrelevant events but they also believe that the events are motivated by others' attitudes and feelings towards them.
>
> (Beck *et al.* 2008, pp. 76–77)

In a very recent volume on the shape that paranoia takes in contemporary life, Freeman and Freeman (2008) consider possible reasons why more and more parents prefer their children to stay in front of the TV or the computer and get no fresh air, rather than go out and play. One plausible explanation is that parents worry about car accidents and about abductions leading to violence and sexual abuse. Although these are understandable concerns, the risks to which children are exposed by giving up socialising and exercising are much more likely to affect their physical and psychological health than parents are willing to concede. Statistics on obesity suggest that many children in industrialised societies lead lives that are too sedentary, gain weight and become vulnerable to serious diseases, such as diabetes and arthritis. Our fears and judgements are dominated by events that are very unlikely to happen (e.g. abduction) rather than by events that are very likely to happen (e.g. bad health due to lack of exercise), because 'we are not good at comparing risks' (Freeman and Freeman, 2008, pp. 4–5). In the rest of the book, the authors mention many non-pathological beliefs that sound moderately paranoid, and that are extremely common. Often we refuse to believe a scientific theory that is well-supported by the evidence and prefer a 'conspiracy' theory. For instance, many reject the view that AIDS is a condition caused by the HIV virus that developed in monkeys and was then accidentally transmitted to humans, believing instead that it is a virus created artificially to wipe out a specific group of people. We also tend to hypothesise that other people intend to exclude us or that they want to harm us, even if we have no robust evidence in support of these hypotheses. For instance, if a friend answers the phone, says on the phone that he is in our company and then starts laughing, we most likely will come to believe that he is laughing at us. These everyday examples make it vivid how mistaken attributions of causal relations concerning physical and mental events also characterise non-delusional thinking.

### 3.3.3 Self-serving beliefs

Inaccurate judgements of causality with respect to external events or intentional actions are not the only instances of epistemic irrationality in normal cognition. Motivational factors can interfere in judgements as well. Here are some examples of signalling, selected recall, and other self-serving biases.

Quattrone and Tversky (1984) asked a group of students to hold their arms in very cold water for as long as they could. Half of the group was told that people can tolerate cold water for longer if they have a healthy heart, while the other half was told that a healthy heart causes lower tolerance. Students in the first group withstood the water longer than students in the second group, even if all subjects claimed that they had not been influenced by the information about healthy hearts and resistance to cold temperatures. This phenomenon is called 'signalling' and some argue that it is a form of self deception (Sloman 2008): a test with potentially diagnostic value is invalidated by the behaviour of the subjects who act driven by their desire to fit a certain profile, without being aware that they are doing so. In the experiment, participants 'signal' that they have a healthy heart to themselves and others. Where is the mark of epistemic irrationality? Participants come to believe that they have a healthy heart on the basis of the observation that their arms tolerate cold water for a long time, but their beliefs are not genuinely supported by the available evidence – the evidence has been manipulated.

Self-serving biases in the consideration of evidence are operative when people think about their past as well (Miller and Ross, 1975). People 'rewrite' past experiences, neglecting evidence of bad performance, concentrating on evidence of good performance, and emphasising their contribution to success-ful enterprises.

> There is a large amount of evidence that people's recollections of their past actions and performances are often self-serving: they tend to remember (be consciously aware of) their successes more than their failures, reframe their actions so as to see themselves as instrumental for good but not bad outcomes, and find ways of absolving themselves by attributing responsibility to others.
>
> (Tirole 2002, p. 639)

Some hypotheses have been suggested to explain selective attention and memory with respect to autobiographical memories. One possibility is that we remember the events we like to think about the most, and thus we 'train' ourselves, albeit unknowingly, to recall pleasant experiences that do not threaten our self-esteeem.

> The basic idea is that the individual can, within limits and at a cost, affect the pro-bability of remembering a given piece of information. Recall that people (consciously or unconsciously) try to remember good news (self-enhancing information) by pay-ing more attention when they receive them and then by rehearsing them [...]. Conversely, when receiving self-threatening information, people tend to pay limited attention and to create distractions [...].They seek contradictory evidence and excuses ('the referee is biased or incompetent', 'I was tired when I gave that seminar in which I was criticized') and rehearse them. And they avoid negative cues later on. (Tirole 2002, p. 647)Memories are distorted in a self-enhancing direction in all sorts of ways. Men and women alike remember having had fewer sexual partners than they really did, they remember having far more sex with those partners than they actually had, and they remember using condoms more often than they actually did. [...] If memory is a central part of your identity, a self-serving distortion is even more likely.
>
> (Tavris and Aronson 2008, p. 79)

These are instances of violations of the principle of total evidence. When attempting to answer the question whether we are successful or talented, as epistemically rational agents we should recall all the available evidence from our history. Instead, we selectively rely on positive events which are likely to support an excessively optimistic assessment of our skills and capacities. In this context as in the context of judgments of causality for external events, subjects who are prey to self-serving biases are the statistical norm, although some differences in the manifestation and strength of the biases can be observed between Western and Eastern cultures (Heine and Hamamura, 2007; Yan and Gaier, 1994; Muramoto and Yamaguchi, 1997; Sedikides *et al.* 2003; Sedikides *et al.* 2005). The epistemic faults of self-serving thought are not different from the epistemic faults we observed in the assessment of scientific hypotheses on the basis of data: people are prone to confirm the hypothesis they initially accepted, or the most desirable hypothesis, and are disinclined to disconfirm it. In addition, people adopt different standards for desirable and undesirable hypotheses: for instance, much more evidence is required to accept the hypothesis that a new acquaintance dislikes them than the hypothesis that she likes them but she is just shy in their presence.

> [...] with biased hypothesis testing, the hypothesis under consideration prompts a search for specific, hypothesis confirming information to the neglect of hypothesis disconfirming information. In contrast, with different standards of proof, people do not necessarily search for some information to the neglect of other information. Rather, they vary in the quantity of information required to accept or reject their hypothesis. People require more information to accept an undesired hypothesis than they require to accept a desired hypothesis.
>
> (Shepperd *et al.* 2008, p. 903)

Some psychologists have attempted to unveil the causes of self-serving biases: do they have an adaptive function by benefiting the agent psychologically? It is plausible that such biases promote individual well-being, and enhance self-confidence which impacts positively on social interactions (Leary 2007; Tirole 2002).

> The mentally healthy person appears to have the enviable capacity to distort reality in a direction that enhances self-esteem, maintains beliefs in personal efficacy, and promotes an optimistic view of the future.
>
> (Taylor and Brown 1988, p. 34)

Although pragmatically the preservation of a good self-concept might have a number of advantages, it is epistemically suspect, as it does lead to the endorsement of beliefs about the self that are badly supported by the evidence. For instance, estimation of risks can be skewed if predictions are based on selective evidence; and beliefs due to self-serving biases can misfire. In some social contexts, audiences can challenge overly optimistic self-accounts, thereby threatening the positive self-image and the authority of the self narrator.

## 3.4 **Unrevisable beliefs**

Even ordinary beliefs present serious deviations from norms of epistemic rationality and, once formed, they are not easily abandoned even if evidence against them becomes available.

It is difficult to talk about epistemic rationality in terms of principles that must be obeyed, because the mark of rationality is often a healthy balance between tendencies that can conflict with one another, as the tendency to change beliefs in response to evidence and the tendency to maintain well-established and well-connected beliefs. Whether the balance is healthy depends on the context: both the impact of the available evidence on the belief, and the quality and reliability of the evidence need to be evaluated. A scientist who stubbornly defends her own hypothesis against the arguments of the dissenting scientific community can be described as a truly original thinker who is not easily swayed by peer pressure and conventional wisdom, or as a fool who doesn't see the errors of her ways and hangs on to unpromising ideas. Often the difference between these two judgements does not lie in the rationality of the beliefs, but in the verdict of history. Similarly, in everyday reasoning, maintaining a belief in the face of counterevidence is not necessarily irrational, especially if good reasons are offered to discount conflicting evidence. In this section, I consider both beliefs with an empirical basis that resist counterevidence and beliefs that are not revisable on the basis of empirical evidence because they have no empirical content. Both categories may put pressure on the notion that responsiveness to evidence is a necessary condition for beliefs.

### 3.4.1 Racial prejudice

Are we affected by racial prejudice in our judgements and decisions? This question can be answered either by listening to what people say about their own attitudes or by inferring their attitudes from the observation of their behaviour. Often, different methodologies lead to different answers. People tend to present themselves as anti-racist and egalitarian in their self-reports, but then the behavioural evidence psychologists gather about their interactions with people of different races tells a different story. Tim Wilson (2002, Chapter 9) reports a study conducted in 20 different locations in the United States in which assistants contacted estate agents and presented themselves as people who wanted to either rent or buy a property (Yinger, 1995). The profiles of these assistants were roughly the same, but some of them were white, some black, and some Hispanic. Estate agents behaved differently towards the minority clients by showing them fewer properties and avoiding contact after the viewings to obtain feedback. This type of behaviour is very likely to generate inequalities in the house market. Another classic study (Word et al. 1974) reported and discussed by Snyder (1984) shows similar behavioural patterns in job interviews, where non-white candidates are given shorter interview times, and less immediate non-verbal responses, leading to poorer performance and the hiring of white candidates. Prejudiced beliefs give rise to self-fulfilling prophecies: the belief that a non-white candidate will perform badly causes in the interviewer a type of behaviour that undermines the performance of the non-white candidate thereby 'confirming' the initial (prejudiced) beliefs.

Another epistemic feature of prejudiced beliefs against a specific race is that they are very resistant to revision, even when convincing counterevidence comes about.

> Miguel might say, 'I don't know what makes them lazy. Maybe it's their genes; maybe it's their culture; maybe it's some metaphysical spirit. Maybe it's none of these. I have no idea. What I know is that they *are* lazy.' If Miguel is further pressed, not so much for a rational basis for his belief but simply for an account of how he arrived at it, he might cite his own experience. Of course it is illegitimate to infer from a small sample in one's experience to an entire group; and in any case, people's interpretation of their own experience [...] is itself often suspect, driven by very stereotypic generalizations it purports to provide evidence for. Nevertheless, just as familiarly, people do engage in such unwarranted generalizing all the time.

> (Blum 2002, pp. 136–137)

This passage can help us clarify one possible connection between the two epistemic faults we chose to focus on in this chapter, lack of empirical support, and resistance to counterevidence. In the case of prejudiced beliefs such as the one Miguel is reporting in the passage given earlier, lack of support contributes to the phenomenon of resistance to counterevidence. If Miguel could identify a source of epistemic support for the belief that a racially defined group is lazy, then his interlocutor could attempt to challenge Miguel's belief by attacking the source of its epistemic grounding (e.g. laziness is not encoded in genetic information or does not seem to be a cultural trait of a specific human group). But because Miguel is not committed to any specific reason for his belief, the belief becomes more difficult to challenge on the basis of evidence. When Miguel cites his own limited experience as a reason for his general belief, the situation does not improve. Whatever evidence we might present to Miguel that people from a certain racially defined group are not lazy, it will always be our experiences against his, and no agreement is likely to be found. Faced with these (unfortunately very common) instances of bad reasoning, we should no longer doubt that there is continuity between delusional reports and irrational beliefs: not only can beliefs, just like delusions, be epistemically irrational on multiple grounds (e.g. lack of support combined with resistance to counterevidence), but the very structure of the epistemically faulty reasoning we observed in Blum's example can be observed in delusional reports and confabulations. Reference to personal experience is extremely common as a justification of a delusional report with bizarre content ('It's happening to *me*'; '*I* know what *I* see. I'm not crazy'.)

The phenomenon of racist beliefs and racist behaviours is not a thing of the past—recent social psychological studies have shown that racist beliefs are routinely expressed and acted upon in everyday settings. Rusche and Brewster (2008) studied the behaviour of a small sample of white servers with respect to black patrons in large restaurants in the United States, and found a variety of firmly held and widespread beliefs which affect the service provided. By means of field work in 2002 (involving no deception) and in-depth questionnaires in 2004, the study revealed that the great majority of white servers in the sample believe that black patrons have unreasonable expectations, that they treat them badly and that they do not tip. For these reasons, they often avoid attending their tables, and share racist comments with other servers, often by using a code. It is interesting that this *tableside* racism, as the authors call it, involves beliefs that are formed on the basis of very limited or no evidence (new servers are 'brought up' into the racist culture by their more experienced colleagues and form racist beliefs about black patrons in the absence of personal evidence). Moreover, the so-formed beliefs become extremely resistant to counterevidence and are self-perpetrating:

> [A] server held firmly to performance expectations based on status characteristics: 'Blacks and Hispanics don't tip above $3.00 no matter how large the bill.' Not only did this server generalize behavior of two racial/ethnic groups, but also associates customers' race with a concrete dollar amount. Essentially, servers say 'I do not expect blacks to perform well as tippers and therefore my service will reflect this expectation.' We argue that white customers are expected to leave fair tips and are therefore given service that merits them. Black customers, on the other hand, are expected to tip poorly and are therefore given poor service that merits bad tips. These performance expectations can thus become *self-fulfilling prophecies* if expectations shape service quality, and service quality influences tip size. In other words, if servers anticipate a poor tip, they may receive a poor tip, not because the customers are inherently bad tippers, but because they were given inferior service. In short, server discrimination is, in part, a function of the interaction between servers' cognition and the social climate in which they work.

(Rusche and Bewster 2008, p. 2021)

When black patrons do tip well, servers usually attribute the 'surprising' event to their own excellent performance in serving them—the surprise does not convert into a piece of counterevidence that shakes the prejudiced belief (Fiske 2000, 2004; Fiske and Taylor, 1984). Given that the racist belief is socially shared in the workplace (often endorsed by restaurant managers as well as by other servers), it is harder to challenge or to abandon.

### 3.4.2 **Religious beliefs and religious delusions**

Although there can be arguments for and against religious beliefs, and some of these arguments have premises that can be empirically tested, it is not uncommon for some religious beliefs (for instance, those involving the existence or causal efficacy of supernatural beings or powers) not to be grounded on observable phenomena and to be held in the face of current scientific theories. Thus, religious beliefs are a good example of mental states that play a role in people's mental economies and influence people's behaviour, but are not necessarily responsive to evidence. Other examples spring to mind: the content of metaphysical or ideological beliefs might also be such that no empirical evidence is relevant to their acceptance. What type of experience would lend direct empirical support to the claim that Platonic forms exist or that every citizen should be treated equally?

Those who have studied religious beliefs and religious delusions have noticed many elements of continuity between the two phenomena, including a general tendency to ascribe responsibility of events (especially negative events) to external factors of a religious nature.

> [R]eligious beliefs are fairly common and are not pathological. Religious people demonstrate an external attributional bias. A proportion of people will experience psychotic experiences, some of which will involve auditory hallucinations. There will be an attempt to make sense of these experiences and the religious people in particular are more likely to make sense of their psychotic experiences by developing religious delusions. These religious experiences and delusions may help the person to deal with the negative life events which they are faced with.
>
> (Siddle *et al.* 2002, p.131)

The most common religious delusions consist of hearing voices and having a hallucination, combined with the attribution of these voices or visions to the intention of God or the devil to communicate. In comparison to other delusions, religious delusions have been found to be more strongly held and less amenable to revision: subjects with religious delusions score particularly low in the hypothetical contradiction test which measures responsiveness to evidence (Brett-Jones *et al.* 1987).

The presence of religious delusions is much more marked in cultures with a strong religious tradition, but criteria aimed at telling religious beliefs apart from religious delusions have been identified. Religious delusions can be distinguished from religious beliefs because: a) both the reported experience of the individual and her ensuing behaviour is accompanied by psychiatric symptoms; b) other symptoms are observed in areas of the subject's experience or behaviour that are not necessarily related to the subject's religious beliefs; c) the individual's lifestyle after the event giving rise to the report indicates that the event has not been for the subject an enriching spiritual experience (Siddle *et al.* 2002, p. 131). Interestingly, none of the criteria concerns epistemic features of the report (unless we believe that the diagnosis of other psychiatric symptoms is made on the basis of epistemic considerations alone) and most of the observations refer to the well-being of the individual as the central criterion of demarcation. The assumption seems to be that the experience leading to the reporting of a religious belief has a comforting and positive effect on subsequent behaviour, whereas the experience leading to the reporting of a religious delusion has a disruptive and negative effect. The approach revealed by these assumptions speaks in favour of there not being a clear epistemic demarcation between religious delusions and religious beliefs which are by virtue of their content less grounded on or less responsive to empirical evidence than other types of beliefs.

### 3.4.3 Conservatism

When psychologists reflect on the mechanisms responsible for the resilience of ordinary beliefs, they identify a number of strategies, and they are worth mentioning here. One of these is *selective exposure*: our beliefs guide the way in which we gain information, so that the information we process is more likely to reinforce our beliefs. This is obvious with political or ideological beliefs: my political beliefs are likely to determine which newspaper I read, and the interpretation of the news I am exposed to is likely to fit my initial beliefs. I am likely to associate with people who have similar ideas to mine, and conversing with them will rarely provide me with a radically different point of view on issues that are important to me. Another similar phenomenon is that of *self-fulfilling prophecies*: we saw earlier that a certain way of treating non-white job candidates during interviews is likely to cause them to perform worse than white candidates, which contributes to the reinforcement of prejudiced racial beliefs. But there are many other contexts in which our expectations, even when unreasonable, lead to events that seem to confirm them. One such case is that of superstitious beliefs: traffic accidents are more frequent on Friday the 13th, because people's belief that the date brings bad luck causes anxiety and stress and is responsible for their driving less carefully.

Further, the order in which evidence is presented influences its perceived importance. *Primacy effects* tell us that the evidence that is presented first is likely to have a more robust impact on belief formation and is also more difficult to dismiss at a later stage than evidence that is presented second. Serial daters soon realise that first impressions determine the success or failure of a date, and trial lawyers are also very aware of primacy effects: when jurors form a belief, that belief becomes resistant to further evidence. Critical attitudes towards already presented and accepted evidence are not commonly expressed or manifested in behaviour, but critical attitudes towards evidence that supports our initial beliefs are even more rare (this is often called the *polarisation effect*). In an influential study, Lord and colleagues (1979) wanted to see whether the presentation of evidence contributes to changing people's attitudes towards a controversial issue. Subjects were exposed to mixed evidence on whether capital punishment is effective in crime reduction. The evidence on both sides of the issue was balanced, but at the end of the experiment subjects endorsed more strongly their initial position for or against capital punishment. They regarded evidence that supported their initial belief as convincing, whereas they were critical of the evidence that spoke against their initial belief.

> People who hold strong opinions on complex social issues are likely to examine relevant empirical evidence in a biased manner. They are apt to accept 'confirming' evidence at face value while subjecting 'discontinuing' evidence to critical evaluation, and as a result to draw undue support for their initial positions from mixed or random empirical findings. Thus, the result of exposing contending factions in a social dispute to an identical body of relevant empirical evidence may be not a narrowing of disagreement but rather an increase in polarization.
>
> (Lord *et al.* 1979, p. 2098)

These many examples of resistance to cognitive probing in normal cognition lead us to accept that rigidity is a common feature of certain types of beliefs, such as beliefs concerning ourselves or beliefs defining who we are and what we value. In the light of this, the resistance to counterevidence manifest in delusions is less perplexing and easier to predict.

## Summary of chapter 3

In this chapter our purpose was to review and assess the following objection to the doxastic conception of delusions: delusions are not beliefs because they are epistemically irrational. I have considered two influential arguments: delusions are not beliefs because they lack evidential support; and delusions are not beliefs because they are resistant to evidence. From the start, we have acknowledged that most delusions are epistemically irrational. They are often both unsupported by the available evidence and unresponsive to counterevidence and counterarguments. But many typical beliefs present the same deviations from norms of rationality. Thus, it is not a good strategy to argue that delusions do not deserve belief status on the assumption that epistemic rationality is a necessary condition on the ascription of beliefs.

In Section 3.1, we highlighted the importance of the notion of epistemic rationality for current definitions of delusions. We also discussed the implications of the idea that delusions are impervious to cognitive probing for the effectiveness of cognitive behavioural therapy. Is cognitive behavioural therapy successful in reducing the subject's preoccupation with the content of her delusion and the rigidity of the delusion itself? In the same section we sketched some arguments for the view that delusions are other than beliefs. Berrios argues that delusions are not beliefs, because there are no facts that the subject wants to explain with the delusion, and even if the delusion could be conceived as the potential explanation of a state of affairs, it would not be regarded by the subject herself as more probable than alternative explanations. Currie and Jureidini argue that delusions are not beliefs because they are not updated on the basis of evidence. We briefly commented that these arguments are grounded on a narrow and idealised conception of belief.

In Section 3.2, we asked whether delusions are really epistemically irrational in a way that is incompatible with some version of the rationality constraint on belief ascription. First, we asked whether the violations of epistemic rationality that we find in delusional reports are competence or performance errors. Second, we asked whether the fact that reasoning styles in people with delusions are not epistemically deviant from accepted norms might speak in favour of the rationality of delusions. Both these issues forced us to consider some aetiological questions: how are delusions formed and are reasoning styles a cause or a consequence of delusional thinking? We found that delusions remain epistemically irrational in the light of the background argument: their irrationality cannot be excused as a temporary mishap and is manifested not in a general tendency that subjects with delusions might have to jump to conclusions, but in the maintenance of hypotheses that are badly supported by the evidence available to them and consistently challenged with strong arguments by reliable sources (we illustrated this point with examples from monothematic and polythematic delusions, among which Cotard and Capgras delusions, and cases of erotomania and persecution). Whether delusions are the result of a performance or a competence error, which is difficult to establish given that we lack a conceptually convincing distinction between the two, theorists agree that delusions are formed in similar way as beliefs, and that, in most cases, they are the product of persistent and systematic perceptual and cognitive failures.

In Section 3.3, we developed an objection to the argument that delusions are not beliefs because they are badly supported by the available evidence. We showed that many typical beliefs, including beliefs about causal relationships and about intentionality, are badly supported by the available evidence and thus fail to satisfy the epistemic rationality constraint just like delusions.

In Section 3.4, we challenged the argument that delusions are not beliefs because they are unresponsive to evidence. We observed that many examples of ordinary beliefs are resistant to counterevidence and counterargument, such as prejudiced beliefs, and beliefs whose content is non-empirical. In presenting these examples from normal cognition we also paid special attention to the claim that delusions and beliefs are continuous rather than categorically different, and we established some analogies between the epistemic faults attributed to delusions and those attributed to beliefs.

There is no epistemic rationality constraint on belief ascription. Let's consider an example. Suppose you believe that interest rates will go up next month on the basis of your analysis of the house market. The fact that you have some form of justification for your belief is part of what makes that state a belief rather than an act of imagination or a desire. If you assert that interest rates will go up next month and claim to have some evidence for it, and defend the claim when you are challenged, then you manifest the pattern of behaviour of a *subject with beliefs* and an interpreter will legitimately ascribe to you the *belief* that interest rates will go up. But there is no need to assume on those bases that it is also *rational* for you to have that belief. In order for you to have a *rational* belief, it is not sufficient for you to have some reasons for its content, you need to have *good* reasons. You might lack robust evidence about how many houses are sold and at what prices, etc. or might have neglected some factor which is relevant to your analysis. These considerations affect the rationality of your belief, but should not constitute a reason for the interpreter to doubt that you have that belief.

The example highlights the distinction we made in the previous chapter between determining whether certain beliefs motivate and explain observable behaviour, and determining whether they satisfy norms of rationality. These seem to be two independent enterprises in the study of beliefs, and they should be regarded as independent enterprises in the study of delusions too. The examples we have referred to in the course of this chapter are important because they suggest that epistemic irrationality is not a feature of a particular class of beliefs. Among the ordinary beliefs that defy the norms of epistemic rationality, we have listed 'scientific' beliefs (e.g. beliefs about probability and risk and beliefs about causal relations), religious beliefs, and motivated beliefs. This was a deliberate choice whose purpose was to show that less than optimal connections between belief contents and the available evidence are widely observed and do not affect only beliefs that, by their very nature, are expected to be less sensitive to evidence.

Last, we made some observations about the epistemic definitions of delusions. As delusions are epistemically irrational, it is comprehensible that definitions of delusions are centred on their weak evidential support and their unresponsiveness to evidence. But these definitions will never be sufficient to demarcate the phenomenon of delusions from that of other epistemically irrational beliefs—it is telling that authors who wish to tell religious beliefs apart from religious delusions include in their criteria non-epistemic considerations such as the subject's preoccupation with the content of the delusion, and the effects of the religious experience on her well-being and lifestyle.

# Chapter 4

# Agential rationality and belief ascription

Her subjective experience of eating was similarly unreal; she felt as though she were 'just placing food in the atmosphere', rather than into her body. She would not eat, get up in the morning, bath, dress, etc. without being coerced. She reported being scared to do these things. She was similarly scared of urinating or defecating, saying: 'I don't know if my bowels work'.
(Young and Leafhead, *Betwixt Life and Death*)

The real causes of human actions are unconscious, so it is not surprising that behaviour could often arise without the person having conscious insight into its causation.
(Wegner and Wheatley, *Apparent Mental Causation*)

In this chapter I consider two other arguments against the view that delusions are beliefs. This time, delusions are charged with agential irrationality, which concerns the behavioural manifestations of the endorsement of belief states. I first consider the relationship between belief status and action guidance, and then consider the relationship between belief status and reason-giving.

In the argument I discuss first, the conclusion is that delusions are not beliefs because they fail to be action guiding in the appropriate circumstances.

Here is a version of the failure of action guidance argument:

i)   In order for *b* to be ascribed as a belief to a subject, *b* needs to be action guiding in the appropriate circumstances.
ii)  Delusions do not guide action in the appropriate circumstances.
Thus, delusions cannot be ascribed to a subject as beliefs.

In Section 4.1, I draw a distinction between acting on a belief and manifesting behaviourally the endorsement of a belief: whereas behavioural manifestability is plausibly a necessary condition for the ascription of beliefs, action guidance seems too demanding as a constraint. Then, I address the empirical literature on delusions in order to establish to what extent delusions are action guiding in order to assess premise (ii). The answers we find won't be general answers that apply to all types of delusions: although all delusions seem to be manifested behaviourally to some extent, not all delusions are consistently acted upon.

In Section 4.2, I assess the agential rationality constraint on belief ascription expressed in premise (i) by looking at whether non-pathological beliefs guide action in the appropriate circumstances. If there are beliefs that seem to be held with conviction but not acted upon—as the psychological literature on attitude-behaviour inconsistencies suggests—then the failure of action guidance argument is seriously compromised.

In the remainder of this chapter I consider another argument based on the agential rationality constraint on belief ascription, which concerns the impact of delusions on observable behaviour *of a specific type*, the deliberation or endorsement of a belief content via reason-giving. The conclusion is that delusions are not beliefs because either they fail to be formed by the subject on the basis of intersubjectively good reasons (deliberation), or because they fail to be endorsed by the subject on the basis of intersubjectively good reasons (justification).

Here are the two versions of the failure of reason-giving argument:

i) In order for $b$ to be ascribed as a belief to a subject, $b$ needs to be formed on the basis of (intersubjectively) good reasons.
ii) Delusions are not formed on the basis of (intersubjectively) good reasons.
Thus, delusions cannot be ascribed to a subject as beliefs.

i) In order for $b$ to be ascribed as a belief to a subject, $b$ needs to be supported by the subject with (intersubjectively) good reasons.
ii) Delusions are not supported by the subject with (intersubjectively) good reasons.
Thus, delusions cannot be ascribed to a subject as beliefs.

In Section 4.3, I address the central motivation of the failure of reason-giving arguments. Then I attempt to establish whether delusions really fail to be formed or supported by the subject with good reasons and assess premises (ii) of the above arguments, by looking at the empirical literature on delusions. Although there is great variability in the answers to this question, depending on the type of delusion and the circumstances in which the subject's endorsement of the delusion is manifested, delusions are generally neither formed nor supported on the basis of (intersubjectively) good reasons.

In Section 4.4, I consider the relationship between delusions and framework beliefs which is relevant both to the assessment of agential rationality in subjects with delusions, and to the claim that there is discontinuity between delusions and beliefs. One view is that delusions are not supported with reasons because the subject attributes to them a foundational role with respect to her other beliefs, and thus treats them as beliefs that do not need to be justified. Another view is that, instead of playing the role of framework propositions, delusions *defy* previously accepted framework propositions. When delusional states are defended with reasons, such reasons are incompatible with a general background of beliefs and practices (the 'bedrock') shared by the rest of the linguistic community. Both arguments rely for their success on the notion that there is a substantial gap between subjects with delusions and other people in their linguistic community, as subjects committed to different framework beliefs play with different ground-rules. I challenge that notion and maintain that delusions neither behave as framework beliefs nor conflict with framework beliefs—attempts at justifying the content of a delusion do not necessarily involve a detachment from common beliefs and practices.

In Section 4.5, I assess the agential rationality constraint based on the capacity for reason-giving—premise (i) of the above arguments—by looking at whether non-pathological beliefs are formed or supported with good reasons. The psychological literature offers striking examples of the mismatch between the reasons people use to justify their attitudes and the likely causes of their attitudes, undermining the myth of the pervasiveness of rational deliberation. Even *post-hoc* justification of attitudes is often far from rational, and episodes of confabulation can be identified in many dimensions of normal cognition.[1]

At the end of this chapter, I suggest that we should give up the idea of a necessary constraint on the ascription of beliefs based on agential rationality and challenge those positions according to which agential rationality serves as a demarcation criterion between delusions and beliefs.

## 4.1 Delusions and failure of action guidance

The notion of agential rationality bridges the traditional gap between the theoretical and the practical sphere of rationality. Thus, it is particularly useful in the context of an analysis of the nature of delusions whose perplexing nature has been sometimes identified with a pragmatic, rather than cognitive, failure (see Fulford 1998). We saw in Chapter 2 that double-bookkeeping in delusions

---

[1] As we shall see, there are a number of things we might mean by giving 'bad' reasons for an attitude: giving reasons that fail to rationalise the reported attitude; giving reasons that are not meaningfully linked with the reported attitude; giving reasons that are not representative of what the subject thinks, or of the mechanisms responsible for the formation of that attitude.

can refer to the endorsement of attitudes that seem inconsistent, but another, very common, form of double-bookkeeping is the inconsistency between reported attitudes and behaviour. More than procedural and epistemic rationality, agential rationality captures the relationship between having beliefs and other things one can do, from defending a particular standpoint on the basis of evidence, to manifesting one's conviction in instances of observable behaviour. Thus, agential rationality is a very useful notion to explore for its potential contributions not only to debates about intentionality, but also to debates about self knowledge and autonomy. Are delusions intentional states of a doxastic nature? Are subjects with delusions mistaken about whether they believe the content of their delusions? Are they responsible for their actions when they act on their delusions?

### 4.1.1 Are delusions action guiding?

Agential rationality primarily concerns the manifestations of the commitment that a subject has towards the content of her thoughts. In order for a subject to be agentially rational with respect to a belief that $p$, the subject needs to be in a position to endorse $p$, by being able to defend $p$ with good reasons and by behaving in a way that is consistent with and can be explained by her acceptance of the truth of $p$. For the purposes of a detailed discussion of agential rationality, I address action guidance first and reason-giving second, but obviously both are behavioural manifestations of the endorsement of the content of a belief-like state.

Is an agential notion of rationality a plausible source of constraints on belief ascription? Some would argue that it is, because agential rationality requires one to exercise the capacity to act on one's beliefs, and influencing action is a mark of beliefs. If I genuinely take it as true that *pad thai* is a mildly spiced dish, I am in a position to give reasons why I take that to be true (e.g. by reference to samples of *pad thai* that I have tasted in the past, or by reference to the recipe for the dish), and to behave in a way that is guided by that belief (e.g. I will recommend the dish to a friend who likes mildly spiced dishes). My giving reasons in support of my reported state, and my acting on it are evidence that the state I reported is a belief of mine. According to the failure of action guidance argument, delusions fall short of belief status if they are candidates for guiding action (that is, they have the type of content that can lead a subject to act on it in the appropriate circumstances), but fail to guide action. The notion of failure of action guidance needs to be unpacked a little.

Acting on a belief is one way of manifesting the endorsement of the content of that belief—there are other behavioural effects of having or reporting a belief that do not amount to leading to a specific action in the appropriate circumstances. There is a sense in which all clinical delusions are manifested in behaviour: minimally, they are reported and are diagnosed *as delusions* partially for the negative consequences that follow from the subject's conviction that the content of the delusion is true. These consequences are often detectable in the subject's health conditions and lifestyle (in terms of stress, depression, preoccupation, social withdrawal, and so on). Freeman and Garety, who adopt a multidimensional approach to delusions, emphasise the effects on behaviour that delusions have, and consider them as important criteria for establishing whether a report is delusional. As they write, it is often the case that 'the person is preoccupied with (emotionally committed to) the belief and finds it difficult to avoid thinking or talking about it' and that 'the belief is a source of subjective distress or interferes with the person's occupational or social functioning' (Freeman and Garety 2004, p. 7). There are also manifestations that are specific to a type of delusion: subjects with persecutory delusions manifest *safety behaviours*, that is, they avoid situations that they perceive as threatening given their delusions, and they are emotionally distressed with respect to the content of their delusions (Freeman *et al.* 2001). If we ask whether delusions manifest in behaviour, the answer needs to be yes. But agential rationality seems to require more than the presence of some behavioural effects, and so does the constraint on the ascription of beliefs. Agential rationality requires that a belief leads to and guides action, in a way that allows interpreters to describe the subject's behaviour as intentional because explained by the subject's belief (together with other cognitive or motivational states).[2]

> She got to the station at 8:30, because she thought that the train was due to depart at 9.
> I recommended pad thai to Sean, because I thought he didn't like hot food.
> ...

The belief about the time at which the train departs is what explains the fact that the agent got to the station at a prior time. The belief about Sean's disliking hot food is what explains why I recommended pad thai to him. For our purposes here, I shall not regard mere behavioural effects of reporting a delusion as sufficient for action guidance. Rather, a delusion will count as action guiding if the subject engages in actions that are consistent with and explicable by the subject's acceptance of the content of the delusion. In this more demanding sense, the anti-doxastic argument goes, delusions fail to have the action guiding role we would expect them to have if the subjects genuinely endorsed them.

[2] For a discussion of whether mental states explain or cause intentional action, see Davidson (1974b), and the ensuing debate on mental causation.

There is a tension in the empirical and theoretical literature on whether delusions are action guiding. On the one hand, it is part of the definition and understanding of delusions and of the way in which they are discriminated from other pathologies that they lead to action as beliefs do. Both Freud (1917) and Young (2000) make sense of delusions as beliefs by stressing their action-guiding character.

> It [the delusion] belongs first to that group of illnesses which do not directly affect the physical, but express themselves only by psychic signs, and it is distinguished secondly by the fact that 'fancies' have assumed control, that is, are believed and have acquired influence on actions.

(Freud 1917, p. 173)

> Some of these [Capgras] patients do act in ways which can be seen as consistent with their delusion.

(Young 2000, p. 49)

The action-guiding nature of delusions can have dramatic consequences: Taylor (1985, 1998) and Skodol (1998) report violent offending in subjects with delusions, especially passivity experiences.[3] Admittedly, it is often difficult to establish whether an act of violence or a crime has been motivated *specifically* by the delusion, but further evidence seems to suggest that, although it is not common, it is definitely possible for a delusion to lead to violence or criminal action. Link and Stueve (1994) observe that thought control, thought insertion and delusions of persecution are more likely to be correlated with acts of violence, and offer some explanation for this phenomenon:

> [V]iolence is more likely when internal controls that might otherwise block the expression of violence break down. From this perspective the nature and content of the psychotic experience becomes important. If the psychotic experience involves the removal of self-control [...], routine, self-imposed constraints on behaviour are more likely to be overridden, and violence becomes a greater possibility. Further, if the afflicted person believes that he or she is gravely threatened by someone who intends to cause harm, violence is again more likely.

(Link and Stueve 1994, p. 143)

Later studies (Appelbaum *et al.* 2000; Stompe *at al.* 2004) did not support these conclusions. Results of correlation between delusions and violence were less significant when anger and impulsivity were controlled for. Threat related symptoms were found to associate with severe violence, but

---

[3] Passivity experiences involve deficits of self-recognition: subjects find it difficult to distinguish between self and others and come to believe that there are external influences on their thoughts and actions.

control-override symptoms were not. On a smaller scale, violent behaviour and some delusions have been correlated: in a study by Junginger and colleagues (1998) on 54 inpatients a few subjects with delusions were found to have committed at least one act of extreme violence which was motivated by their delusion; in another study by Förstl and colleagues (1991) on subjects with delusions of misidentification, 18% of a group of 260 was found to engage in violent behaviour relative to their delusion. Additional support for the action guiding role of delusions comes from individual case studies. Cases of Cotard delusion have been reported where people stop eating and bathing themselves as a consequence of believing that they are dead (Young and Leafhead 1996).

> Patients not only claim that they are dead or non-existent and that their bodies have been replaced by corpses, but they might also act dead. They may be mute or speak in sepulchral tones. Along with saying that they have no feelings, they might not respond to obnoxious stimuli and threatening gestures [...]. They are akinetic and often refuse to eat.

> (Weinstein 1996, pp. 20–1)

Here are some other examples of people who behave in accordance with their delusions. Capgras patients often act on their delusions by showing hostile or aggressive behaviour towards the alleged impostors. One often reported case is that of Ms. A., who killed her mother after having suffered for 5 years the delusion that her parents were impostors (Silva *et al.*, 1994). Affected by perceptual delusional bicephaly, the delusion that one has two heads, a man who believed that the second head belonged to his wife's gynaecologist attempted to attack it with an axe. When the attack failed he attempted it to shoot it down—as a consequence he was hospitalised with gunshot wounds (Ames 1984). A woman who believed that people were trying to harm her by occult powers assaulted her parents and her sisters and then went to the police to complain that they had been using diabolic powers (Wessely *et al.* 1993). The life of a woman with Frégoli delusion, the belief that people the patient sees are actually the same person in disguise, was dominated by her conviction that her adulterous neighbour was following her to prevent her from telling others about his extra-marital relationship.

> Betty allowed herself little time either to sleep or to eat: instead she constantly watched the street, noting the time and the number plates of passing cars. She sometimes confronted the drivers, demanding that they reveal their true identities and intentions.

> (Ellis and Szulecka 1996, pp. 40–1)

On the one hand, psychologists emphasise the extensive behavioural effects of delusions (see Kopelman 1987), and psychiatrists use the correspondence between subjects' reports and their actions as diagnostic of delusions. On the other hand, subjects with delusions have been found to engage in different behaviour from the behaviour that would be expected of them if they did genuinely believe the content of their delusions.

> According to the boast of one young male patient, 'This evening, in one of the best hotels in the city, my wedding to a leading actress is going to be held.' However, when evening came, he behaved quite calmly as if nothing special was going to happen.
>
> (Komiyama 1989, p. 18)

Bleuler (1924) notices that patients who claim to be a dog don't bark like dogs, and they behave as if their delusion were to be taken metaphorically. In a later paper, Bleuler (1950) argues that there is double awareness in schizophrenia. Subjects with schizophrenic delusions may fail to act in accordance with their delusions and behave in a way that reflects how things really are. Sass (2001) talks about the notion of double-bookkeeping which we briefly introduced in Chapter 2, and suggests that subjects with delusions are at least implicitly aware that their delusions do not represent reality. These ideas have been recently re-elaborated by Gallagher (2009) who suggests that delusions are disconnected from the subject's relevant behaviour and often fail to guide action. This is reason to think, according to Gallagher, that delusions are not erroneous beliefs, but alternative realities occasionally inhabited by the subjects.

> The level of detachment from everyday reality [...] may vary from one form of delusion to the next. [...] The Cotard patient is dead and rotting in the delusional world, but eats and lives in everyday reality.
>
> (Gallagher 2009, p. 259)

> A patient can view doctors and nurses as poisoners (in delusional reality) but happily eats the food they give her (in everyday reality).
>
> (Gallagher 2009, p. 260)

In a very interesting and revealing study, the behavioural manifestations of delusion have been studied by considering both the perspective of the subject with the delusion, and the perspective of a relevant third person, such as a relative, carer, social worker, or nurse (Wessely et al. 1993). In the study no association between first-person and third-person answers was found. In some cases, subjects reported not having acted on the delusion, whereas informants said that subjects had acted on the delusion, and viceversa. The results showed that having delusions was making it more likely that subjects acted in a way that could be seen as delusional, but did not demonstrate that specific delusional contents were being acted upon. The exception seems to be the case of persecutory delusions, which have pervasive effects on people's behaviour that are specifically related to the content of the delusions.

There are some difficulties in deriving a definite conclusion on whether delusions are action guiding on the basis of mere observation of the behaviour of subjects with delusions. However, one thing to keep in mind when assessing anti-doxastic arguments is that, if ascribing a cognitive state is not sufficient to explain the subject's action, but a motivational state also needs to be ascribed, then there is a missing step in the failure of action guidance objection to the belief status of delusions. My failing to recommend a *pad thai* to Sean might be explained by my lack of commitment to the belief that *pad thai* is a mildly spiced dish, or by my intention to get back at Sean whose April's Fools joke against me ruined my reputation at work. In general terms, failing to act on a delusion is not necessarily a sign that the subject with the delusion lacks commitment to the content of the delusion. What if the failure to act tells us something about the subject's motivational states, rather than about the nature of her delusion? This is certainly a suggestion that needs exploring, although it might give us additional reasons to detect deviations from agential rationality in subjects with delusions, such as the failure to be motivated to act on one's beliefs.

Another difficulty is that some delusions do not have a clear behavioural correlate—if someone were to believe that thoughts are put into her mind from spaces in the air, how would you expect her to act?

### 4.1.2 Are delusions acceptances?

Agential rationality seems to be a plausible constraint on belief ascription, because action guidance is regarded as a core feature of beliefs. Thus, it is not a surprise that many arguments against the belief status of delusions are based on the so-called 'behavioural inertness' of delusions. Behavioural inertness would show that subjects with delusions are not *really* committed to the content of their delusional states.

> Perhaps the strongest objection to the doxastic account is that delusional patients fail to demonstrate the kind of *commitment to the content of the delusional state* that they would if they believed it. This lack of commitment can manifest itself in theoretical reason, practical reason, and in affective responses.
>
> (Bayne and Pacherie 2005, p. 183, my emphasis)

One view is that, if delusions are (often) behaviourally inert, then they should not be regarded as beliefs but as *acceptances*. Keith Frankish (2009) identifies behavioural inertness as one of the greatest challenges for doxastic accounts of delusions, and points to empirical literature indicating that subjects with delusions make 'assertions [that] are often at odds with their non-verbal behaviour' (p. 270). His argument is of particular interest, even if he does not explicitly endorse a rationality constraint on the ascription of beliefs, because he contributes to the debate on the nature of delusional states by reserving a fundamental role to what I called the 'agential rationality constraint on belief ascription'. The view is that, in one sense of 'belief', the possibility of ascribing a certain belief to a subject depends on the subject's belief meeting rationality constraints by being consistent with the subject's behaviour.

> Even if we allow that deluded subjects do in some sense believe their claims, it is doubtful that we could form any empathic understanding of their state of mind if these beliefs are not subject to the usual rational constraints and do not have the usual sensitivity to evidence and influence on action.

(Frankish 2009, p. 271)

There is a charming ambiguity in talking about the 'usual' rationality constraints pertaining to epistemic and agential features of beliefs. These rationality constraints are *usually* taken to apply to beliefs by philosophers of mind who are sympathetic to interpretationism and tend to idealise beliefs, but, as we saw, they are not *usually* satisfied by beliefs. Frankish has a diagnosis for the discrepancy between reported beliefs and behaviour which is at odds with the principles of interpretation upheld by theorists of belief ascription. He convincingly argues that there are two main functions played by the states to which the folk-psychological notion of belief applies. Accordingly, there are two types of beliefs: level-1 beliefs are 'nonconscious, passive, graded, dispositional states' which are ascribed to others on the basis of rationality constraints; level-2 beliefs are 'conscious, controlled, binary, functional states' that are subject to failures of activation and are not ascribed on the basis of rationality constraints. Level-1 beliefs are consistent with behaviour and action guiding, whereas level-2 beliefs are not.

Level-2 beliefs have been previously referred to in the literature as opinions or acceptances, although the three notions are not equivalent. To illustrate this distinction with an example, consider a study by Aronson (1999). College students attending the university swimming pool endorse the general principle that one should not waste water (level-2 belief, or policy) but take unnecessarily long showers behaving as if they believed that water were not a scarce and precious good (level-1 belief, or disposition). Another example comes from the study of moral attitudes (Haidt 2001). People often condemn behaviours that are socially unacceptable (e.g. incest) because driven by a basic unconscious emotion of disgust (level-1 belief), but in their explanations for their moral judgements they cite violations of moral principles they take themselves to endorse (level-2 belief). In the account developed by Frankish, delusions are acceptances, in that they behave as general policies that subjects consciously adopt and not as pre-conscious behavioural dispositions. Some delusions will be bound by sensitivity to evidence, and thus count as *doxastic* acceptances, whereas other delusions will not be, and thus count as *non-doxastic* acceptances.[4]

The apparently anomalous features of delusions seem to receive an explanation if we acknowledge that delusions are acceptances: they are consciously reported, they are available to reflection, they have limited influence on behaviour, and they are not often ascribed on the basis of a rationalisation of the observable behaviour, but on the basis of subjects' verbal reports.

> [The actions of deluded patients] are understandable qua manifestations of the premising policies in which those states consist, and interpreting a deluded patient will involve forming and testing hypotheses as to the character of these policies.

> (Frankish 2009, p. 281)

We have previously commented on the limitations of talking about 'beliefs' and 'delusions' as if they were homogeneous categories. Frankish is right that there are different types of beliefs, and different types of delusions, and he successfully identifies some interesting dichotomies. Nonetheless, I wonder whether the distinction he proposes between two levels of beliefs really provides a neat solution to the debate on the nature of delusions. First, there seem to be no necessary connections between the listed features of, respectively, level-1 and level-2 beliefs. It is not necessary for unconscious, passive and graded states to manifest in behaviour, nor is it necessary for conscious, functional and binary states to be behaviourally inert. Delusions, which for Frankish are level-2 beliefs if they are beliefs at all, are available to conscious control and personal-level inference, but can be graded and can manifest in behaviour, as we saw in previous examples and vignettes.

Once these possibilities are acknowledged, the distinction between level-1 and level-2 beliefs appears less theoretically useful, and is itself an idealisation. This can be seen clearly in the discussion of rationality: Frankish seems to think that level-1 beliefs do not conflict with one another, and do not cause attitude-behaviour inconsistencies. But there is nothing in the description of level-1 beliefs that exempts them from irrationality of the procedural, epistemic or

---

[4] For another formulation of the notion of acceptance, and of the problem of epistemic sensitivity, see Paglieri (2009). Also, see Paglieri and McKay (2006).

agential type and thus makes them more amenable to interpretation. People can have conflicting behavioural dispositions (where conflicts are often explained on the basis of contextual or situational factors), and in those cases interpreting behaviour on the basis of rationality constraints would fail, with or without the additional 'interference' of level-2 beliefs. Further, people might have behavioural dispositions which they refrain from acting upon. This is relevant to claims about agential rationality and action guiding. A possible explanation of double-bookkeeping in delusions is that the delusion motivates action ('My wife has been kidnapped and an impostor has taken her place, I need to go to the police') but a policy suggesting that the content of the delusion would not be believed by others blocks the action ('If I go and tell them what happened, the police would think I'm crazy'). If this is ever a plausible account of what might happen with delusions, the delusion is a behavioural disposition which is not acted upon because there is a level-2 belief, a policy, modulating its potential behavioural effects.

Even if such an account of double-bookkeeping in delusions is rejected, the possibility of level-2 beliefs having behavioural efficacy is an important point (which we shall come back to before the chapter is over, and in the next chapter). Some beliefs might have a less immediate impact on behaviour than other beliefs, without being causally inert. Even when the policies we verbally commit to ('One should not waste water'; 'Incest is morally wrong'; 'One should not go to the police to report stories about identical replicas'; 'I am not responsible for failing the driving test') are confabulatory reconstructions with limited evidential bases, they do affect our behavioural dispositions and ultimately our actions—not all our actions are hostage to unconscious and passive states. The impression one gets from the literature against the doxastic account of delusions is that behavioural inertness is postulated because verbal reports are regarded as less representative of people's behaviour than other observable manifestations. But this needs not be the case.

> It is important to realize that attitudes and personality traits can express themselves, and therefore can be inferred from, verbal as well as non-verbal responses. This point is often misunderstood. Many investigators assume that verbal responses reflect a person's attitude or personality trait, whereas non-verbal ('overt') actions are measures of behaviour. In point of fact, however, both verbal and non-verbal responses are observable behaviours.

> (Ajzen 2005, p. 134)

Here are examples of how 'level-2' beliefs have a behavioural impact that goes beyond mere verbal reports: subjects who are alerted to the discrepancy between their policies and their behaviour often change their behaviour in order to be faithful to their policies, or confabulate to explain away the apparent conflict between behaviour and policies. Once this causal impact on behaviour is acknowledged, the distinction between level-1 and level-2 beliefs does little to ease the worry about the alleged behavioural inertness of delusion. The dichotomies Frankish pointed to (conscious/unconscious, binary/graded, inert/action guiding, and so on) should always be kept in mind when making general claims about beliefs (or delusions) but they do not give rise to two neat categories of mental states.

This might leave us with an unsatisfactory explanation of the alleged behavioural inertness of delusions, but I think there is nothing to worry about. The behavioural inertness of delusions is a philosophical myth rather than a fact needing explanation. As we argued, delusions might fail to guide action in some of the appropriate circumstances, but do always manifest in behaviour, or they could not be detected, diagnosed, and considered as harmful to the person reporting them. Moreover, when action guidance is compromised, we need to remind ourselves that often delusions are accompanied by other pathologies that are likely to affect the subject's motivation to act.[5] A satisfactory argument for the view that delusions are not acted upon because they do not have the causal power of beliefs cannot be made without keeping this in mind.

## 4.2 Beliefs and failure of action guidance

If I sincerely state a preference for chocolate ice-cream over crème caramel, but systematically choose crème caramel over chocolate ice-cream when I order dessert, which preference should an interpreter ascribe to me? The preference I am committed to when I declare my love for chocolate ice-cream, or the preference implied by my choice of crème caramel? Lack of attitude-behaviour consistency makes things really difficult for the ascription of intentional states such as beliefs and preferences, and is regarded as a serious violation of agential rationality. The constraint can be applied with varying strength: in Chapter 2, on procedural rationality, we considered the argument according to which bad integration among attitudes compromises the ascription of beliefs with determinate content. A similar argument could apply to cases of epistemic or agential rationality: where attitudes fail to respond to evidence or to guide action, those attitudes cannot be ascribed as beliefs with determinate content, and explanation and prediction of behaviour in intentional terms is thus compromised.

---

[5]  I thank Matthew Broome for making this point clear to me.

There are many sources of evidence for the case of reported beliefs (and other doxastic attitudes) that fail to guide action—research programmes in psychology with different objectives seem to converge on this point in their results. In this chapter I focus on instances of attitude-behaviour inconsistency which were observed in the course of studies on cognitive dissonance and introspective reflection. The take-home message is that some beliefs have the capacity for guiding action, but action guidance should be listed among the desiderata for rational beliefs, and not among the necessary conditions for belief ascription.

## 4.2.1 Hypocrisy

According to the cognitive dissonance theory, put forward by Leon Festinger (1957), pairs of 'cognitions', if relevant to one another, can be either consonant or dissonant. In the original formulation, cognitions are consonant if one follows from the other and dissonant if the opposite of one cognition follows from the other. The thesis is that, in the presence of dissonance, the subject feels psychologically uncomfortable and attempts to reduce it. In brief, when there is tension between two mental states within the subject, the subject is disposed to reduce or eliminate this tension. It is a consequence of the theory that people will be likely to appreciate and stick to those activities in which they have invested much of their time, energy, and resources, because the thought that such activities have no value conflicts with people's previous involvement in them. Elliot Aronson is responsible for applying the theory to dissonant cognitive elements concerning conceptions and justifications of the self. He claims that one can make accurate predictions about dissonance reduction when one considers the behaviour of subjects who come to believe something about themselves that does not cohere with the idea they have about the kind of people they are. The prediction is that subjects will attempt to reduce the dissonance by revising their behaviour in accordance with their self-concept.[6] Our interest is in the data about dissonant attitudes and not in the adequacy of the predictions psychologists can make about dissonance reduction. Let me consider the case of dissonant 'cognitions' about the self as evidence that subjects 'do not practise what they preach', as Aronson puts it, and thus that there is a widespread phenomenon of attitude-behaviour inconsistency.

---

6  Furthermore, studies on reasoning suggest that people desire to have attitudes that are compatible with their values and commitments. Chaiken *et al.* (1996) who worked on defence motivation found that one is more likely to defend with reasons attitudes that are consistent with one's previous core or self-definitional attitudes.

Aronson became interested in the use of condoms by college students in the States, because it looked as if students were endorsing a general principle but not acting in accordance to it. Surveys and interviews had shown that sexually active young adults were in favour of people using condoms to prevent AIDS. Still, other evidence was available to the effect that the great majority of college students were not using condoms regularly. When asked about the reason for their behaviour, they replied that condoms were a 'nuisance'. The outcome of the surveys seemed to imply that students were concerned about the dangers of unprotected sex but did not think the dangers 'applied to them in the same way as they applied to everyone else' (Aronson 1999, p. 114). Aronson predicted that, if the college students had been alerted to the fact that they were in a state of hypocrisy, then they would attempt to change their behaviour, since the belief that they were hypocrites surely would not match their self-concept. To test this hypothesis, Aronson devised an experiment during which students were divided in two groups and had to make a video about the dangers of not using condoms. One group only was asked to think about the circumstances in which they found it particularly difficult or impossible to use condoms in the recent past. At a distance of a few months, those students who participated in Aronson's experiment and were made aware of their hypocrisy, reported to have used condoms at a higher percentage than the students who were in the other group. Also, a greater percentage of the students in the first group took advantage of a condom sale in the college.

Leaving aside the question whether the results of the experiment we have described confirm the thesis of dissonance reduction, the patterns of behaviour observed in the experiment should be familiar. In everyday life outside the lab, we all experience similar instances of inconsistent pairs of attitudes and behaviour in ourselves and others. For my purposes here, the interesting aspect of the case presented by Aronson is that the subjects in the experiments were having, and some will have continued to have, an attitude-behaviour inconsistency. One might have ascribed to the students inconsistent beliefs on the basis of considerations about their reports and their behaviour. They seemed to believe that there was danger in unprotected sex but behaved as if they did not need to worry about unprotected sex themselves. They endorsed condom use as a general principle whereas their own behaviour showed little concern for safe sex.

## 4.2.2 Poor self prediction

In the psychological studies attitude-behaviour inconsistency is established on the basis of prediction. Typically, a subject's attitude is measured, her future behaviour is also measured, and then consistency is assessed on the basis of the correlation between reported attitude and behaviour. Fabrigar and colleagues (2005, p. 105) notice that a distinction needs to be made between prediction and influence[7]: the attitude might influence the subject's behaviour even when it does not predict it, because the success of the prediction is hostage to other factors apart from the robustness or causal efficacy of the attitude (e.g. background knowledge, accessibility of the attitude, ambivalence). Keeping these methodological caveats in mind, it is fascinating to learn about cases in which reported attitudes do not seem to match observed behaviour, and thus subjects can be charged with agential irrationality. In the classic review paper by Allan Wicker (1969, p. 75), we read that there is 'little evidence to support the postulated existence of stable, underlying attitudes within the individuals which influence both his verbal expressions and his actions'. More recently, others have endorsed a similarly pessimistic account of the role of attitudes and traits as predictive of behaviour:

> [B]y the late 1960s empirical research has failed to provide strong support for behavioural consistency or predictive validity of traits and attitudes. People were found neither to behave consistently across situations, nor to act in accordance with their measured attitudes
>
> (Ajzen 2005, p. 38)

The history of empirical evidence on attitude-behaviour inconsistencies seems to have started in the thirties. The sociologist LaPiere found in 1934 that restaurants and hotels around the US had an explicit policy not to serve Asian people but would actually serve an Asian couple in the great majority of circumstances. In a similar vein Corey in 1937 found that knowing students' attitudes about cheating in an exam does not help predict whether they would actually cheat given the opportunity. In the study, the great majority of students who had expressed a very disapproving attitude towards cheating did actually cheat when asked to self-assess their exam papers, especially if the exam papers were difficult. Subsequent studies lead psychologists to ask whether the construct of an 'attitude'—which was defined in terms of predictability of behaviour—was useful (Abelson 1972; Festinger and Carlsmith 1959). Suggestions were made that reliable causal relations could be observed from behaviour to attitude, especially when the behaviour was repeated many times, but not viceversa.

Fazio and Zanna (1981) argue that this pessimism is not warranted by all research studies, and that reported attitudes can be used to predict behaviour

---

[7] Compare this distinction with the distinction we made earlier between an action being guided by a belief and a belief having behavioural effects.

reliably in some domains, including voting. Rather, they suggest that behaviour follows more reliably the correspondent attitude if the attitude has been formed on the basis of greater direct experience. Attitude-behaviour inconsistencies can be reduced by manipulating the conditions in which the subjects' attitudes are elicited. Following Bem's self-perception theory, Zanna and colleagues (1981) have shown that attitude-behaviour correlations are more consistent if subjects are invited to think about their past behaviour (how many times they privately prayed or attended a religious service) before expressing an attitude (about whether they are religious). This means that attitudes can accurately predict future behaviour if they have been inferred from past behaviour. This conclusion has been recently confirmed by a series of studies by Fabrigar and colleagues (2006), who found that background knowledge has a positive impact on attitude-behaviour consistency when it is knowledge of highly behavioural relevance. (In Frankish's terminology, level 2 beliefs are more likely to be consistent with one's behaviour if formed on the basis of the observation of one's previous behaviour, allegedly caused by level 1 beliefs).

Very recently, Eric Schwitzgebel has investigated the question whether moral philosophers behave morally – not entirely unsurprisingly, he has found that they are more likely to steal books from libraries and that they are not perceived as more moral than other philosophers by their colleagues (Schwitzgebel, forthcoming; Schwitzgebel and Rust, forthcoming).

The vast philosophical literature on attitude-behaviour inconsistency may not lead us to reject the very notion of 'attitude' as the expression of a behavioural disposition that can give rise, within the same individual, to other consistent behavioural dispositions—but certainly such literature offers some convincing examples of beliefs that are endorsed with conviction and not acted upon in the relevant circumstances. This is all we need to challenge the idea that only within psychopathology we are tempted to ascribe beliefs that are not consistent with some of the subject's behavioural dispositions.

## 4.3 Delusions and failure of reason-giving

Reason-giving is a capacity that is central to agential rationality: the subject's capacity to give good reasons in support of the content of her beliefs is a personal-level capacity that tracks the subject's explicit commitment to the beliefs she reports. According to the failure of reason-giving objection, agential rationality is a precondition for the ascription of beliefs. Delusions that are candidates for endorsement via reason-giving present a failure of agential irrationality because subjects either do not form them on the basis of good reasons, or do not support them with good reasons. Thus, delusions fall short of belief status. Here I explore the relationship between reason-giving, authorship and agential rationality, with special attention to the elements of continuity and discontinuity between delusions and beliefs. Further implications of authorship and agential rationality for self knowledge, in delusions and beliefs, will be explored in more detail in the next chapter.

### 4.3.1 Authorship and agential rationality

Authorship is the capacity to endorse the content of a conscious mental state on the basis of what one takes to be one's best reasons (see Moran 2001). Authorship does not apply to all conscious mental states. Some mental states are not candidates for authorship or can be authored only to a very limited extent, as one does not typically deliberate upon or justify the content of a merely perceptual belief or a drive. (Of course, there are exceptions. In the context of a philosophy class on scepticism or a conversation with a solipsist, a defence of the content of one's perceptual experiences with reasons may be expected.)

Andrew would not be the author of his belief that studying law is the best option for him, unless he were in a position to defend that claim with reasons. But the same would not apply to other conscious mental states of Andrew. His being hungry or his seeing his bike leaning on the front gate of the school are states that he can authoritatively report without giving reasons for them; it is not so clear what it would mean to 'endorse' them, other than acting in a way that is consistent with them. Even if we restrict our attention to beliefs only, variation can be observed. Consider the belief that I need to cross two busy roundabouts on my way to work. There is very little about that belief that is *up to me*. If challenged, I can support the belief by appealing to the accuracy of my perceptual experiences and the reliability of my memory. On an everyday basis, I can act in a way that is compatible with my having that belief. But in no other significant way can I be said to endorse the belief that there are two roundabouts on my way to work. I manifest my authorship potential to a greater extent with respect to those beliefs whose content I am prepared to defend on the basis of reasons, such as opinions, or with respect to other attitudes, such as intentions and motivated desires (see Carman 2003). The belief that the debt of developing countries should be cancelled, for instance, is the type of belief that I can endorse with reasons. I can argue for the claim that cancelling the debt would have significant benefits for people in developing countries by allowing their governments to invest more resources in education. The belief is authored by me, because it is up to me what to believe, and I take responsibility over its content by having formed it or defended it on the basis of what I consider to be my best reasons.

Judgements of authorship will be affected by the type of reported attitude, and by the significance of the content of the attitude for the subject reporting it. Some beliefs are such that, when a subject reports them, it is expected that she can offer some justification for them. For instance, if someone who was born and always lived in England reports the belief that it is best for her to move to Egypt, then we expect her to have some reasons for the belief, as acting on it would constitute a life change with fairly radical consequences. There would be something deeply puzzling about the following exchange:

Bonnie: 'The best thing for me is to move to Egypt'

Adam: 'Why?'

Bonnie: 'I don't know. No reason.'

The phrase 'the best thing' seems to imply some weighing and evaluation on behalf of the speaker, as if the statement made were the outcome of reason, but no reason-giving follows the statement. In this case, the lack of justification in Bonnie's answer could make Adam not only doubt whether Bonnie has authority over the belief she reports, but also whether she *really* believes what she says, i.e. that the best thing for her would be to move to Egypt. (This dialogue leaves us perplexed in a similar way as some dialogues with subjects reporting their delusions.)

How does authorship relate to agential rationality? Authorship of a belief is achieved via reason-giving, that is, a subject is the author of a belief if she is able to provide what she takes to be her best reasons for endorsing the content of that belief, either in deliberation or justification. Authorship typically applies to conscious mental states on whose content one can exercise some control, such as beliefs, preferences and decisions, but some mental states can be authored to a greater degree (e.g. opinions) than others (e.g. perceptual beliefs). The endorsement of a belief can be explicitly or implicitly manifested in several ways, e.g. behaving in a way that is compatible with the endorsed beliefs, but we have an instance of authorship when the belief can be endorsed via reason-giving.[8] Agential rationality applies to all those belief states that are candidates for authorship, but of all the beliefs that are authored, only a subset will be authored *in a rational way*. Agential rationality is a more demanding notion than authorship: whereas authorship requires that a subject is able to endorse the content of her beliefs *on the basis of what she takes to be her best reasons,*

---

[8] As we shall see in Chapter 5, authorship as the capacity a subject has to give what she takes to be her best reasons in support of her reported attitudes gives rise to a form of first-person authority (agential authority) which is an important aspect of self knowledge.

agential rationality requires that the subject is able to endorse the content of her beliefs *on the basis of reasons that are intersubjectively good*. If the subject endorses a belief on the basis of reasons that she does not take to be her best reasons, she is not genuinely engaging in deliberation or justification. If she endorses her beliefs on the basis of reasons that are not good reasons, she may be genuinely engaging in deliberation and justification (and thus be the author of her beliefs) but she is not agentially rational.

This distinction between the conditions for authorship and the conditions for agential rationality is important, because deliberation and justification are not always processes characterised by good reasoning, and do not always have as outputs rational formation, or satisfactory justification of beliefs. People can deliberate and justify, without successfully identifying the best reasons available to them. In order to be the author of a belief, all the rationality or reasonableness required is the endorsement of the belief on the basis of what the subject takes to be her best reasons. It is neither necessary that the belief be optimally rational nor that the processes of deliberation and justification which lead one to endorse the belief be themselves optimally rational. But for agential rationality the bar is raised. A subject is agentially rational with respect to a belief if the belief is a candidate for authorship and she forms it or endorses it on the basis of good reasons.

Here is how the conditions for authorship and agential rationality compare by reference to an example:

> **Authorship:** In order to be the author of the belief that he should study law at university, Andrew needs to be able to endorse the content of his belief on the basis of what he takes to be his best reasons for it.
>
> **Agential rationality:** In order to be agentially rational with respect to the belief that he should study law at university, Andrew needs to a1) form the belief on the basis of (intersubjectively) good reasons or a2) support the belief on the basis of (intersubjectively) good reasons, and b) act upon the belief in the appropriate circumstances.

Now that the conditions for authorship and agential rationality have been spelled out, we can see how these notions can apply to the reporting of delusional beliefs.

### 4.3.2 Are delusions authored?[9]

It is a hard task to determine whether delusions are authored, and whether they conform to the standards of agential rationality, because one needs to

---

[9] Arguments in this section have been developed with Matthew Broome. See Bortolotti and Broome (2008) for details.

examine detailed reports in order to come to a conclusion about whether the content of a delusion is genuinely endorsed and defended with reasons. Authorship draws attention to the form rather than the content of delusional reports.[10] It can be difficult to determine whether a delusion defies understanding, because cultural and individual differences can affect the plausibility of the delusional content itself or the type of reasons offered in its defence. How articulate the subject is in reporting the delusion is also an important factor, as information that is salient to the subject might not be entirely accessible to others, or communicated in a fragmented and unsatisfactory way. But these difficulties impact on intelligibility to a lesser extent if we concentrate not on plausibility of content, but on the extent to which subjects with delusions are prepared to defend the content of their delusion. What seems to be at issue is not whether others are willing to accept the delusion as true when it is reported, but whether the very subject reporting the delusion endorses its content.

Consider the following textbook examples of delusions:

> A 21-year old man has sudden conviction that certain songs played on the radio used his voice in the role of lead singer. He cannot explain why.

> (Yager and Gitlin 2005, p. 978)

> A man believes his wife is unfaithful to him because the fifth lamp-post along on the left is unlit.

> (Sims 2003, p. 119)

In the first two cases, subjects make the reports with conviction but offer no explanation or reason to believe that what they say is true. The inability or unwillingness to provide evidence for what they claim is somehow at odds with the subjects' apparent high degree of conviction and with the personal references contained in their reports. When no further elaboration is offered, such cases illustrate delusions that, in Jaspers' terminology, are deemed 'ununderstandable'.[11]

Now consider other two cases:

> A woman claims her blood is being injected out of her body in her sleep because she has spots on her arms. The interviewer says that they are freckles and that he has them

---

[10] The distinction between 'form' and 'content' of a delusion derives from Jaspers (1963) and is revisited here.

[11] Some distinguish between delusional beliefs and delusional experiences, and would class this type of delusion, reported but not defended with some relevant reason, as mere experiences. For insightful discussion of this point, I thank Flavie Waters.

too – and shows her. She agrees they are similar, but still maintains that she is being injected.

(Sims 2003, p. 123)

A woman fails to recognise the man who drives the family car and pays the bills as her husband, although she concedes that he looks very much like her husband. She notices that he is just a bit 'fatter'.

(Sims 2003, p. 123)

Here subjects are able to defend their delusions by appealing to events that have some meaningful connection to the content of their delusional states. These reports do not differ qualitatively from ordinary belief reports in which subjects do not have good or sufficient reasons to justify or maintain their beliefs. As I previously noted, there are considerable methodological limitations in this analysis, as establishing the degree of endorsement is a complex endeavour and textbook cases do not come with sufficiently detailed information to allow for some measurement of endorsement. Only further examination of a subject's set of beliefs via carefully directed questioning could tell us whether the reasons adduced for endorsing the content of the delusional state are regarded by the subject herself as good reasons; and to what extent the subject would maintain conviction when probed. Whether a reason is good is likely to depend on measures of procedural and epistemic rationality, and especially on the inferential and evidential connections that can be identified between the content of the delusion and other intentional states the subject is committed to, and the sensitivity of the delusional content to the evidence available to the subject. Thus, tailored evidence needs to be provided to answer these questions satisfactorily.

Here are two more detailed reports that can serve as the basis for assessing authorship in subjects with delusions. The first case was brought to my attention by Max Coltheart[12]: a young man was affected by memory deficits following a severe head injury. He experienced feelings of familiarity towards TV programmes when he saw them for the first time (*déjà vecu*). He felt like he had seen the programmes before, not at any indefinite time in the past, but at the

---

[12] This case has been discussed in a presentation by Max Coltheart entitled 'Déjà vecu for News Events but not Personal Events' at Memory Day, Macquarie Centre for Cognitive Sciences, 28th November 2008. Other cases of recollective confabulation in persistent déjà vecu have been recorded in the literature. Subjects have a persistent feeling that they have experienced a certain situation before, when the situation is present and novel. The condition often leads to 'confabulations and dysfunctional behaviour in everyday life' (Moulin *et al.* 2005, page 1364).

time when he had been hospitalised in the city, years earlier, for the accident that caused him the memory deficits. In a recorded interview, he was asked to explain how he could have seen before even live programmes, such as the news or sport events, and he provided a very elaborate explanation. He claimed (correctly) that in the rural location where he lived with his family there were fewer channels than in the city where he had been hospitalised. From this he developed the delusional explanation that in the countryside they broadcast programmes that were shown years earlier in the big city for the benefit of those who could not see them at the time (this was incorrect). The interviewer gently probed him with questions such as 'Does this make sense to you?'; 'How do you think this is possible?', and so on. As a result, the man further elaborated his views, although at some stage he admitted that the situation was confusing, and that he no longer talked to others about it, because they tended not to believe him.

The second case is described by Komiyama. It is the report of a young man with schizophrenia, MF:

> 'They are saying things that concern me on television and in the newspapers. The neighbors have a very strange attitude towards me. I can hear sounds coming from the ceiling, and it seems that someone is eavesdropping. After something happens at home, people are talking about it the next day at work. I'm sure that the construction company that we have dealings with has bugged my house. I think that it's all been done on the orders of the factory manager, but it's not clear.' After a time, he started saying things like the following: 'In the office, the boss and the people who work with me make two noises, or sometimes just one. I've thought a lot about what they mean. If two sounds are made, it means that I must make the girl I lived with before my marriage my mistress. One sound means make a date with her. But they don't say it clearly in words, so I don't understand what they want me to do. I can't understand what I should do about the girl.'

> (Komiyama 1989, p. 15)

These kinds of detailed case reports or descriptions allow to 'measure' degrees of commitment to a delusional report, or at least form some hypotheses about the extent to which the subject endorses the content of the delusional state on the basis of the reasons he can offer in its support. Although the man with déjà vecu had a bizarre belief content, and some of the explanations he offered in its support were inconsistent with one another and implausible, his line of reasoning suggests that he was committed to the content of his belief. In the narrative of the man with schizophrenia who attributes significance to sounds from neighbours and colleagues, there do not seem to be (intersubjectively) meaningful connections between such sounds and the personal events he links them to. A provisional analysis suggests that in these cases there might be authorship, but there is no agential rationality.

For the earlier vignettes, a detailed analysis of the subjects' responses is not available. For the case of the man who reports that his wife is unfaithful due to the lamp-post being unlit, and the case of the man who hears his voice on the radio, there are two possible scenarios to be considered. In the former scenario, say, the man who reports to believe that his wife is unfaithful (*hypothesis*) because the lamp-post is unlit (*evidence*) cannot provide any further explanation of the relation between the two. The relation between evidence and hypothesis, therefore, remains mysterious. In the latter scenario, the man reports the same delusion but also elaborates a complex theory about the connection between the hypothesis and the evidence. Typical explanations could invoke intervention from a third party—for instance, he could claim that the government is trying to warn him of his wife's infidelity by leaving clues that only he can decipher, such as that particular lamp-post being unlit. When an explanation of the connection between evidence and hypothesis is available, the delusion appears as more understandable to an interpreter, even if the plausibility of the hypothesis given the evidence remains highly questionable and suggests a violation of epistemic rationality. In the latter scenario, one could say that the interpreter gets a better sense that the speaker *believes* the content of the reported delusion and is in a position to offer some reason for attributing that particular significance to an apparent random event.

To provide a distinction between cases in which no reasons for a belief are offered and cases in which bad reasons are offered is not always easy. When does a very bad reason cease to be a reason altogether? The difference between some of the examples we considered are striking in this respect: for the subject with Capgras, the fact that an observed man is fatter than how she remembers her husband to be can be conceivably regarded as a reason for denying that the observed man is her husband. In contrast, the lamp-post being unlit would seem to bear no meaningful relation with the fidelity of one's spouse, unless additional explanations were offered. The case of the woman with spots in her arm is an intermediate case: there are meaningful links between blood being injected out of an arm and visible spots on the arm, but the type of spot identified as evidence for the injections is not of the right kind. As rationality (i.e. having intersubjectively good reasons for endorsing a belief content) is not a requirement for authorship, delusions could be regarded as authored if an attempt to engage in reason-giving is made. But these delusions would fail to meet the standards of agential rationality when the reasons offered by the subjects are not (intersubjectively) good reasons. When the type of delusion involved would demand justification and an expression of commitment, because its content has potentially very significant and disturbing implications for the subject, and no attempt at reason-giving is made, then delusions neither satisfy the demanding conditions for agential rationality, nor are they authored.

### 4.3.3 Giving reasons: deliberation and justification

Considerations about reason-giving can motivate various arguments against the doxastic nature of delusions, which can be classed as *failure of reason-giving* objections. So far, I have considered two versions of the constraint, one that focuses on the act of forming a belief on the basis of reasons and one that focuses on the act of justifying beliefs on the basis of reasons. The latter does not require an explicit act of deliberation but focuses instead on the endorsement of a belief content, independent of the process of belief formation. Whereas justification via reason-giving can apply to the majority of belief types, only a small subset of the attitudes that we commonly regard as beliefs are formed via explicit deliberation. Some reflective evaluations and some opinions are formed as a result of explicit deliberation, but a much wider set of beliefs are not formed this way. Even if a subject is not fully aware of what caused her to have a certain attitude (e.g. her preference for a certain artwork), she can always 'search for reasons' at a later stage and come to endorse her attitude on the basis of reasons that might not coincide with the reasons for (or the causal mechanisms responsible for) the formation of that attitude.

In the debate on the doxastic conception of delusions there is a tendency to view the inability to provide a personal-level account of how delusions are formed as an argument against their status as beliefs. This is due to an idealisation of the notion of belief, where it is taken for granted that the paradigmatic belief is formed on the basis of reasons. The endorsement of a delusion as a result of deliberation is seemingly supported by some accounts of delusion formation: in Ellis (1998), subjects are represented as scientists looking for a plausible explanation of a strange phenomenon, and Stone and Young (1997) apply a similar account to instances of Capgras. My husband looks different to me and this fact demands an explanation. To explain it, I consider several hypotheses and endorse the hypothesis that the man in front of me is not my husband but an impostor. I end up endorsing the delusional hypothesis because this is not inhibited even if implausible. The main problem with this account (when generalised to the formation of all delusions) is that it is not likely that the event giving rise to the formation of delusional hypothesis is open to introspection and reflection.

Another argument against the doxastic nature of delusions can be based on the principle that, even if a belief is not formed via an explicit act of deliberation, the psychological causes of the formation of the belief must be available to the subject as reasons for the belief and have a role in the justification of the belief. If the psychological causes of the formation of a delusion are not available to the subject as reasons for the delusional state and do not play a role in the justification of the delusional state, then delusions are not beliefs. There are concerns with the principle on which this argument is based: some beliefs are such that we can offer reasons for endorsing their content, but these reasons do not make reference to the psychological mechanisms that are causally relevant to the formation of the beliefs. We shall see some examples of this phenomenon—when the psychological mechanisms responsible for the formation of our attitudes are not open to introspection. Delusions are no exception. When I report that the man looking a lot like my husband is an impostor, I cannot refer to the lack of autonomic responses as the cause of my report because autonomic responses are not experienced. The lack of affective response responsible for the experience of unfamiliarity is not conscious and accessible to me as evidence for the hypothesis that the man standing in front of me is not my husband but an impostor, and is not likely to play a role in the *post-hoc* justification of my delusion either.

To say that affective responses are not accessible is not to say that no conscious experience relevant to the formation of the delusion is accessible, or that there cannot be a personal-level account of delusion formation. It seems important to distinguish the view that subjects are aware *that they lost their affective response to the familiar face* from the view that subjects are aware that *the familiar face looks different*. The personal-level account does not need to be committed to a description of the subject's experience in terms of 'affective responses'. Subjects with Capgras may be aware of the fact that their spouse or relative looks different without necessarily being aware of the fact that the affective response is missing. We do not seem to be aware of our affective responses in the great majority of cases, and sometimes only skin conductance can reveal whether the response is present. But it is sufficient that I am aware that my husband's face looks different to me in order for me to have something to explain (and something to refer to in *post-hoc* justifications of the delusional state).

One question is how we should conceive the content of experience that is available to introspection and reflection in this case. There are at least three cases in which an object of experience can turn out to be unfamiliar to the subject of experience.

a) One can fail to re-identify the object and sees it as novel—as if one had not experienced it before. A typical reaction to this failure, when acknowledged, would be to say: 'I've never seen this before.'

b) One can fail to re-identify the object because one sees it as if it were different from how one experienced it before or from how one would have expected it to be. A typical reaction to this failure, when acknowledged, would be to say: 'It is not x, because it looks different from *x*.' The element of comparison is important in this case. It signals that a similarity or continuity with a previously known object of experience is detected but that the similarity or continuity is not sufficient for the re-identification to succeed.

c) One can re-identify the object but fail to have the emotional response toward it that usually accompanied one's previous experiences of it. In this case, one would say something like: 'I feel differently toward this object.'

(Bortolotti and Broome 2007, pp. 39–40)

What happens in cases of Capgras? The Capgras patient does not recognise that person as the person dear to her, so the recognition that is taking place is just a partial one and its cognitive and affective components cannot be entirely made independent of one another. The experience of Capgras patients cannot be characterised purely as (c). Their reaction to the abnormal experience is not exhausted by their feeling estranged from the object of experience. If I had awareness that my emotional reactions or feelings toward my husband had changed, but could recognise him as my husband, I would not fail to re-identify him and I would not postulate the presence of an impostor. Rather, I would attempt to find an explanation for the radical change in my emotional response. But Capgras patients do offer explanations such as those mentioned in (b), where they claim that the person as they currently experience her does not entirely correspond to the person they know. The recognition of another person implies an affective response—as Matthew Broome puts it, if we did not care, we would not notice. In the Capgras case, recognition is not likely to be a two-step process ('I recognize him as my husband but I don't have the relevant affective response and I feel estranged from him'), but a unitary radically novel and disorientating experience ('It's not him').

According to the subpersonal-level account of the formation of delusions, the content of the subjects' experience is neither consciously accessed by the subject nor analysable. The delusional state is formed as the effect of the subject's experience, but the experience does not lend any epistemic support to the content of the delusion. The delusion is the 'output of a modularized affective subsystem' (see Gerrans 2000, p. 115). I have no conscious access to my experience of there being something wrong with how my husband looks, and given that the experience is not something for which an explanation can be found, there is no weighing up of evidence. There are no *reasons* for the formation of the delusion, just causes that cannot be cashed out in psychological or intentional terms.[13] This account would explain why delusions are much more resistant to counterevidence than typical beliefs: the subject might recognise

---

[13] For a discussion of this point, see Campbell (2009).

the implausibility of the delusional hypothesis, but cannot give it up, because it is not amenable to reason. Against the sub-personal level account of delusion formation, it has been noted that often subjects attempt to describe the difference between the impostor and the spouse or relative in terms of slight discrepancies in the physical appearance, such as 'the eyes are too close' or 'she's too tall'. This could be taken as supporting the personal-level account, as subjects provide evidence based on their perceptual experience for the plausibility of the report. The obvious response is to regard these references to the physical appearance of the 'impostor' as confabulatory attempts to justify one's conviction in the face of external challenges. The physical difference might be something that played no role in the formation of the delusion and to which the subject appeals in order to provide a *post-hoc* rationalisation of her commitment to the implausible content of the delusion. According to this view, once the subjects find themselves with the delusion, they try to make it sound plausible to themselves and others by reference to perceptible differences between the physical appearance of their spouses or relatives and that of the alleged impostors.

There are two issues emerging from the debate about whether the formation of delusions can be better accounted for in personal or subpersonal terms. One issue is which account (personal-level or subpersonal-level) is most plausible given the available evidence. This is an empirical issue to be settled by science, and different accounts might apply to different types of delusion (see Aimola Davies and Davies 2009). The other issue is whether settling this issue has any implications for the doxastic account of delusions. If we accept the personal account, there is no reason why we should deny that delusions are beliefs. The delusion would be formed in the same way as idealised beliefs are, as an explanation for a fact that is relevant to the subject. If the subpersonal-level account for the formation of the delusion prevails, there seems to be nothing intrinsically incoherent in the view that some beliefs are not the product of personal-level hypothesis formation. Arguably, our everyday perceptual experience is also the effect of a modularised system and lends support to our beliefs in a retrospective fashion. A typical perceptual belief is not produced through a conscious deliberative process of hypothesis formation. It isn't the case that one sees a chair and, by a conscious deliberative process, one forms the hypothesis that there is a chair. Rather, what happens is that the perception of the chair gives rise to the perceptual belief that there is a chair independently of any hypothesis formation.

The notions of authorship and agential rationality allow us to revisit these debates on reasons, delusion formation and belief status. In all cases of beliefs, endorsement of belief contents is a core notion, but the type of endorsement that applies to one type of belief might not be relevant to another type. Agential rationality with respect to explicit deliberation is a suitable notion of rationality for some beliefs, such as considered opinions. Agential rationality with respect to justification of belief contents has a wider scope, including beliefs that are not formed via deliberation, such as beliefs about likes and dislikes. Naturally, the mere fact that a belief has not been produced in a way that is open to introspective analysis does not prevent subjects from providing reasons for it at the stage of justification. Once we have formed a perceptual belief about there being a broken chair in the living room, we can justify it by appealing to our perceptual experience of the chair. Once the subject with Capgras delusion finds herself with the thought that her husband has been replaced by an impostor, she will justify it by reference to differences in appearance between the man in front of her and her husband. This account of attempted justification where the reasons for the reported attitude do not necessarily coincide with the psychological causes of its formation, does not compromise authorship of the attitude, unless the subject's reasons are not what she takes to be her best reasons. The account would not compromise agential rationality either, if the reasons provided by the subject were (inter-subjectively) good.

## 4.4 Delusions and framework beliefs[14]

One might convincingly argue that the notions of authorship and agential rationality should not be applied to delusions, because, if beliefs at all, they are *framework* beliefs. Framework beliefs are foundational beliefs, beliefs one is committed to without necessarily being able to offer independent reasons for having them. The belief that the earth existed prior to one's birth is a good example. Some philosophers have discussed whether subjects who are typically very committed to such beliefs are in a position to engage in the game of justification with respect to them (Wittgenstein 1969; Campbell 2001; Eilan 2000; Thornton 2008; Bortolotti 2002). Most reasons speakers could offer to justify the believed proposition that the earth existed before their births are reliant upon the same proposition being true. Thus, the acceptance of framework propositions is usually not questioned and is considered to be immune from doubt.

---

[14] Arguments in this section were developed with Matthew Broome. For more details, see Bortolotti and Broome (2008).

### 4.4.1 **Can we author framework beliefs?**

Let's think about what it would be like to justify the belief in a framework proposition. Given the nature of framework beliefs, their endorsement is more likely to be manifested behaviourally than by reason-giving. For instance, a sign of *implicit* endorsement is the use of a shared language that presupposes the truth of the relevant framework proposition. Many linguistic terms, including the terms 'parent' and 'history', would acquire different meaning if it turned out to be false that the earth existed before our births. Such belief can be defended only on the basis of coherence with other beliefs we have and not on the basis of there being more basic reasons to support the conviction that the proposition is true. But a defence based on epistemic conservatism or coherence is still a form of justification. We are usually not asked to justify framework beliefs, but if we were, we could do so.[15] The reasons adduced in support of framework beliefs would probably not persuade the sceptic of the truth of framework propositions, but authorship is not about grounding conceptually sophisticated beliefs onto more basic ones or answering sceptical challenges. It is about the potential for endorsement via reason-giving.

Some attempts at explaining what causes failures in reason-giving invite us to draw an analogy between beliefs in propositions such as 'The earth existed long before our births' and delusions. A subject reports her delusion with great conviction but cannot offer reasons for it, because she believes that the fact reported is more certain than any of the facts she might mention in its support. Not to believe the content of the delusion is, for the subject, out of the question. The analogy lies in the fact that neither the delusion nor the framework belief is justified because there is a sense in which they cannot receive any independent justification. John Campbell makes this point on a much discussed paper. He defends the analogy on the basis of the certainty with which the relevant proposition is believed:

> The kind of status that we ordinarily assign to propositions like 'The world has existed for quite a long time' ... is assigned by the deluded subject to propositions like 'I am dead' or 'My neighbour has been replaced by an impostor.' That is, they are treated as

---

15 The account of fundamental aspects of our world-view ('hinges') in terms of hinges as framework propositions has been challenged in recent work. According to Moyal-Sharrock (2004), the endorsement of a hinge is deemed as necessarily ineffable. If the endorsement of hinges cannot be reason-based and cannot be articulated or verbalised, then it may not allow for authorship, as the type of endorsement that usually characterises authorship involves the capacity for justification via reason- giving. On this alternative account, the endorsement of a hinge would be manifest primarily in a way of life, via non-verbal behaviour, rather than via the capacity for arguing for the content of a belief.

the background assumptions needed for there to be any testing of the correctness of propositions at all.

(Campbell 2001, p. 96)

Another element of continuity is that changes both in framework beliefs and delusions determine changes in meaning. The subject with delusions sometimes offers reasons that appear to have no meaningful connection to the content of the delusion, because the connection she identifies is based on a meaning relation that is salient to herself only and, as a result, her endorsement of the delusion is not appreciated by others. The analogy lies in the fact that the rejection or acquisition of a framework proposition has the same effect as the rejection or acquisition of a delusional belief. They both cause the subject to review meaning connections between previously used terms. As we could no longer make sense of what the words 'parents' or 'history' meant if we did no longer assume that the earth existed before we were born, so we cannot define death in terms of complete absence of experience if we endorse the Cotard delusion.

> Sometimes the patient will say that she is disembodied. The patient may claim to be dead despite being able to walk and talk. Indeed, the patient may say that she is dead even though she realizes that no one else would accept this claim. The trouble is, how can the patients really be said to be holding on to knowledge of the meanings of their remarks when they are using the words in such a deviant way?

(Campbell 2001, p. 91)

It is certainly true that are the content of some delusional beliefs signals a redefinition of meaning relations and implies an attribution of special significance to events that might appear irrelevant or casual to anybody but the subject of the delusion. The lamp-post being unlit *means* infidelity. Having freckles on one's arms *means* that injections were made. Maybe 'death' no longer *means* death. The analogy between delusions and framework beliefs appears to be working and to support the view that, whatever we say about the authorship of framework beliefs, we should also say about the authorship of those delusions which share these fundamental features with them. But the analogy is far from water-tight at a closer look.

First, the refusal or incapacity to provide a justification for delusions on the basis of their being absolutely and undoubtedly true is not sufficient reason to claim that delusional states play the role of background assumptions in reason-giving—that would be a very implausible claim especially where delusions are relatively circumscribed (Broome 2004). We would expect a framework proposition to be perfectly well-integrated in the belief system. Indeed, the framework proposition should be one of its unshakeable pillars, and to be relied upon in the justification of beliefs that are much more open to doubt and to revision. Many un-authored delusions do not behave that way. They are isolated from the other beliefs in the system and no reason-giving exercise employs them as assumptions. Second, there is a problem with the analogy when we consider different types of delusions. Bayne and Pacherie (2004a) have argued convincingly that, in some versions of the Capgras delusion, the example originally used by Campbell in the first quotation we reported, delusions cannot be regarded as playing the same role as framework beliefs. Subjects with Capgras often recognise that the content of their delusion is implausible, sometimes even unbelievable, but they would not find the content of framework beliefs implausible or unbelievable. Third, it is right that the adoption of a delusional belief leads subjects to identify new meaning relations or reject previously accepted ones with respect to the Cotard delusion, where the subject claims to be dead. But the same phenomenon is totally absent in other delusions, such as Capgras. As Broome (2004) argued, the explanation of what happens to subjects with Capgras does not usually need to rely on the introduction of new meaning relations. It is because subjects understand what the word 'impostors' means that they find it disturbing that their dear ones have been replaced by such impostors. It is because psychiatrists understand what subjects report that they are able to diagnose the delusion as a version of Capgras and engage in conversation with their patients. Meaning always needs to be shared to some extent. Arguably, only in the most acute stages of mental illness, characterised by marked thought disorder, bizarre behaviour, and catatonia, are the subject's thoughts are private and incommunicable to others.

### 4.4.2 **Are delusions framework beliefs?**

Objections to the analogy between delusions and framework beliefs can be reformulated by using the notion of authorship. The analogy fails because the nature of the commitment to a framework proposition is different from the nature of the commitment to the content of a delusion, and this seems to be true across the board, independent of what type of delusion we are considering.

Let's start with the *intersubjective* dimension of the relation between the subject and the proposition and consider both the issue of the redefinition of meaning relations and that of the verbalisation and communication of reasons. The analogy between delusions and framework beliefs would have it that both belief-like states are such that 1) changes in the commitment to their content give rise to changes in meaning relations, and that 2) the commitment is not usually properly articulated or verbalised. These commonalities are only apparent though, because there are different explanations for how delusions and framework beliefs determine meaning relations and for their being rarely verbally endorsed.

Why do we think that giving up a framework proposition would lead us to redefine meaning relations? Just like language, the commitment to framework propositions is usually shared by an entire community—sometimes as large as that of all humans. Campbell (2001) offers the same answer to this question: abandoning a framework belief makes a difference to other beliefs and causes a redefinition of relevant terms in the language of the community that undergoes this often radical change. The idea that meanings are shared is conveyed in slogans, such as 'meanings ain't in the head', or 'there cannot be a private language'. Why do we think that endorsing a delusion would bring about changes in meaning? There is a sense in which meaning relations revealed in the reports of delusions can be private to the subject with the delusion. The delusional belief is typically rejected by the people surrounding the subject, and the subject is acutely aware of that. This is a first important disanalogy between framework beliefs and delusions: they both determine meaning relations, but the former do so within a community, whereas the latter do so for a subject in isolation from, and often in opposition to, the community of which the subject is a member (Thornton 2008; Gallagher 2009). Not all delusions are the same, as I suggested in the previous section. Endorsing the content of a delusion does not always bring about a change in meaning relations. The case of Cotard is interesting because when subjects with the delusion offer reasons for believing that they are dead, we suspect that they use the word 'death' differently from how other people in their community use it (or differently from how they would use it in other contexts). But in other cases, the endorsement of a delusion causes no evident shifts in meaning relations. People with paranoia and persecutory delusions use the words 'government', 'spy' or 'terrorist' in the same way as everybody else around them. In those cases, the delusion might still bring alienation, but meanings are not private to the subject. The analogy between persecutory delusions and framework beliefs is thus not convincing with respect to the notion of meaning renegotiation. The content of such delusions is reported and communicated successfully to others, but not endorsed by others.

Why are delusions rarely endorsed with intersubjectively good reasons? The subject's endorsement of a delusion can be difficult to verbalise or articulate clearly and therefore it is seldom communicated to others. The subject with delusions might be resistant to talking about her delusions for fear of meeting people's incredulity and hostility, and because she wants to avoid being made fun of. Indeed, these are some of the causes of distress and social alienation that often accompany the experience of subjects with delusions. For framework beliefs, the story is radically different. A framework belief is almost never explicitly reported within a community and opportunities for expressing a commitment to it are rare. But the reason why the commitment to the content of a framework belief is not explicit is that the subject endorsing a framework belief sees no need to express her commitment to the content of that belief. She expects everybody else around her to be committed to the same belief content, and she does not need or want to state the obvious. The content of the framework belief is taken for granted. The commitment to a framework proposition is not always explicit and verbalised, but, when it is expressed in behaviour and in the endorsement of beliefs that rest on it, it brings social inclusion and participation in social practices. Endorsing the content of a delusion seems to have the opposite effect. It brings social exclusion and initiates a renegotiation of meanings that leads to a drastic revision of the belief system when the delusion is elaborated, or a drastic compartmentalisation when the delusion is circumscribed. In short, in the case of delusions regarded as un-understandable either the reason-giving exercise required to author a delusion is not present, or the endorsement of the belief is 'private', that is, deprived of its social dimension. When reasons are given, they are not recognised as (good) reasons by others.

Let's consider now the *intrasubjective* character of the commitment to a belief and concentrate once more on the manifestations of authorship as reason-giving. Within the subject holding onto a belief, there are significant differences between the attitude towards a framework belief and the attitude towards a delusion. The commitment to framework proposition is pervasive and manifested in many instances of behaviour, although the belief remains in the background and may never be explicitly reported or justified. Not only is the believed proposition compatible with other propositions believed by the subject, but it brings cohesion within the system by supporting them and making their acceptance possible. In other words, framework beliefs are used in reason-giving when the commitment to other beliefs is tested. What happens in the case of delusional reports? Differences emerge between subjects with elaborated and with circumscribed delusions. It is possible that to some extent subjects with elaborated delusions behave towards their delusions as subjects with ordinary beliefs behave towards framework beliefs, by taking them for granted, employing them in reason-giving and reserving to them a pronounced action-guiding role. But for the subjects affected by those delusions that are heavily circumscribed, the delusion does not give rise to the behaviour that would naturally ensue from believing with conviction the content of the delusion and the endorsement of the delusion is not implicit in the endorsement of other beliefs. Rather, the delusion often explicitly conflicts with other accepted beliefs, generating tensions and sometimes even inconsistencies in the belief system.

To bring together inter- and intrasubjective considerations, the analogy between framework beliefs and heavily circumscribed delusions works if confined to observations about meaning change and gaps in the verbalised attempts to support the belief, but it fails to account for the intersubjective dimension of the acceptance of a framework proposition. The analogy between framework beliefs and more elaborated delusions makes sense of the continuity in the behavioural manifestations of the commitment to the belief at the intrasubjective level, but it is implausible at the intersubjective level where the changes of meaning relations required to make sense of the delusion are not shared by the rest of the subject's community and are not as easily communicated to others, and delusions fail to play the foundational role of framework beliefs.

### 4.4.3 Do delusions conflict with framework beliefs?

In the previous section I argued that the analogy between delusions and framework beliefs is not successful, due to marked differences in the inter- and intrasubjective dimensions of the commitment that subjects manifest to the content of their delusions. There is another view according to which reference to framework beliefs can improve our understanding of delusions—delusions are not like framework beliefs, but are puzzling in so far as they involve the rejection of framework beliefs. Rhodes and Gipps (2008) claim that delusions are distinctive because the subjects who report and endorse them do not share the *bedrock* with other members of their community.[16] What do they mean by 'bedrock'? Where Wittgenstein introduced the notion of hinges, or framework propositions, in *On Certainty* (§§96-99), he compared belief systems to a river, to describe how we know the things we know.

> But I distinguish between the movement of the water on the river-bed and the shift of the bed itself; though there is no sharp division of the one from the other. [...]
> And the bank of that river consists partly of hard rock, subject to no alteration or only to an imperceptible one, partly of sand which now in one place now in another gets washed away, or deposited.

> (Wittgenstein 1969, §97 and §99)

---

[16] Also see the commentaries to Rhodes and Gipps' paper by Giovanni Stanghellini and Nassir Ghaemi in *Philosophy, Psychiatry & Psychology* 15(4), 2008.

In the river, there is sand and there are rocks. The sand gets moved around, is subject to change. The hard rock is more stable, although of course it is subject to erosion and can change too. When Rhodes and Gipps talk about the bedrock, they refer to those beliefs we have that are close to certain and play a foundational role with respect to other, less certain, beliefs. Their idea is that the puzzling features of delusions can be explained as a change in the belief system, such that subjects with delusions come to have a different foundation for what they believe and no longer share the bedrock with other members of their community. As a consequence of this shift in basic beliefs, subjects with delusions operate outside the set of dispositions and cultural assumptions, the *background*, which is reflected in everyday practice and makes successful communication and mutual understanding possible.

Is it plausible to argue that subjects with delusions have lost their grip on the shared bedrock? Unexciting as my thesis might sound, I suspect that the answer to this question depends on the type of delusions we wish to explain. Many cases of delusion do not require any suspension of or deviation from expected norms. My main concern is that invoking discrepancies in the bedrock would lead us to see delusional beliefs as radically discontinuous from false and irrational beliefs. But naïve interpreters are to some extent successful in making sense of the behaviour of subjects with delusions. Although mutual understanding can be and often is compromised, interpretation of behaviour on the basis of beliefs and other intentional states does not seem to be affected by even pervasive and radical breakdowns of rationality.

Rhodes and Gipps, who want to show that delusions are not based on the same bedrock as ordinary beliefs, illustrate their view with some examples, such as that of Katie:

> Katie repeatedly claimed that everyone thought that they had the right to 'tell her off'. Furthermore, she said, everyone had a 'device' that transmitted information about her. If something happened to Katie in one place, then information about these events was transmitted to other places. She would hear comments on a topic at work, and hear references to these when she entered a shop.
>
> (Rhodes and Gipps 2008, p. 295)

Katie claims that people have a device that can transmit to others information about herself and she supports that claim with evidence (from the brief extract, we would say that she is the author of her delusion). Moreover, the reasons she offers for believing in the existence of that device are not intersubjectively good reasons—she is not agentially rational—but they 'make sense', that is, they stand in the right relation with the belief content that she endorses, even if we would probably not consider them sufficient reasons for forming or maintaining that belief. Is Katie's belief really so puzzling?

## 4.4.4 Can framework beliefs be justified and revised?

The bedrock is constituted by framework beliefs. These beliefs are accepted without doubt and they function as the starting point for any attempt at justifying other beliefs, which are less basic and more susceptible to change. In Rhodes and Gipps' words, framework beliefs 'convey our direct, pre-reflective and practical *grasp* of the world, rather than express *judgements* we make *about* it' (p. 298). Rhodes and Gipps argue that in subjects with delusions there is a shift in framework beliefs. In their diagnosis, we are taken aback by subjects with delusions if their beliefs conflict with our bedrock certainties. The puzzlement is due to the fact that we don't even know whether we can argue them out of their delusion, given that we have radically different starting points and we might not agree on what is a good reason for what.

The phenomenon that the notion of the bedrock wants to capture is real and relevant to the way in which delusions might appear not just false, but occasionally defy prediction and explanation in intentional terms. That said, the description of the bedrock put forward by Rhodes and Gipps raises some questions. First, is the grasp of the content of framework beliefs necessarily 'pre-reflective'? It is true, and a point that Wittgenstein made a few times when he introduced the notion of framework beliefs, that we don't usually express judgements about whether the Earth existed before our births or whether we have hands, and we don't often mention reasons for endorsing those belief contents. Yet, we *can* endorse the beliefs verbally, and provide reasons for them, in situations in which our hold on such beliefs is ever so slightly shaken by unusual circumstances, or when we engage in a reflective exercise about what we are committed to. For instance, in a philosophy class on scepticism, we do exactly that, we reflect upon those basic beliefs about reality that we usually take for granted. For the time of the discussion, we seriously consider the possibility that our experiences are the result of electrically stimulated brains in vats, and not the result of causal interactions between our bodies and the external world. While we take seriously these sceptical scenarios, it is not obvious that framework beliefs are true: do we really have hands?

Second, is it right to claim that framework beliefs cannot receive justification? It is true that they do not usually require justification, but this does not mean that they cannot be justified or endorsed with reasons. The thought that basic beliefs are not amenable to justification derives from a narrow conception of acceptable forms of justification, according to which beliefs can be justified only if they are grounded in other beliefs that are necessarily more basic. The way in which we show our commitment to framework beliefs is by acting in ways that are compatible with believing their content, and by endorsing other beliefs that are consistent with them and supported by them.

Framework beliefs are embedded in a coherent set of beliefs and in a practice that gives us better reason to endorse those beliefs than to doubt them or reject them. This is not a type of justification that would satisfy the sceptic, I grant that, but the mere possibility of a form of justification should be sufficient to reject the claim that the bedrock is just an otherwise ineffable 'form of life'. I think it should be seen instead as something that is constituted by beliefs that can turn out to be either true or false.

Wittgenstein did stress that there are some beliefs that are more basic and less open to revision than others. But he fully recognised that there is no sharp distinction between the hard rock at the bottom of the river and the sand: both are subject to change. We would be mistaken if we took his description of the bedrock to mean that some beliefs *cannot* receive justification or can *never* be revised. Wittgenstein observed that some religious beliefs contradict framework propositions: Catholics, to use his example, believe that Jesus had only one human parent, whereas he firmly believed that every human being has two human parents (§239). Depending on how we intend the phrase 'having two human parents', the framework belief can now be regarded as much less certain in the light of the possibilities created by some reproductive technologies, such as IVF or reproductive cloning.

Here is another example. In the 1950s Wittgenstein himself used as an example of a bedrock certainty two beliefs that we have come to consider as false: that nobody could ever fly to the moon, and that the very possibility of flying to the moon would defy physics.

> If we are thinking within our system, then it is certain that no one has ever been on the moon. Not merely is nothing of the sort ever seriously reported to us by reasonable people, but our whole system of physics forbids us to believe it. For this demands answers to the questions 'How did he overcome the force of gravity?' 'How could he live without an atmosphere?' and a thousand others which could not be answered.
>
> (Wittgenstein 1969, §108)

Now we do have answers to Wittgenstein's questions: we know how to overcome gravity and how a human being can live (temporarily) without an atmosphere. Religious beliefs and scientific progress can shake our bedrock. Neil Armstrong was walking on the moon in the same year in which 'On Certainty' was published (posthumously).

With these clarifications in mind, let's go back to Katie and her delusion. Does she reject a framework belief when she expresses and endorses her delusional belief? She believes many of the things that people around her also believe: that strangers would have no reason to tell her off or be hostile to her unless they had some (negative) information about her; that personal information about herself that she did not pass on to other people must have reached them in other ways; that hostility should be avoided; that it is better not to be around people who tell us off; etc. There is nothing in Katie's delusional set of beliefs that defies our bedrock certainties, apart from (maybe) the belief that there exists such a device that can transmit personal information about us without our consent. But surely that's not such an incredible belief to have. Some people think that surfing the internet or using a store loyalty card is unsafe, because such practices allow third parties to access one's personal information and are a violation of privacy. Sophisticated versions of the device Katie talks about can be easily imagined and may become real in a not-too-distant future. As Wittgenstein taught us, the science fiction of one generation is the reality of the next.[17]

Once we have made the notion of bedrock more plausible, and conceded that different beliefs can be subject to revision and justification to a different extent, the bedrock could be used to explain the strange content of some delusions, where the beliefs reported are internally incoherent, clash dramatically with shared conceptions of what is possible and what isn't, or are not endorsed on the basis of any reasons, not even bad ones. But in most cases, framework beliefs are shared by subjects with and without delusions, and the shift in the bedrock required to make sense of the behaviour of subjects with delusions is minimal (e.g. Katie's belief in the 'device'). There is no compelling reason to believe in a radical discontinuity between delusional and non-delusional thought. The idea that subjects with delusions and subjects without inhabit different worlds seems to contrast with the occurrence of circumscribed delusions and with the capacity naïve interpreters have to make sense of the behaviour of subjects with delusions by ascribing intentional states to them. The bedrock can be shaken and shifted in ways that are more or less rational, and more or less destabilising for the other beliefs we hold dear.

## 4.5 Beliefs and failure of reason-giving

The question whether beliefs are supported by *good* reasons is a tricky one to answer, as there are different types of beliefs, some of which are not generally

[17] Other types of delusions seem to fit better the view that there is loss of common background and meanings are no longer shared. As we already discussed, people who are affected by Cotard delusion, and believe that they are dead, behave in such a way that make us doubt whether they really understand the concept of 'death' and seem to have conflicting beliefs or attitudes about their own situation and experience. In these cases postulating a meaning renegotiation or a little shift in the bedrock might be necessary in order to understand the subjects' reports.

supported with reasons. In this section my purpose is to consider some examples of failure of reason-giving in normal cognition, in order to challenge the application of the agential rationality constraint on belief ascription to the case of delusions. According to the evidence we shall look at, some reported attitudes (beliefs, preferences, evaluations) are neither formed by subjects on the basis of intersubjectively good reasons, nor supported on the basis of intersubjectively good (*post-hoc*) reasons. That is, there are observable failures of reason-giving independent of whether we take agential rationality to apply both to deliberation and justification, or exclusively to justification.

It is interesting that on the basis of the studies of the effects of reason-giving on reported attitudes psychologists have argued not only that people ordinarily lack agential rationality and authorship (as they provide reasons that are not intersubjectively good reasons, and are not even their best reasons) but also self knowledge (as measured in terms of consistency between reported attitudes and other attitudes, or consistency between reported attitudes and subsequent behaviour). Here we focus on whether people to whom we ascribe beliefs meet the standards of agential rationality, but in the next chapter I shall extend the analysis to whether people can obtain knowledge of their own attitudes by giving reasons for endorsing them. I shall maintain then that the practice of reason-giving has epistemic benefits, although being the author of one's attitudes does not guarantee the rationality and stability of the reported attitudes or the knowledge of the psychological mechanisms causally responsible for the formation of those attitudes.

### 4.5.1 Bad reasons for attitudes

Some interesting data on reason-giving come from experimental evidence obtained in the course of a series of studies on the effects of introspective deliberation and justification. Results indicate that research participants are very likely to shift their commitments when they are asked to give reasons for their previously held attitudes (Wilson and Hodges 1994); they are more vulnerable to the effects of evidence manipulation when they are asked to give reasons for their attitudes (Wilson *et al.* 1993); the quality of the decisions and predictions made on the basis of reflective introspection or reason-giving is inferior to the quality of decisions and predictions made otherwise (Wilson and Schooler 1991; Halberstadt and Levine 1999); and when making a decision, looking for reasons slows down research participants' information processing and reduces their capacity to discriminate among important factors (Tordesillas 1999). What has been observed in these studies is that research participants' initial attitudes often differ from their final attitudes after they have engaged in an analysis of reasons, and this generates issues about self knowledge that I will address in the next chapter: when the attitude endorsed after analysing reasons is different from the attitude reported at the start, which of the two attitudes represents the participant's genuine standpoint?

Here are some examples: people provide bad, confabulatory reasons for their choices (Nisbett and Wilson 1977; Wilson 2002, Chapters. 5–6) and attempt to justify their moral judgements on the basis of general principles that cannot be applied to the scenarios whose moral properties are being evaluated (Haidt 2001). Carruthers summarises the implications of the study by Nisbett and Wilson (1977):

> Subjects in a shopping mall were presented with an array of four sets of items (e.g. pairs of socks, or pantyhose), and they were asked to choose one of them as a free sample. (All four sets of items were actually identical). Subjects displayed a marked tendency to select the item on the right-hand end of the display. Yet no one mentioned this when they were asked to explain why they had chosen as they did. Rather, subjects produced plainly confabulated explanations, such as that the item they had chosen was softer, it had appeared to be better made, or that it had a more attractive colour.

> (Carruthers 2005, p. 142–3)

Nisbett and Wilson (1977) argue that verbal introspective reports are often driven by judgements of plausibility, rather than by direct knowledge of the mechanisms by which one selects the preferred items. It is more plausible for me to think that I chose a nightgown due to its qualities, for instance, its softness and colour, rather than due to its position on a rack. But in the context of the experiment, people who ignore the effects of the relative positions of the examined items, provide reasons for their choices that are not good reasons. Notice that this is an excellent example, because the charge of agential irrationality can be made on the basis of two distinct versions of agential rationality. People endorse their preferences on the basis of reasons that have nothing to do with the psychological mechanism that is responsible for those preferences; moreover, they provide reasons for their attitudes that are not intersubjectively good reasons. We are told that the samples people had to choose from were actually identical, so it is not plausible that a nightgown or a pair of socks was chosen because of their superior quality, texture or colour.

Another example comes from experiments on the origins of moral reasoning, but is in fact very similar to the experiment on the causes of one's choice of socks and nightgowns. People report an attitude (a moral judgement) towards something (a situation, in this case), but their explanation as to why they have that attitude does not fit with what is likely to have caused the attitude (given the manipulation of the experimenter) and is not a good explanation. To illustrate, consider a study by Haidt (2001, p. 814) where people were asked about the following scenario:

> Julie and Mark are brother and sister. They are travelling together in France on summer vacation from college. One night they are staying alone in a cabin near the beach. They decide that it would be interesting and fun if they tried making love. At the very least it would be a new experience for each of them. Julie was already taking birth control pills, but Mark uses a condom too, just to be safe. They both enjoy making love, but they decide not to do it again. They keep that night as a special secret, which makes them feel even closer to each other. What do you think about that, was it OK for them to make love?

The reaction of the great majority of subjects is to answer that it was not OK for Julie and Mark to make love. Interestingly, when asked to justify their answer, subjects attempt to connect some aspects of the story to a violation of a moral principle, but the story has been constructed in such a way that their attempts are often unsuccessful. For instance, the argument that making love was wrong for the two siblings because it would have caused bad psychological consequences and ruined their relationship is not supported by the details of the scenario.

> Most people who hear the above story immediately say that it was wrong for the siblings to make love, and they then set about searching for reasons. They point out the dangers of inbreeding, only to remember that Julie and Mark used two forms of birth control. They argue that Julie and Mark will be hurt, perhaps emotionally, even though the story makes it clear that no harm befell them.
>
> (Haidt 2001, p. 814)

Haidt argues that what determines people's moral attitudes is a basic emotional reaction to which they have no introspective access. Then, a more articulate but confabulatory explanation is offered, which does not seem to reflect either the real reasons for the judgement, or the specific features of the case to evaluate.

> In the social intuitionist model one feels a quick flash of revulsion at the thought of incest and one knows intuitively that something is wrong. Then, when faced with a social demand for a verbal justification, one becomes a lawyer trying to build a case, rather than a judge searching for the truth.
>
> (Haidt 2001, p. 814)

Haidt (2001) and Haidt and Bjorklund (2008) conclude from these experiments that people's judgements are actually driven by inaccessible moral intuitions[18] which give rise to moral beliefs that are difficult to revise. People explain their judgements on the basis of general moral principles they take themselves to have, even if these are not supported by the situations they were asked to evaluate, and do not recognise the all-important role of their basic emotions and intuitions. As in the previous case, the choice of socks and nightgowns, we have two potential failures of agential rationality. People do not recognise what determines their judgements, but quite independently of that, when they come up with reasons in support of their attitudes, their reasons do not concern the relevant features of the environment they were asked to express a judgement about.

### 4.5.2 Dating couples

Consider this intriguing case. People dating for a few months are asked to give reasons why they are attracted to their partner, and then rate the commitment to the relationship and the likelihood that they will live together or get married in the future (Seligman *et al.* 1980). Participants' responses are elicited via questioning. Guided by the formulation of the questions, some couples are invited to offer *intrinsic* reasons for their being together ('I date X because. . .'), whereas others are invited to offer *extrinsic*, more instrumental reasons ('I date X in order to. . .'). Research participants invited to give extrinsic reasons end up rating more negatively their attitudes towards their partners and tend not to predict living together or getting married in the future. They do not seem to realise that their reports are biased by the way in which the questioning was conducted: the fact that they give reasons for their attitudes does not guarantee that they report an attitude that accurately represents how they feel and what they think about the relationship.

Wilson and Kraft (1993) designed a similar study on attitudes towards one's partner (but without evidence manipulation). Participants were first asked to report their attitude towards their relationship, then they were divided in two groups, and finally asked for their evaluations again, and for a prediction about the future of the relationship. In one group, the intermediate task was to list reasons for the success or failure of the relationship. In the other group,

---

[18] It is of course possible to present good reasons for resisting the claim that Julie and Mark did something wrong (e.g. by appealing to the notion of some actions contributing to a person's moral corruption, or affecting negatively a person's self-image etc.), but Haidt's point is simply that the reasons offered by the participants were not the reasons latching onto the causes of their moral disapproval and they were not compatible with certain features of the vignette.

they were given a different task. Results show that the participants who were asked for reasons for the state of their relationship experienced an attitude shift between the former and latter reports.[19] In a study where a follow-up interview was included, Wilson *et al.* (1984) found that participants who evaluated their relationship and made a prediction without being asked for reasons made a more successful prediction than the participants who were asked for reasons.

In the original dating couples study, research participants form their attitudes and make their predictions on the basis of evidence for and against the likelihood of success of their relationship, but the evidence most accessible to them is constituted by their answers to the experimenter's questions. These answers were framed so as to promote a certain perspective on the relationship, either as something worthy in itself, or as something which is instrumental in order to achieve other goods. This manipulation in the experimental design leads research participants to a one-sided evaluation of their relationship and to a prediction that does not take into account all the factors which affect the success of the relationship. The reasoning process by which they arrive at their attitude is far from epistemically rational: they can be charged with the violation of the principle of *total evidence*, which both Carnap and Davidson considered as a fundamental principle of rationality. According to this principle, all the relevant available information should be taken into account when forming an attitude. This breakdown of rationality is largely responsible for the prediction that the participants' reported attitudes will not be consistent with their future behaviour. The hypothesis here is that the participants' future behaviour will be affected by all the important factors relevant to the success of their relationships, and not just by those factors which research participants have been asked to consider during their interview with the experimenter.

The participants in these studies are guilty of agential irrationality. As agential rationality concerns endorsement via reason-giving, and endorsement can be manifested in deliberation and *post-hoc* justification, it is not a surprise that agential rationality is compromised. Deliberation and justification are reasoning processes, and they are affected by biases as any other reasoning process is (Nisbett and Wilson 1977; Kahneman *et al.* 1982; Stanovich 1999).

Given the results of the further studies by Wilson and colleagues (1984), it is safe to project widespread failure in the predictions made on the basis of the

---

[19] See Tiberius (2008) for a detailed analysis of these studies and of their implications for the relationship between reflection and well-being.

attitudes reported by the participants who engaged in reason-giving and whose evidence was manipulated. It is likely, then, that participants will have experienced an attitude-behaviour inconsistency, by acting in a way that is not compatible with their reported attitude. I shall address more explicitly the connection between authorship, intentionality and self knowledge in the next chapter. For our purposes here, it is sufficient to notice that ordinary beliefs and other attitudes with doxastic components (such as preferences and value judgements), just like delusions, can fail to be endorsed on the basis of inter-subjectively good reasons.

In most of the discussion so far, we have been considering possible demarcation criteria for delusions, a reason to claim that they should be in a different category from ordinary beliefs. We started with the thought that delusions are not beliefs because they fail to satisfy norms of procedural, epistemic and even agential rationality. But then we noticed that beliefs exhibit qualitatively similar failures. An alternative thought is that delusions are irrational in a more disturbing and puzzling way: what Campbell (2001) and Rhodes and Gipps (2008) were trying to do is to diagnose the feeling of unease that people encounter when they are faced with delusional reports. But possible explanations of such puzzlement—that delusions are like framework beliefs, or that they conflict with framework beliefs—have also failed to provide us with a satisfactory demarcation criterion. The studies on bad reasons for attitudes further undermine the project of characterising delusions as different from beliefs because of their puzzling nature. For the dating couples studies seem to deliver *very* puzzling results: people do not seem to know why they have the attitudes they have, and behave in ways that are not consistent with the things they say. More importantly, it is sufficient to change the format of a question to induce them to report diametrically opposed attitudes towards their dating partners.

## Summary of chapter 4

In this chapter I wanted to assess another set of objections to the doxastic nature of delusions, inspired by the agential rationality constraint on the ascription of beliefs. Delusions are often deemed as categorically different from beliefs because they do not guide action as we would expect beliefs to do; they are not formed on the basis of intersubjectively good reasons (endorsement by deliberation); and they are not supported by intersubjectively good reasons (endorsement by justification). I have attempted to show that the features we attribute to beliefs in terms of guiding action, being deliberated about, and being the object of justification, are often idealised, or apply only to some types of beliefs. In this chapter as in the previous two, the conclusion is that delusions do not satisfy the demanding conditions for agential rationality, but most beliefs do not satisfy them either. Thus, the *failure of action guiding* objection and the *failure of reason-giving* objection we have discussed fail to challenge the doxastic conception of delusions.

In Section 4.1, I have briefly distinguished behavioural manifestability from action guidance. Although there are many ways in which the endorsement of a belief content can be manifested in behaviour, guiding action requires that the subject engages in actions that are consistent with and explicable by the subject's acceptance of the content of the belief as true. In this sense of action guidance, delusions often fail to guide actions in the appropriate circumstances, and this is one of the reasons why philosophers have argued that they cannot be beliefs. In particular, I reviewed the notion of 'double-bookkeeping' introduced by Sass and developed by Gallagher, according to which subjects with delusions are aware that their delusions are not representations of reality; and I have assessed Frankish's recent suggestion that delusions should be regarded as acceptances.

In Section 4.2, I asked whether beliefs always guide action and the answer (unsurprisingly) has been that they do not. There are beliefs that are verbally endorsed but not acted upon in everyday life (hypocrisy) and cases in which inconsistencies are noted between attitudes and behaviour, to the point that the very notion of an attitude being manifested in stable behavioural dispositions has been criticised by experimental psychologists since the 1950s.

In Section 4.3, I started developing the failure of reason-giving objection. This argument needed to be explained and motivated as the notion of agential rationality with respect to reason-giving is not as common and as explicitly discussed in the literature on belief ascription as that of procedural or epistemic rationality. To argue for the relevance of reason-giving to the debate on the nature of delusions, I described what it means to author a belief, that is, being able to provide what one takes to be one's best reasons for the content of that belief, in deliberation and justification. Then I characterised agential rationality as the capacity to provide intersubjectively good reasons for a belief content, and I considered arguments according to which delusions are not beliefs because they are either formed on the basis of reasons that are not good reasons, or supported by reasons that are not good reasons. I presented a number of examples of delusions, and showed that some are authored and some are not, but most of them can be charged with agential irrationality.

In Section 4.4, I assessed two arguments that do not explicitly reject the doxastic conception of delusions but could be interpreted as defending a categorical distinction between beliefs and delusions. What these arguments have in common is that exploit the notion of framework belief. Framework beliefs are those basic beliefs that we regard as certain and that they play a foundational role with respect to other, less certain, beliefs. The first argument I considered was a defence of delusions from the charge of agential irrationality: delusions are not defended with reasons because they regarded as certain and immune from doubt—there is no need to provide a justification for them. The second argument suggests that delusions conflict with framework beliefs—this would explain why we found them more puzzling than non-rational beliefs. People who report delusions do not regard as certain what other members of their community do, and thus are less involved in shared practices and forms of life. (If either of these arguments were convincing, then the unwelcome consequence would be that subjects with delusions and subjects with beliefs subscribe to different certainties, and communication and debate between them would be really difficult if not impossible). Contrary to these arguments, I suggested that a careful examination of the notion of a framework belief shows that delusions neither play the role of framework beliefs nor necessarily conflict with framework beliefs.

In Section 4.5, I considered examples of beliefs and other attitudes that are neither formed nor justified on the basis of intersubjectively good reasons. These examples included instances of normal confabulation, where people justify their choices with reasons that do not reflect the psychological mechanisms responsible for the formation of their choices, and instances of attitudes supported by reasons that are not stable or plausible from a third person point of view. In presenting examples from normal cognition I deliberately chose paradigmatic cases of belief (beliefs about whether a certain scenario is immoral and beliefs about the success of a relationship) which are candidates for reason-giving. These examples lead us to abandon an overly idealised conception of the processes of deliberation and justification—and recommend a straight-forward rejection of the agential rationality constraint on the ascription of beliefs.

# Chapter 5

# Beliefs and self knowledge

I: Are thoughts put in your head which you know are not your own sometimes?

L: Yes.

I: How do you know they are not your own?

L: They tell me to put on clothes. They check my bath water for me, with this hand.

I: Who checks your bath water?

L: Whatever her name happens to be, whatever I choose her name to be, she does it for me.
(McKay *et al.*, *Severe Schizophrenia*)

Precisely because Actors must often consider the necessity of convincing others of the reasonableness of the causal argument selected, they need to create accounts, narratives, or mini-theories that enrich the central reason(s) guiding and justifying their position.
(Zimbardo, *The Discontinuity Theory*)

The previously discussed argumentative strategies against the belief status of delusions have not succeeded. In the analysis of three possible constraints on belief ascription we found that norms of rationality governing relationships among beliefs, between beliefs and evidence, between beliefs and action guidance, and betweens belief and reason-giving are routinely violated. Thus, many of the most influential arguments aiming at denying belief status to delusions on the basis of their failing to satisfy norms of rationality for beliefs have been found wanting. In this chapter I want to leave behind the issue whether and to what extent delusions and beliefs are irrational, and start exploring another line of argument in order to explain why some delusions strike us as puzzling, to the extent that they may resist interpretation.

Let's grant (on the basis of the conclusions reached so far) that delusions can play the same role as beliefs in interacting with other intentional states, responding to evidence, guiding action, and being formed or supported by reasons. Although delusions rarely conform to norms of rationality, ascribing them as beliefs helps us make sense of the behaviour of others, predict their future behaviour, and empathise with their outlook on themselves and the shared environment—John Campbell (2009) would say that delusions, just like beliefs, are 'control variables' in that they can be 'systematically mapped onto specific psychological outcomes' (p. 147). We can explain in intentional terms why a subject with Cotard stops engaging with people and things around her, and we can also explain why subjects with persecutory delusions are suspicious of strangers. Some of our predictions of the behaviour of subjects with delusions will succeed, other predictions will fail, but making the predictions is, on the whole, both useful and necessary. Nonetheless, there are other delusions that remain deeply perplexing—delusions that even when ascribed as beliefs to subjects do not help us understand the subjects' point of view or explain and predict their behaviour in intentional terms.

Here is a proposal. As it is misleading to claim that all types of beliefs have to satisfy certain criteria (such as being supported by empirical evidence or being action guiding), so it is misleading to engage in the debate on the nature of delusions by generalising over different types of reports that can be regarded as delusional. It is perfectly possible that some delusions are belief states and other delusions aren't. One suggestion is that those delusions that defy interpretation don't do so because of their irrationality, but because they fail to exhibit some of the core features of beliefs, and signal a failure of self knowledge in the subjects reporting them. In order to flesh out this proposal we need to concentrate on two capacities that subjects can exercise with respect to some of their beliefs: ownership and authorship of thoughts.

We saw in the previous chapter that reason-giving allows one to become the *author* of one's thoughts. By being able to justify a belief with reasons that the subject regards as her best reasons, the subject acquires control over the content of what she believes and obtains a form of first-person authority over the reported thought. When the subject has the capacity to ascribe a belief to herself, by introspection, inference or an act of authorship, then she becomes the *owner* of her belief. Ownership and authorship allow subjects to develop a sense of entitlement to their thoughts (see Moran 2001). But when ownership and authorship fail, and the subject shows no commitment to the content of her report in behaviour, then the report resists intentional characterisation. 'Inserted' thoughts are an example of a case in which the subject reports thoughts that she does not endorse: these are thoughts to which the subject has first-personal access but that are rejected by the subject as alien to herself. These thoughts are not ascribed as beliefs. By failing to recognise whether a thought is their own and failing to endorse the content of the thoughts they report, subjects with delusions can elude interpretation and may also become *unreliable biographers* of their own life (Gerrans 2009), and inaccurate and incomplete narratives are likely to affect autonomous thought and decision-making (Kennett and Matthews 2009).

In Section 5.1, I establish some important connections between authorship and a certain type of first-person authority. I argue that the results of the psychological studies on introspective reflection and attitude-behaviour inconsistency that we mentioned in chapter 4 as example of failures of agential rationality do not necessarily constitute a failure of authorship. Even if research participants do not offer good reasons for their attitudes, they offer *some* reasons and (as far as we know) they take those reasons to be their best reasons. They can be said to own and author their attitudes, independent of whether those are the attitudes that they would report if they were fully rational agents. In the process of assessing authorship of thoughts in these cases, I discuss the conditions for first-person authority.

In Section 5.2, I present a case that is significantly different from the case of research participants giving bad reasons for their reported attitudes, and from most of the cases of delusions we discussed in the previous chapters. Thought insertion is a condition in which, with respect to the 'inserted' thought, ownership and authorship fail and this makes interpretation impossible. My purpose is to argue that thought insertion is puzzling in that it presents a radical failure of self knowledge and the 'inserted' thought is (rightly) denied belief status not because it is irrational, but because it is not manifest in the subject's behaviour.

In Section 5.3, I consider some of the implications of failed ownership and authorship with the integration of beliefs into the subject's self narrative. Depending on their importance and centrality in the subject's cognitive life, the beliefs the subject feels entitled to become part of her self concept. However, marginalised beliefs and disowned thoughts do not have the chance to contribute to the subject's self narrative. This leads us to consider another characterisation of delusions, as unreliable biographies, and explore some of the implications of failures of ownership and authorship of thoughts for the construction and preservation of a sense of self, and for autonomous thought and decision-making.

## 5.1 **Authorship and first-person authority**

We introduced the notion of authorship in Chapter 4, as the capacity a subject has to give reasons that she regards as her best reasons for those of her attitudes

whose content can be endorsed via reason-giving, such as opinions and intentions. This capacity is typically exercised in deliberation and justification,
when the subject takes a stance about a particular issue, or is asked to defend
her point of view against a potential objection. Here we are going to explore
the close relationship between authorship and knowledge of the self, and argue
that failures of agential rationality do not necessarily undermine self knowledge, but failures of authorship do.

### 5.1.1 Routes to knowledge of the self

What is the relationship between authorship and self knowledge? There are
many methods by which I can obtain knowledge about myself. For instance,
I could acquire information about myself by perception ('My legs are crossed');
by inference ('I constantly avoid meeting Jenny, this must be because I dislike
her company'); by self-shaping ('What do I think about the death penalty?
After considering statistics about crime in countries where there is death
penalty, I resolve to be opposed to it'); by attending to conscious experience
('I was very sad when I read about the accident').[1] Distinctions among these
methods of acquiring self knowledge are very important, but for the present
discussion, I offer a simplified account of the way in which we can come to
self-attributions which fits with the traditional philosophical debates about self
knowledge and first-person authority. A subject can ascribe mental content to
herself as a result of *direct epistemic access* to the content of her mental states or
as a result of *inferences based on evidence* about her own behaviour. When she
has direct epistemic access to her mental states, she does not need to rely on
behavioural evidence to work out what the content of those states is and therefore she has a *prima facie* advantage over external observers (e.g. Burge 1988;
Heil 1988; Peacocke 1998). Even when the subject lacks direct epistemic access,
she can often rely on more and better evidence about her own behaviour than
a third person, and generally she can make more successful inferences from
her behaviour to the content of her mental states (e.g. Ryle 1949). The route to
first-person authority that is based on the subject's capacity to obtain better
access to her mental states than a third person is an *epistemic* route.

A subject can gain control over her attitudes by *deliberation*, when she forms
an attitude on the basis of reasons that are regarded by the subject as her best
reasons for endorsing its content; or *justification*, when she defends the content

---

[1]  For these distinctions, I am indebted to Eric Schwitzgebel's paper, 'Introspection, what?',
presented at the Introspection and Consciousness Workshop at the Australian National
University in Canberra, on October 31st, 2008.

of her attitude on the basis of reasons that she takes to be her best reasons. In these circumstances, the subject can ascribe an attitude to herself on the basis of an act of *authorship*. She is the author of a belief if she forms it or justifies it on the basis of what she takes to be her best reasons. Moran (2001) argues that authorship provides a route to first-person authority that is distinct from the epistemic one. In order to appreciate the distinction we can reflect upon the common practice of ascribing beliefs on the basis of observed behaviour. There are circumstances in which it makes sense to say that, as interpreters of the behaviour of others, we might come to know what their beliefs are better than they do themselves. Even if one has direct epistemic access to one's beliefs or richer evidence about one's own behaviour, one is vulnerable to self deception or self attribution biases, or may have beliefs that cannot be attended to. But not even a very competent interpreter can ever *author* someone else's belief, because authorship requires the capacity to endorse the belief on the basis of what one takes to be one's best reasons. This type of first-person authority does not derive from a privileged form of epistemic access, but rather from a series of actions that one can perform with respect to the content of that belief. The subject can deliberate, justify, endorse, manifest a commitment.[2] This is the *agential* route to first-person authority which is manifested via authorship.

> If it is possible for a person to answer a deliberative question about his belief at all, this involves assuming an authority over, and a responsibility for, what his belief actually is. Thus a person able to exercise this capacity is in a position to declare what his belief is by reflection on the reasons in favor of that belief, rather than by examination of the psychological evidence. In this way [...] avowal can be seen as an expression of genuine self knowledge.

> (Moran 2004, p. 425)

Andrew's story about why he applied to study law at university is different from the way in which his friends explain his decision. He justifies his decision by claiming that studying law is a good move for his future career, whereas his friends suspect that he chose to study law at his father's insistence. First-person and third-person accounts of behaviour diverge for at least two important reasons. Andrew knows things about what he thinks and how he feels that others can only derive by observing his behaviour and making inferences

---

[2] For a similar account of self knowledge, where one comes to know what one believes by considering the reasons for what one believes, by looking outward rather than inward, see Fernández (2003). In Fernández (forthcoming) you find an application of this account of self knowledge to the case of thought insertion which you might want to compare with my own (Bortolotti and Broome 2009).

from it. He has some prima facie epistemic advantage over his friends, given by direct access to the content of some of his mental states. Moreover, Andrew is vulnerable to different attribution and reasoning biases from the ones that affect third-person observers. For instance, he will be exposed to self attribution biases when he reflects upon his own dispositions, personality traits, past history, likelihood of success, and so on. Hence, access to the content of his mental states is not entirely transparent, but rather, his knowledge of his own reasons is refracted through such biases. It is not easy to determine which story is the correct one if conflict between first- and third-person accounts emerges, because dispositions, traits, and even biases are subject to change. Authorship captures what is special about Andrew's own explanation for his decision. Andrew takes an *agential* perspective on his decision by endorsing it as the right decision, whereas his friends can only be observers of his behaviour and interpreters of the reasons for his decision. Whatever story he tells about it, Andrew is 'authoritative' about his decision, because he can do something that his friends cannot do; endorse the decision on the basis of his sense of his best reasons for it. In other words, by being able to offer a justification for it, Andrew is in a position to take *responsibility* for his decision.

### 5.1.2 The deliberative stance

Following what Moran says about the conditions for authorship of a belief, I author my belief that *p* if I am in a position to endorse that belief on the basis of reasons that I take to be my best reasons for *p*. Authorship does not require that the belief itself be true or rationally formed. It does not even require me to have better reasons in favour of, rather than against, the content of the belief. After all, I can be misled about what my best reasons are. But I must see myself as endorsing the belief for my best reasons in order to be its author. If this condition is not met, according to Moran (2001), the process leading to the endorsement of the belief cannot be seen as a process of genuine deliberation or justification. When I engage in deliberation or justification I do not report my belief or explain my behaviour from a neutral stance; to some extent, I determine what the content of that belief is going to be and I exercise control over the belief I report. My stance towards the belief I author is different from your stance towards it, when you, as an interpreter, ascribe to me that belief on the basis of the observation of my behaviour. In the interpretive stance, beliefs are ascribed to oneself or others in order to explain or predict behaviour. In the *deliberative stance*, beliefs are either formed or justified on the basis of how things are according to the subject's best judgement and are expected to determine the subject's future behaviour. This distinction is useful in order to map some of the asymmetries between first- and third-person knowledge.

The explanation of behaviour provided in interpretation is not compromised if the beliefs ascribed are false or unreasonable by the standards of the interpreter. You can ascribe to me the intention to keep drinking in the pub until closing time, in order to explain instances of my behaviour, but that does not mean that from your point of view my intention is a reasonable one. Suppose that I don't want to leave the pub early because I don't want to disappoint my friends who only respect heavy drinkers. Suppose that I am actually bored to death by their unintelligible conversation, that I am tired, and that I have an important job interview in the morning. You can no doubt explain my behaviour (that I want to stay till closing time because I don't want to disappoint my friends) without being at all persuaded that my reasons are overall good reasons. From the point of view of the deliberator, having reasons for an attitude is not sufficient to author that attitude. I need to believe that continuing to drink in the pub until closing time is the best thing to do, and I need to be able to support my intention to stay in the pub and keep drinking with reasons that I take to be my best reasons. It is possible that I am the kind of person who considers obtaining the approval of her friends more important than being in top form at a job interview. But now suppose I do believe that the best option for me would be to go home and get some sleep, and I decide to stay in the pub nonetheless. Maybe I am weak-willed. I really should go home, I know that, but I cannot make myself leave. If asked to justify my decision the next day, when I get up with a serious hangover and puffy eyes, I can put together some reasons why staying in the pub was a good idea. If challenged, I can say that it was the best pub in town, that I have rare opportunities to spend quality time with my friends, and that I needed to relax before such a big day.

In the context of justification leading up to authorship, how good I take my reasons to be does matter to whether I succeed in authoring my attitudes. But in the context of a *post-hoc*, half-hearted rationalisation of my attitudes[3], it seems that standards have dropped. I myself know (or part of me does, depending on the preferred analysis of the situation) that the reasons I come up with are not my best reasons. In this latter version of the example, I no longer qualify as a deliberator or a justifier. The rules of the game of deliberation and justification don't permit it.

---

[3] Tiberius (2008, p. 125) refers to the phenomenon of making something false fit facts about oneself as 'self-fabrication'.

### 5.1.3 **Authorship challenged**

Nothing in the way in which the context of deliberation and justification are described suggests that reason-giving needs to occur in ideal conditions in order to play a role in the acquisition of knowledge of one's own states. However, the claim that reason-giving provides an additional route to first-person authority is controversial. The relation between the capacity for reason-giving and first-person authority has been attacked on the basis of the same psychological evidence that we reviewed in chapter 4 as examples of agential irrationality. The evidence about the limitations of introspection in deliberation and justification has been interpreted as an illustration of how the reflective process of analysing reasons for attitudes undermines rather than promotes self knowledge:

> It is common for people to analyze why they feel the way they do [...]. It is usually assumed that such reflection is beneficial, leading to greater insight about how one feels. We will argue the reverse; that is, that this type of self-analysis can mislead people about their attitudes, thereby lowering attitude-behavior correlations.

> (Wilson *et al.* 1984, p. 5)

Psychologists have found that analysing reasons for attitudes causes subjects to 'change their minds', that is, the attitudes reported after the reason-giving exercise are not consistent with the attitudes previously reported by the subjects; the attitudes reported as a consequence of engaging in reflective exercises are not found to be representative of the subjects' future behaviour; when providing reasons for their reported attitudes, subjects are blind to the 'real reasons' for those attitudes which indicates that the exercise of giving reasons does not provide any genuine insight into the workings of their own mind; the attitudes reported after analysing reasons tend to be 'less optimal' than those reported without analysing reasons (e.g. subjects make worse choices with respect to expert judgement, are more prone to evidence manipulation in evaluations, or are more vulnerable to inconsistencies).

Findings revealing an inconsistency or instability of attitudes, or an inconsistency between attitudes and behaviour are taken to be evidence for a failure of first-person authority. Recall the examples of attitude-behaviour inconsistency reviewed in Chapter 4. In the dating couples study (Seligman 1980), where research participants are asked to think about reasons for dating, their reasons are manipulated by the format of the questions. Those who are asked for their instrumental reasons for dating are going to assess their relationship as less promising than those who are asked for their intrinsic reasons for dating. As participants report attitudes that are not likely to be manifested in their future behaviour, the evidence speaks against the quality and reliability of first-person ascriptions made when analysing reasons. In the experiment by Seligman and colleagues, participants endorse a belief that they are prepared to justify with reasons, e.g. that their relationship is not satisfactory and will not last. But we suspect that their other attitudes and future behaviour will be at odds with their reported attitude (and with the prediction they make on the basis of it).

The evidence that shows a failure in identifying the 'real reasons' for reported attitudes and the evidence disputing the quality of reported attitudes after reason-giving are a challenge to the view that reason-giving has the epistemic advantage of providing an insight into the workings of one's own mind. The idea that people often lack awareness of the 'real reasons' for their attitudes is at the core of the view that judgements about the morality of certain behaviours are due to basic affective responses conditioned by societal pressure and not to the application of general moral principles (Haidt 2001). As we saw, the view is that we have an immediate reaction to a scenario (e.g. disgust) and as a consequence we come to believe that the actions in the scenario are immoral (e.g. incest). But when asked to explain why we made that judgement, we provide reasons that have nothing to do with the emotional responses that caused our judgement. When we engage in reasoning, we search for arguments that will support our already made judgements in an attempt to disguise moral dumbfounding.[4] If these results could be generalised, they would mean that people are not aware of what really causes their moral judgements to be the way they are and 'make up stories' when required.

The observation that the attitudes that are reported after engaging in reason-giving are less than rational or optimal is relevant in the context of attitude shifts. There are studies on preferences for jams which have been used to illustrate the effect of reason-giving on attitude change. For instance, see Wilson and Schooler's 'Jam Taste Test' (1991). In the study, people express preferences that are aligned with those of experts when they do not think about reasons for their attitudes. But if they are made to think about reasons why a jam is superior to another, they tend to change their mind and provide a rating which does not match those of experts. The comparison with expert judgement rules out the possibility that subjects endorse different attitudes after thinking about reasons, because the search for reasons has made them realise what attitude is better supported by the evidence available to them. If the attitude reported after engaging in reason-giving is different from the previously reported one, less rational or less consistent with future behaviour, then the

---

[4] For a discussion of the evidence see Clarke (2008).

implication seems to be that searching for reasons leads subjects astray. The standard interpretation of the psychological evidence on analysing reasons, or on reasons-based judgements and evaluations (Wilson 2002; Lawlor 2003), invites us to see deliberation and justification as obstacles to the attainment of self knowledge. Here is a possible reconstruction of the argument against the contribution of authorship to self knowledge:

- If giving reasons in support of one's attitudes contributes to first-person authority over those attitudes, then people who have the opportunity to analyse their reasons in support of their attitudes should enjoy first-person authority over those attitudes.[5]
- Research participants who are given the opportunity to analyse reasons for their attitudes systematically fail to exhibit first-person authority over those attitudes.
- Therefore, giving reasons in support of one's attitudes does NOT contribute to first-person authority over those attitudes.

The argument could also be presented as a comparative claim between the performance of research participants who have the opportunity to engage in introspective deliberation and justification, and research participants who don't.

- If giving reasons in support of one's attitudes contributes to first-person authority over those attitudes, then people who have the opportunity to analyse their reasons in support of their attitudes should be more authoritative with respect to their attitudes than people who are not given the same opportunity.[6]
- Research participants who are given the opportunity to analyse reasons for their attitudes are systematically less authoritative with respect to their attitudes than research participants who are not given the same opportunity.
- Therefore, giving reasons in support of one's attitudes does NOT contribute to first-person authority over those attitudes.

When research participants who engaged in introspective deliberation or justification attempt to predict their own behaviour on the basis of their reported attitudes, their predictions are less successful than those of a well-informed third person or of the self predictions of research participants who did not engage in introspective deliberation or justification. The interpretation of these findings is that reason-giving undermines rather than promotes self

---

[5] For the purposes of the present discussion I will not distinguish the effects of *spontaneous* reason-giving (when the subject endorses the content of a belief via reason-giving without being asked to do so) from those of *prompted* reason-giving (when the subject is asked to provide reasons for a reported belief).

[6] Notice that this premise does not seem to be justified on the basis of Moran's account of authorship. Moran suggests that reason-giving provides an additional route to first-person authority (different from privileged epistemic access), and thus does not claim that epistemic and agential authority are cumulative.

knowledge. Lawlor (2003, p. 558) claims that in the studies on dating couples research participants lack first-person authority, because their attitudes are unstable and because participants are likely to behave towards their partners in a way that is not consistent with or explicable by their reported attitudes. And yet, they were invited, in the course of the experiments, to think about the reasons for their reported attitudes. The suggestion is that the reason-giving exercise did not bring out the *real self* in the research participants: the attitudes endorsed as a consequence of analysing reasons for dating were not manifested in the participants' subsequent behaviour and did not reflect their commitment to the relationship.

There is something very unsettling about the pattern of the research participants' responses, and about the ease with which their responses were manipulated by the experimenters. However, it is not obvious that the participants experienced a failure of first-person authority over their attitudes. For Lawlor's argument to go through, we need to agree that research participants meet the conditions for authoring their reported attitudes and yet fail to gain authority over them. Lawlor is right that participants qualify for authorship. The evidence shows that they are not alienated from the attitudes they report and, when asked to do so, they give reasons for endorsing those attitudes which they take to be their best reasons. We must conclude, then, that they meet the criteria for authorship with respect to the attitudes they report. Their reported attitudes are up to them and are 'answerable to their explicit thinking about the matter' (Moran 2001, p. 123). The next question is whether research participants fail to gain authority over their reported attitudes. Those who argue that research participants in the psychological studies on attitude shifts and in those on attitude-behaviour inconsistency fail to exercise authority over their reported attitudes must assume that certain conditions need to be satisfied for first-person authority. In order for a subject to have first-person authority over an attitude endorsed with reasons: 1) the attitude needs to be stable and consistent with other relevant attitudes and with future behaviour; 2) the reasons for endorsing the attitude need to be also the reasons why the attitude was formed; 3) the subject needs to know why she has that attitude. Are these requirements sensible conditions on first-person authority?

## 5.1.4 Rationality and stability of attitudes

The mismatch between reported attitudes and long-term behavioural dispositions does not necessarily undermine first-person authority. Inconsistencies between attitudes and behaviour can be due to a variety of factors, such as a genuine and motivated attitude change or instability caused by an unresolved tension among conflicting attitudes. As Ferrero (2003) puts it, temporal stability of reported attitudes is not necessarily a precondition for first-person authority, and attitudes do not need to be persistent in order to be the object of knowledge. For instance, within a constructivist account of the self, as that described by Dan Zahavi, it would not make sense to deny research participants knowledge of their own attitudes on the basis of claims about attitude-behaviour inconsistencies:

> Self knowledge is [...] a dynamic and unending process. The same, however, can be said for what it means to be a self. The self is not a thing; it is not something fixed and unchangeable, but rather something evolving, something that is realized through one's projects, and therefore something which cannot be understood independently of one's self-interpretation.
>
> (Zahavi 2003, p. 58).

Referring to empirical studies showing how inaccurate people's predictions of their own future emotions are, Valerie Tiberius emphasises the potential instability of both attitudes and commitments and the constructive nature of self knowledge.

> Because our commitments are disorderly, uninterpreted, and changeable in these ways, there is an inevitable element of creation in the process of acquiring self knowledge.
>
> (Tiberius 2008, p. 117)

The question whether stability of attitudes matters to self knowledge with respect to those attitudes depends (to some extent) on the nature of the attitudes we are considering. Stability might not seem a very important factor for evaluative judgements that are marginal to the core of our conception of our self (e.g. which jam we like best). But it might become a very important factor for attitudes that are, to some extent, self-defining, such as judgements about what makes life worthwhile, ideological or political affiliations, and so on. These attitudes are of a more dispositional nature and represent things about ourselves that we take to be less open to revision, less fleeting. We take it as part of what it is to have such attitudes that they are to some extent stable. How to consider the results of the dating couple studies? We should keep in mind that research participants in these studies had been dating their partners for a relatively short period of time, and this may be part of the reason why their attitudes and predictions could be manipulated so easily via a particular style of questioning. Yet, one could argue that attitudes towards dating partners are very important aspects of the self concept, and thus they should be regarded, as ideological and political commitments, as attitudes that we expect to give rise to long-term behavioural dispositions.

As we argued in the previous chapter, the belief that a relationship is doomed to failure, due to the fact that no intrinsic reason for dating can be recalled at the time, is not a rationally formed belief. But this does not mean that the belief should not be ascribed to oneself or genuinely endorsed as one's own. Even if the belief is not formed rationally, or no rational justification is available for it, the belief content is reliably self ascribed when it represents the participant's *current* state of mind. In other words, research participants should not believe that their relationship is doomed to failure only because they have been asked to think about extrinsic reasons to date their partners. But, if the research participants really believe that their relationship will fail at that time, first-person authority is not compromised by their ascribing that belief to themselves. There is no simple algorithm to determine what someone's genuine state of mind is, but there is behavioural evidence to be taken into account: if participants report an attitude and give reasons for it, this is evidence that they have that attitude. The fact that they later act in a way that is not compatible with that attitude, may be evidence that they never had it, or simply that they no longer have it.

To sum up, neither the rationality nor the stability of the reported attitudes should be a precondition for first-person authority. In order to maintain that research participants lack first-person authority over their reported attitudes, we would need to show that, at the moment of reporting their attitudes, they did not know what the content of their attitudes was or did not know that they had those attitudes. If participants reported something that they did not believe, but sincerely, then they would be mistaken about what they thought or felt, and they would experience a failure of first-person authority over their attitudes in spite of apparently meeting all the conditions for authorship. This would be a problem for a view such as Moran's, according to which authorship gives rise to first-person authority. But if they reported what they believed, it seems that, based on considerations about the rationality and stability of the reported attitudes, we have no reason to deny first-person authority to them.

## 5.1.5 Causal efficacy

Psychologists often complain that philosophers see deliberation everywhere, and idealise it. When people are asked to deliberate upon a case, express a judgement, or justify with reasons an already formed attitude or judgement, they are often vulnerable to evidence manipulation and biases. Moreover, it is possible that, even when a certain reasoning process sounds like an act of deliberation, where subjects weigh up evidence to decide on, say, whether the death penalty should be abolished, we are faced with a *post-hoc* justification of

a judgement that has been formed otherwise, hostage to unconscious dispositions and basic likes and dislikes. In this vein, Haidt (2001) suggests that most
of our attempts at arguing for the truth of our reported attitudes are not a
causally efficacious exercise in deliberation, but a rationalisation. He compares
the job of a judge to that of a lawyer. In deliberation we are like judges who
have to weigh up the evidence in favour and against a case, and make up our
minds by that process. But when we engage in *post-hoc* rationalisation we are
like lawyers trying to build a case, and we are no longer interested in the truth
of the matter.[7]

One argument for the view that reason-giving does contribute to first-person
authority is that by weighing up evidence subjects are able to determine
what their attitudes are. This claim is disputed in the interpretation of the
psychological evidence. Giving reasons is presented as largely causally inert.
When reason-giving is a causally inert process, I *discover* rather than *determine*
the content of the attitudes I report, even when I endorse them on the basis of
reasons. The upshot is that there is no *agential* route to first-person authority:
reason-searching is merely a heuristic and not a deliberative process, given that
the content of the reported attitudes is established independent of the process
of reason-giving and is not affected by it. The distinction between the interpretive and the deliberative stance collapses and there is no need to distinguish
between reasons contributing to the formation of an attitude and reasons
offered in confabulation, because there are *no* reasons of the former type.
I acquire beliefs about which beliefs I have in much the same way in which
I acquire beliefs about what other people believe, and reason-giving is epiphenomenal. Philosophers stress the role of reason-giving in deliberation whereas
psychologists argue that reason-giving is largely irrelevant to attitude
formation. Moran emphasises the active causal role of reason-giving for
the formation of attitudes, whereas Wilson opts for a deflationary account of
reason-giving as an ineffectual add-on. Who should we believe?

I suspect that very few cases will fall neatly into the two categories described
by Haidt (2001): searching for the truth or deceiving oneself (and others).
If what makes the reason-giving *post-hoc* is that the reasons adduced to support the attitude do not coincide with the reasons why the attitude was formed
in the first place (or better, do not coincide with the causes of its formation, if
no explicit deliberation was involved), then the conclusion that no first-person
authority can ensue from the reason-giving exercise seems rushed. If what
makes the reason-giving *post-hoc* is that the reasons adduced to support the

----

[7] See Section 4.5.1.

attitude are not regarded by the subject herself as her best reasons, then the conclusion that no first-person authority can ensue from the reason-giving exercise is more plausible. The comparison between the context of interpretation and the context of deliberation (or first-person justification) is useful no matter how we adjudicate controversial cases of confabulation, self deception and weakness of will. It shows how by deliberating and justifying one can take responsibility over the content of one's own thoughts and how the first-person perspective is not exhausted by direct access.

There are situations in which attitude formation occurs almost entirely below the level of conscious reflection, and in those situations psychologists are right that reason-giving plays at best the role of advocacy. There are beliefs that just pop up in our belief box independent of a process of deliberation, and whose causal history is not transparent to introspection (Wilson 2002, pp. 97–8). A belief, say, has been formed, and one provides reasons for that belief that are aimed to show oneself and other agents how the belief makes sense within a certain narrative of the self. 'This is me, I don't like compromises'. 'It would have been silly to ignore her advice'. 'I never spend time with my friends, I could not have left the pub earlier'. This tendency to construct a coherent self is well-supported by the psychological evidence: as we saw in chapter three, people are more likely to preserve rather than challenge their previously identified values and commitments. But even in the circumstances in which attitudes are the result of gut reactions, or subjects find themselves with attitudes they haven't explicitly formed by weighing up evidence, giving reasons is valuable, and is still an act of authorship. Subjects are not always epistemically blameworthy for not having access to the mechanisms responsible for the formation of the attitudes they find themselves having. Reason-giving cannot always contribute to uncovering the causes of those attitudes, but, when the reasons offered are good reasons, it has other epistemic benefits: it enhances awareness of having those attitudes, and it is instrumental to creating connections between those attitudes and other attitudes subjects have, either allowing subjects to develop a coherent narrative or highlighting a clash that can give rise to the revision of their new or prior attitudes. Think about cognitive behavioural therapy as an example of how this process can be beneficial to the subject, even when the attitudes reported and defended with reasons are not 'optimal' or rational, and when it is not at all clear to the subject how they were formed.

Analysing reasons brings about changes in the self: even the psychological evidence concedes this, although it suggests that those changes are usually for the worse. The point is that the attitudes endorsed as a consequence of the reason-giving exercise might be significantly different from (and less desirable than) the ones reported at the beginning, but they are not necessarily less representative of the self. Even if the initial attitudes were not formed via deliberation, the opportunity for reason-giving enables subjects to endorse the attitudes they find themselves as having on the basis of the reasons they take themselves to have. Whether the results of this reason-giving exercise are epistemically desirable depends on the details of each case. There are circumstances in which it might be more beneficial to be at the mercy of one's unconscious dispositions than to endorse attitudes that are based on non-rational processes of deliberation and justification (which I take to be the message of part of the introspection-effects literature). In other circumstances, reason-giving will contribute to a greater awareness of one's attitudes, priorities and values, and will provide to subjects the resources to include their attitudes in a general narrative of themselves. This narrative, in turn, will play a causally active role in shaping explicit acts of deliberation and justification, by which the subject will be able to determine, and not just subscribe to, future attitudes (Velleman 2005).

### 5.1.6 Knowing why

The behaviour of the dating couples in the experiment by Seligman and colleagues can be interpreted as follows. They knew what their attitudes were at the time when they reported them, no matter how representative of their future behaviour those attitudes would have turned out to be. But they did not know *why* they had those attitudes. They did not realise that they formed those attitudes on the basis of partial evidence about their relationship, evidence that had been manipulated by the experimenter. Can we regard these research participants as authoritative with respect to the belief that their relationship is not going to be long-lasting, if they ignored the reasons for their prediction? Described in these terms, the experimental results seem to be a good example of failure of first-person authority, because in this context a well-informed third person (e.g. the experimenter) could answer the why-question more reliably than the first person (e.g. the research participant). But this move assumes very demanding conditions for knowledge of one's attitudes (again). If self knowledge must include not just knowledge of the content of one's conscious attitudes and knowledge of who is having those attitudes, but also knowledge of *why* the person having those attitudes has them, then self knowledge is made close to unattainable. In those cases in which there is no introspective access to the mechanisms responsible for forming or endorsing ttitudes, self knowledge seems to require formal training in scientific psychology!

This implicit condition for first-person authority can be formulated in two ways:

a) In order to have knowledge of my having an attitude, *I cannot be mistaken about* the reasons why I report and endorse that attitude.

b) In order to have knowledge of my having an attitude, *I need to be aware of* the reasons why I report and endorse that attitude.

Condition (a) sounds more plausible than condition (b). Condition (a) says that in order to have knowledge of my attitudes, I cannot have false beliefs about the reasons for my having those attitudes; no 'mistakes' are tolerated. Condition (b) says that in order to have knowledge of my attitudes, I must know what there is to know about the reasons for my having those attitudes; ignorance is not tolerated. But what could be the motivation for thinking that (a) and (b) are plausible conditions on first-person authority? One motivation could be that intentions and other attitudes are identified (also) on the basis of why subjects have them. Not knowing why I have an attitude, then, would mean not knowing *which* attitude I have. Let's the recall the example we discussed earlier. I intend to stay in the pub until closing time. Having true beliefs about why I have that intention, or being aware of the reasons for having it, may be necessary for me to know that I have that particular intention as opposed to another. I might not be fully aware of the reason why I intend to stay in the pub until closing time, because I might not recognise the extent to which obtaining my friends' approval is important to me. When I endorse my intention to stay in the pub until closing time on the basis that I am having a good time, I am referring to a new attitude which happens to have a lot in common with the attitude caused by my unconscious desire to obtain my friends' approval. The content of the intention (*to stay in the pub*), and the commitment to that content expressed by the attitude (*intending* to stay in the pub) are the same, but the reasons for forming or endorsing the attitudes are different.

If the reasons for forming or endorsing an attitude are relevant to establishing which attitude I report, ignoring why I have an intention compromises my authority over that intention. But, in the case at hand, it is open to the friend of authorship to argue that when we provide reasons for an attitude, we form a new attitude. Thus, there are really two attitudes, one acquired for reasons that are not transparent to introspection, and the other formed or endorsed on the basis of reasons. On this view, the attitude I endorse via reasons is not the one caused by the unconscious desire to obtain my friends' approval, but it is the one motivated by the conscious desire to continue enjoying a pleasant evening. What is the role of reason-giving then? Through an analysis of my reasons, I don't gain any further insight into the reasons for my previous intention (the one caused by the desire to obtain my friends' approval), but I come to know that I have an intention that has the same content (the intention supported by my desire to continue enjoying the evening). Notice that when we describe the situation in these terms, my ignorance of the reasons for the initial intention to stay in the pub is not aggravated by reflection. Moreover, depending on whether we think that reason-giving can be causally efficacious, there needs be no deception: I may be right that my desire to continue having a good time in the pub motivates my (further) intention to stay. If the reasons for forming or endorsing the attitude do not matter to which attitude I report, the conditions for first-person authority formulated in (a) and (b) are not motivated, and first-person authority is neither enhanced nor undermined by reflection.

There are two psychological models that attempt to explain the instability of attitudes when subjects are asked to provide reasons for them, and they neatly map onto these two ways of describing the situation. The first account appeals to retrieval mechanisms and the idea that attitudes towards an object or person are constructed mainly on the basis of those aspects of the object or person to be evaluated that are easily accessible to the subjects when they attempt to retrieve the relevant information (Wilson *et al.* 1984). By looking for reasons for a previously reported attitude, subjects justify it on the basis of their most accessible reasons. These reasons might be different from what caused the attitude to be there in the first place. According to the other model, 'attitudes are freshly computed based on available contextual cues' (Sengupta and Fitzsimons 2004, 711). Thus, attitudes are re-formed from scratch as a result of any new search for reasons. Both models explain the effects of evidence manipulation that subjects experienced in the dating couples study, but on the latter model participants do not have a definite set of attitudes that vary according to the retrieval circumstances. Rather, they construct their attitudes as they go along, using a variety of strategies that depend on the context of self ascription (Bettman *et al.* 1998). Research on preference reversals and decision-making also supports this view: attitudes, values and preferences are 'constructed in the process of elicitation' (Tversky and Thaler 1990, p. 210).

The former model assumes that the same attitude can be endorsed for different reasons. In the description of the situation according to which there is only one attitude, there is no real motivation for accepting such demanding conditions as (a) and (b) on first-person authority over reported attitudes. Moreover, the outcome of the reason-giving exercise is to allow the subject to justify her intention on the basis of *some* reasons rather than none, and this process might be beneficial by increasing the subject's awareness of having the attitude and promoting the inclusion of the attitude in a system in which it coheres or clashes with prior attitudes. The latter model argues that attitudes are constantly re-formed if reasons in their support are being analysed. In the description of the situation where there are really two attitudes, reason-giving is not responsible for the ignorance of the reasons for the original attitude, but may be responsible for the formation or at least the genuine endorsement of the second attitude.

I defended the view that there is a route to first-person authority, the agential one, which derives from authorship, and authorship is manifested by the capacity to deliberate on the content of an attitude or to justify an attitude on the basis of what the subject takes to be her best reasons.

### 5.1.7 Authorship rescued

Based on the account of authorship I defended, largely borrowed from Moran (2001), the implications of the psychological studies on introspective reflection and attitude–behaviour inconsistency for first-person authority should not be accepted. The evidence helps us resist the temptation of idealising the capacity for reason-giving: justification and deliberation are not always rational processes, and the attitudes formed on their basis might fail to meet standards of rationality too, as well as being often inconsistent with the subject's other attitudes and behaviour. Moreover, reason-giving is not always an active process of deliberation, and can be just an attempt to mask the absence of reasons. Finally, the fact that a subject has analysed reasons for an attitude does not mean that she is aware of the actual mechanisms causally responsible for the formation or endorsement of that attitude. Authorship is not about *producing* rational attitudes, but it is about *acknowledging* an attitude *as one's own on the basis of reasons*. The arguments against reason-giving as a source of self knowledge work only if we accept very demanding conditions for first-person authority. I have shown that those conditions should be resisted: one can have first-person authority over an attitude even if the attitude is irrational and unstable; even if the reasons given for endorsing it are not the reasons why it was formed; and even if one is not aware, or is mistaken about, the reasons why one has formed or endorsed it.

Limited as it is, both in rationality and causal efficacy, authorship has a very important role to play. The psychological mechanisms that lead subjects to form an attitude can sometimes be partly or wholly unavailable to introspection and subjects often exercise no control over their behavioural dispositions. But by giving what they take to be their best reasons for their attitudes, subjects gain control. At the end of the process of deliberation or justification, they might renew the commitment to the content of a previously reported attitude, but often on the basis of different reasons, or change their attitude and make a different commitment, which might meet independent standards of rationality to a greater or lesser degree, depending on the quality of their reasoning. These effects of introspective reflection should be expected consequences of analysing reasons. Motivated attitude shifts are likely to increase responsibility and self awareness when the processes leading up to authorship are rational processes, e.g. when they take into account all the relevant available evidence and are based on the subject's best reasons. But even when the processes of deliberation and justification that give rise to new commitments are not optimally rational, the undesirability of these attitude shifts should be seen as a consequence of a breakdown of rationality and should not be seen as having negative implications for self knowledge. Reason-giving has additional epistemic benefits: it increases awareness of having the reported attitudes and allows one to include them in a system of other attitudes. In this way, reason-giving constitutes a first step towards the creation of a self narrative that might demand coherence and motivate further attitude shifts.

In conclusion, how should we square the philosophical and the psychological literature on reason-giving? Moran is right that reason-giving provides an additional route to the knowledge of the content of one's own attitudes and to the knowledge of one's having those attitudes. But he presented a far too idealised picture of deliberation as an exercise in rationality. The processes and the outputs of deliberation and justification might not meet standards of rationality, as they are affected by the same limitations that apply to all other reasoning processes, and are hostage to selective memory and attention, poor thinking, evidence manipulation and attribution biases.

> The reasons considered in making a choice may be influenced by the effects of context, salience, compatibility, framing and elicitation procedures, which are manipulable.
>
> (Zimbardo 1999, p. 377)

The studies on introspective reflection suggest that when we think about reasons we can fail both to meet standards of rationality for the formation and justification of our attitudes and to identify correctly the mechanisms which are causally responsible for our own conscious attitudes. Moreover, contrary to some readings of the deliberative stance, not all instances of reason-giving are aimed at making one's mind up about something. The reasons we offer for our attitudes are sometimes just an attempt to mask the absence of justification with whatever reasons seem best to fit our reported attitudes: these instances of normal confabulation are epistemically blameworthy and scarcely conducive to (self) knowledge (Wilson 2002; Wegner 2002). We should remember, though, that making up stories is not the only role for *post-hoc* reason-giving. We might have no introspective access to how our attitudes were formed, and rather engage in a process of rationalisation which allows us to *determine* or *discover* our best reasons in support of the attitudes we happen to have. In this latter scenario, *post-hoc* reason-giving is epistemically praiseworthy as it allows us to gain control over attitudes acquired in ways not transparent to introspection.

My diagnosis of the apparent tension between the philosophical and the psychological literature is that the puzzling results of the studies on introspective reflection are due to a frequent breakdown of rationality, and to the limitations of introspective reports in general. It is not reason-giving in particular that is responsible for failures of self knowledge. The capacity for self ascribing and endorsing an attitude on the basis of reasons is, with respect to some attitudes, necessary for self knowledge. The message often drawn from the introspection literature, e.g. that deliberation and justification get in the way of self insight and that we'd better go with the flow rather than stop and think, is not supported by the evidence. *Bad* instances of deliberation and justification make for the endorsement of attitudes that do not meet independent normative standards of rationality and might lead one to form false beliefs, about the world in general or about oneself. But this is hardly news and does not apply to *good* instances of deliberation and justification.[8] All we need to concede to the standard interpretation of the psychological evidence is that first-person authority over the attitudes we can endorse with reasons does not guarantee the rationality and stability of the reported attitudes, and does not guarantee knowledge of the mechanisms responsible for the formation of those attitudes.

## 5.2 'Inserted' thoughts[9]

In the previous section we explored the relationship between authorship and self knowledge, and I argued that authorship gives rise to a form of first-person authority. Here I want to focus instead on the relationship between ownership and authorship, and intentionality: some thoughts are denied belief status when they are neither owned nor endorsed by the subject reporting them. Here I consider the radical case of 'inserted' thoughts. The main thesis is that, if it is true that 'inserted' thoughts fail the test of intentionality, this is primarily due to a failure of self knowledge, and not to a breakdown of rationality.

---

[8] For a similar point, see Tiberius (2008, p. 127).

[9] Some of the arguments in this section have been developed with Matthew Broome. For more details, see Bortolotti and Broome (2009).

The analysis of thought insertion in terms of ownership and authorship of thoughts has some advantages over previous accounts of thought insertion, according to which the puzzling status of the 'inserted' thought is due to a loss of the sense of agency.

## 5.2.1 What is thought insertion?

There are a number of disorders of the self that might affect the way in which one feels one's thoughts are formed, held, reported, accessed or influenced by other individuals or external forces. In thought insertion subjects experience a thought as foreign. This experience is accompanied by a story about how the thought has been inserted from outside. We need to distinguish between the delusional belief that some third party is inserting thoughts into one's head (*the delusional explanation*); and the thought that is regarded as inserted (*the inserted thought*). The former is a belief that can be authored: the subject is not alienated from it and can offer some (often implausible) explanation of how thought insertion occurred. For example, a subject might explain that the 'inserted' thought has been put in her head via a special device capable of transmitting thoughts. She might go into greater detail as to how the machine can transmit thoughts and elaborate on the magical power or the technology responsible for such a device. The transmission or the 'inserting' process is seen as a *physical* process. It is with respect to the latter thought—the 'inserted' one—that questions of ownership and authorship emerge. The thought is known first-personally by the subject and therefore the subject is aware of the content of that thought independently of behavioural evidence. But the subject regards it as alien and out of her own control (Sims 2003, p. 164).

Not all thinking disorders involve the subject's *total* alienation from a thought that is known first-personally. In some cases, the subject feels that her own thought is shared with others, broadcast without her permission or withdrawn by others, but she maintains a limited sense of attachment to the thought in so far as she recognises the thought as originally her own, as produced by her, or as something she is committed to. In these cases, distress derives from a perceived violation of privacy or breach of personal boundaries. In thought insertion total alienation ensues, and this is the case we are going to concentrate on, because it has the most puzzling theoretical consequences for the philosophy of thought, that is, the divorce between first-personal awareness of the content of a thought, and the possibility of self ascribing that thought. The subject 'experiences thoughts that do not have the feeling of familiarity, of being his own, but he feels that they have been put in his mind without his volition, from outside himself' (Sims 2003, p. 168). Radical alienation can be experienced to the same degree with respect to physical movements as well as to thoughts, when the movement of a limb, for instance, occurs independently of the subject's will to move and is perceived as foreign.

Here are some examples of disorders of passivity:

(a) A university student in her second year believes that her university lecturer has implanted an electronic device in her head that can control her thoughts.

(Lewis and Guthrie 2002, p. 70)

(b) One evening one thought was given to me electrically that I should murder Lissi.

(Jaspers 1963, p. 580)

(c) When I reach for the comb, it is my hand and arm which move. But I don't control them. I sit watching them move and they are quite independent, what they do is nothing to do with me. I am just a puppet manipulated by cosmic strings.

(Graham and Stephens 1994, p. 99)

(d) A 57-year-old woman suffered a stroke and thereafter perceived her left hand as having a will of its own. On one occasion, the hand grabbed her by the throat and choked her, requiring great effort to pull it off. She described the hand as possessing 'an evil spirit' and stated that it did not belong to her: 'Those are two very different people, the arm and I'.

(Scepkowski and Cronin-Golomb 2003, p. 261)

Some of the cases above involve the violation of personal boundaries and the hypothesis of external control. Only (b) is a case of thought insertion. It is difficult to describe thought insertion further without discussing different theories about how best to characterise it, because any description comes with some theoretical assumption. The presence of 'inserted' thoughts is usually analysed in the literature in terms of a subject having ownership of a thought towards which she fails to experience a sense of agency. In other words, subjects introspect and find that there is a thought in their minds which they feel they have not themselves voluntarily produced (Gallagher 2004; O'Brien and Opie 2003; Stephens and Graham 1994). Although very intuitive, the characterisation of thought insertion in terms of a loss of the sense of agency with respect to a reported thought is unsatisfactory,[10] because it assumes that thoughts are ordinarily accompanied by sense that the thought has been 'voluntarily produced' by the subject. This does not seem to be the case: there are non-'inserted' thoughts whose content has not been the object of explicit deliberation or that are perceived as controlled by forces outside the subject. Although these thoughts are not accompanied by a sense of agency, they are

---

[10] For alternative responses to the loss of sense-of-agency analysis of thought insertion, see Gibbs (2000) and Vosgerau and Newen (2007).

not regarded as 'inserted'. That means that, if the sense of agency is part of the explanation of the phenomenology of thought insertion occurs, it is not a complete one.

The claim that ownership is preserved in thought insertion is also problematic, given that the subject affected by thought insertion is often radically alienated from the thought she reports.[11] Those who argue that ownership is preserved in thought insertion deploy a notion of ownership primarily characterised by the spatiality condition, i.e. the capacity to locate a thought within the subject's personal boundaries (Gallagher 2004). This notion of ownership has a number of limitations. It is too weak, as it allows for someone to own a thought that cannot be self ascribed; and it relies for its intelligibility on a metaphor (i.e. the mind as a container with thoughts as material objects occupying that space) that is at best controversial, both as a psychologically realistic image of how the mind works and as a naïve image of how laypeople conceive of their minds as working.

In order to be able to compare different accounts of thought insertion, we need some clarity in the terminology. Let me list five capacities that are mentioned in the literature on thought insertion:

i)   locating a thought in one's personal boundaries (*spatiality* condition for ownership);

ii)  accessing the content of a thought directly and first-personally (*introspection* condition for authorship);

iii) acknowledging a thought as one's own (*self ascription* condition for ownership);

iv)  endorsing the content of a thought on the basis of one's best reasons (*authorship as endorsement*);

v)   being causally responsible for the formation of a thought or producing a thought (*agency with respect to thoughts*).

The notions of ownership available in the literature are defined in terms of the conjunction of (i) and (ii), or in terms of the conjunction of (i), (ii) and (iii): the owner of a thought is taken to be the subject who can locate the thought within her personal boundaries and has direct access to the thought, but in some accounts it is also expected that the subject can acknowledge the thought

---

[11] Other authors challenge the idea that ownership is preserved in thought insertion: Mullins and Spence (2003) describe thought insertion as a condition in which thought possession fails. Graham (2004) argues that self ascription of thoughts is impaired in thought insertion.

as her own and ascribe the thought to herself. Now we have all the conceptual resources to describe thought insertion, and to explain why philosophers find it so puzzling and so interesting. Capacities (ii) and (iv) can come apart in the reporting of both ordinary and delusional beliefs. But (ii) and (iii) seem to come apart only in quite exceptional cases; in thought insertion, the subject is aware of the content of the 'inserted' thought in a first-personal way but does not acknowledge that the thought is her own. Because of the detachment of (iii) from (ii), thought insertion challenges commonsense and it is a puzzle for our philosophical conception of what it is to have a thought.

## 5.2.2 Thought insertion as a failure of ownership

When discussing thought insertion, Gerrans (2001b) and Gallagher (2004) employ a notion of ownership that is characterised by the spatiality condition and the introspection condition. Thus, for Gallagher, it is sufficient for one to own a thought that the thought is experienced first-personally *in one's head*. This experience is independent of any sense of acknowledgement, and of any sense of responsibility for the generation or the maintenance of the thought. If we apply the notions of ownership characterised by introspection and inclusion in the subject's personal boundaries to the case of thought insertion, we find that the subject *owns* the 'inserted' thought, as she can locate it within her personal boundaries and has direct, first-personal access to its content.

This notion of ownership has several drawbacks, though. To start with, it does not seem to vindicate the everyday notion of ownership as having an entitlement to or a legal right of possession over the object that is owned (OED, 2007). Campbell (2002) discusses a more demanding notion of ownership, according to which a subject needs to acknowledge the thought as her own and ascribe it to herself in order to be its owner. To some extent, the notion of ownership as including the self ascription condition does justice to the notion of ownership as entitlement, because the subject can ascribe the thought to herself on the basis of introspection, psychological information about herself or consideration for the reasons in favour of the content of that thought. Although all these sources of entitlement are possible, and in some cases more than one source can be available at once, they are not necessary for self ascription. No additional claims *need* to be made about the thought being endorsed or produced by the subject; ownership remains distinct from authorship and from the sense of agency.

If we apply the more demanding notion of ownership to the case of thought insertion, then we find that the subject *does not* own the 'inserted' thought. The thought is accessed directly and reported first-personally, but it is not reported *as the subject's own thought*. It is 'mineness' as entitlement to the thought which is the crucial and distinguishing feature of this account of ownership; and it is this 'mineness' which is conspicuously missing from the subject's phenomenology. Hohwy (2007) comes to a similar conclusion from a different starting point. In an attempt to characterise what 'mineness' is and where it comes from when it is applied to a perception, a thought or an action being something the subject recognises as her own and feels entitled to, Hohwy talks about the capacity to predict that such an event is happening:

> I propose that we interpret the experience of perceptual mineness as the experience of having predicted, and thus already being familiar with, what one perceives. It is mineness in the sense in which what is experienced as familiar is felt to be mine, even when we cannot place the familiar object in a concrete autobiographical narrative. The contrast is when the perceived causes in the environment are deeply unexpected.

> (Hohwy 2007, p. 8)

For Hohwy, for the sense of ownership to develop with respect to a perception, for instance, the spatial location of the act of perceiving within the personal boundaries of the agent is not sufficient, and inclusion in a personal narrative is not necessary. It is whether the act of perceiving is unexpected or predicted by the agent that affects the agent's sense of ownership of the act.

If we think about the notion of ownership in general, spatial considerations are usually not sufficient to claim ownership. If a neighbour's child throws a ball into your garden, the ball does not become yours in virtue of the fact that it fell within the boundaries of your property. In order to keep the ball and silence the protestations of the weeping child you would have to show that you are entitled to keeping that ball, e.g. show a receipt from a toy shop indicating that you did acquire that ball sometime in the past. Another example which might be more relevant: what happens in successful transplants is that someone else's organ is inserted in one's 'personal boundaries'. The fact that a heart is beating inside you, does not necessarily make the heart *yours*. It is not sufficient for an object to be within one's personal boundaries, or within the boundaries of one's property, to be owned by that person.

Additional reservations could be expressed about the significance of the spatiality condition for the notion of ownership when such a notion is applied to thoughts. All conditions for ownership of thought are to some extent reliant on a metaphorical way of describing thoughts as things that can be possessed. However, the introspection condition seems to take into account the specific attributes of what is owned, that is, thoughts are the type of objects that can be introspected, i.e. mental states, because they have a content that can be accessed first-personally, and that can be ascribed to oneself on the basis of introspection. Instead, the spatiality condition seems to rely for its plausibility on a very controversial conception of the mind as a container where objects are placed. If by looking into the box, a thought is found, then the thought is one's own. Independent of what we think about the ontological status of thoughts, this metaphor is excessively crude.

Proponents of the significance of the spatiality condition might reply that subjects with thought insertion talk about their thoughts as foreign objects unduly pushed into a personal and private space: subjects report thoughts to be *physically inserted* in their minds. Conceptualising thoughts as material objects enclosed in a physical space would then be acceptable, as it is compatible with the reports of subjects with the condition. But this move is problematic for two independent reasons. First, untutored descriptions of mental life might be interesting evidence for psychological theories of belief formation and ascription, but are rarely a good guide to the ontology and epistemology of the mind. Second, if one wanted to take all aspects of the phenomenology of thought insertion at face value, one would also have to take into account that subjects with thought insertion explicitly *disown* and take distance from the thoughts they report, claiming that they are the thoughts *of others*.

These observations about the alleged match between the spatiality-focused account of ownership and the phenomenology of thought insertion raise further concerns. An appeal to the notion of ownership in the case of thought insertion needs to make sense of ownership of thoughts in general and give us the tools to describe what is puzzling about the thought insertion case. If the proposed analysis of ownership fits the case of thought insertion extremely well, but the price to pay is that it cannot be successfully applied to other cases of ownership of thoughts, then it is *ad hoc*. An indication that the notion of ownership as satisfaction of the spatiality and introspection conditions is *ad hoc* is given by the fact that it makes thought insertion lose all of its puzzling features. What seems puzzling about thought insertion is that one can introspect a thought without acknowledging that the thought is one's own. But this is no longer a difficult condition to describe, given that the less demanding notion of ownership vindicates it entirely. The capacity for self ascription is missing, but it is not an integral part of what ownership requires.

In thoughts that can be first-personally accessed, as opposed to other objects, ownership and acknowledgement of ownership seem to go together. One usually knows that a thought is one's own when it is, because ordinarily one would not be in a position to access the content of that thought unless one was the subject of that thought. Introspecting a thought is usually sufficient for ascribing that thought to oneself.[12] This is what makes thought insertion interesting to philosophers: with respect to an 'inserted' thought, you recognise that the thought is in your mind (satisfaction of the spatiality condition), and you can access its content first-personally (satisfaction of the introspection condition), but you don't think the thought is yours (failure of the self ascription condition). You might have a story to explain how the 'inserted' thought ended up in your mind (delusional explanation) in which it is clear that you had no role in bringing that thought about, and that you do not endorse it. Independent of how that thought got into your mind, and what role it now has in your system of beliefs, you don't acknowledge the thought as yours and you don't ascribe it to yourself.

The notion of ownership primarily characterised by inclusion in one's personal boundaries and introspective access is not suitable to account for the experience of the person affected by the delusion, because it cannot capture the conflict that is experienced. For the subject affected by thought insertion, the 'inserted' thought is an unwanted intruder and the very distress lies in the fact that the thought is in their head but also, in a conventional sense, they don't acknowledge it as *theirs*. The exclusion of the self ascription condition from the less demanding notion of ownership makes the experience of thought insertion apparently more tractable, and less pathological, but at the cost of accepting statements of the form 'x is mine, but I don't acknowledge it as mine', or 'x is P's but P does not acknowledge x as hers' that are acceptable when applied to many objects, and yet have the flavour of inconsistency when applied to thoughts.

According to the more demanding notion of ownership, the subject with thought insertion fails to satisfy the conditions for ownership, because she fails to satisfy the self ascription condition. This means that thought insertion is characterised by a failure of ownership. The thought does not belong to the subject; she doesn't acknowledge it as hers. This account gives us the resources to explain what does work in thought insertion (the introspection condition is satisfied), and allows us to make sense of the conflict that is experienced by subjects with thought insertion (due to the fact that the introspection condition is satisfied, but the self ascription condition is not). No role is played

---

12 Sometimes philosophers talk about 'immunity from error through misidentification' (Campbell 2002; Coliva 2002). The idea is that I can be mistaken about what my thought is about, but I cannot be mistaken about who the subject of my thought is.

by the spatiality condition, whose reliance on a dubious model of the mind we have already discussed. Thoughts might be 'seen from the inside' but they are not acknowledged as belonging to the subject. Inserted thoughts are unwanted and unwelcome, and this is one of the key symptoms often linked to violence in psychotic illness.

### 5.2.3 Thought insertion as a failure of endorsement

In some psychological literature authorship is often identified with *intentional causation*: authoring an action consists in being causally responsible for it via the formation of a prior intention (Wegner and Sparrow 2004). This is what I named 'agency with respect to thoughts' in the list of relevant capacities in the previous section. The notion of authorship we have been developing in this chapter and the previous one is different, as it is primarily concerned with the *endorsement* of the content of a mental state, where the endorsement is measured in terms of the capacity for reason-giving. In order to be the author of a belief in this sense, to take responsibility for it and be committed to its content, it is not necessary to assume that the reasons that justify endorsing the belief map onto the psychological causes of its formation.

Let's think about the difference between the following formulations:

F) In order to be the author of the belief that he should file for divorce, Patrick needs to *have formed* that belief on the basis of the best evidence available to him.

E) In order to be the author of the belief that he should file for divorce, Patrick needs to *be able to endorse* that belief on the basis of the best evidence available to him.

Formulations (F) and (E) differ in that (F) is concerned with the process of formation of the belief and (E) with the process of endorsement that could be obtained either via deliberation over or later defence of the content of the belief. In order to make sense of the notion of authorship that I have largely borrowed from Moran (2001), (F) is far too demanding as a condition for authorship. Following Moran, the conditions for authorship can be met by the process of justification only, as it is perfectly conceivable and often the case that one acquires good reasons for endorsing the content of a belief that was initially formed on the basis of very weak evidence; that a belief is justified in a way that is distinct from the way in which it was originally formed—as the results of the introspection effect studies show; and that a belief appears in the belief box as the result of dispositions that are not transparent to the subject via introspection, and then is defended on the basis of reasons after the subject has been made aware of the existence of the belief and challenged to offer a justification for it.

If we took authorship of thoughts to require (F), the attitudes to count as authored in a psychologically realistic account would be so few that the phenomenon might be deprived of some of its interest: it would legitimately apply only to the outputs of explicit deliberation. The process of endorsement via reason-giving is not necessarily a process of thought production, but it is not a causally inert process either. It is a process that, in Moran's words, culminates with the subject taking responsibility over the reported attitude and making a commitment to it that is likely to be reflected in further reported attitudes and other forms of behaviour. This sense of responsibility and commitment is often described by suggesting that *it is up to the subject* what to believe. Authorship of beliefs is not hostage to the way in which beliefs are formed but to whether their content is endorsed on the basis of reasons. Authorship, as we have described it, is not about creation *ex nihilo*; it is about what relation one bears to the content of a belief, in deliberation or justification.

In the literature on authorship processing, instead, authorship is discussed in the context of movements rather than thoughts and it is taken to require intentional causation. Subjects are regarded as authors when they act on their intentions. Wegner and Sparrow (2004) suggest that there are cases in which the self is the author of an action, but does not perceive the action as self-generated (e.g. hypnosis or alien hand syndrome) and there are other cases in which the subject is not causally responsible for an action, but the action is perceived as self generated (e.g. when an instance of behaviour has good con-sequences for the subject, the behaviour is seen as willed and self generated even if it was not). In the notion of authorship I have developed following Moran (2001), there is less scope for a mismatch between *actual* authorship and the *sense* of authorship. If the content of a belief is endorsed by the subject of that belief on the basis of reasons, then she is the author of that belief, no matter how the belief got there in the first place.

Is it possible to develop a notion of authorship as intentional causation for beliefs, a notion that makes sense of the formulation in (F)? If it were possible, then the notion could be appealed to by those who believe that 'inserted' thoughts are puzzling because they are not accompanied by a sense of agency. In order to apply Wegner's analysis of the production of movements to the production of thoughts we would need to assume that the latter works in an analogous way to the former. The sense of authorship Wegner talks about rests on there being an intention prior to a perceived movement that the subject regards as the cause of the movement. But the analogy does not seem to work. The notion of authorship in the authorship processing literature seems to be at home with movements, which are either preceded by intentions or are involuntary, but not with beliefs, which can be formed independently of the presence of explicit intentions and acts of deliberation.[13] The notion of author-ship we find in Moran seems to be better suited to account for intentional states of a certain type, as it requires the presence of a content that can be endorsed on the basis of reasons, rather than for movements that cannot be 'endorsed' independently of the intentions that precede them and sometimes cause them.

According to standard accounts of thought insertion (see discussion in Gerrans 2001b; Gallagher 2004; Gibbs 2000), the subject is aware of a thought in a first-personal way, and recognises that the thought is within her personal boundaries, but lacks something else, which is described as a sense of agency with respect to the thought. This is the sense that the thought was voluntarily produced or brought into existence by the subject. In other words, it is the sense that the subject had a causally efficacious role in the generation of the thought. What is the evidence that the sense of agency is what is missing from the experience leading to reports of thought insertion? The phenomenology of the delusion seems to be compatible with the subject lacking a sense of agency; the subject affected by the delusion typically says that she has the thought because someone else gave it to her, or because some piece of machinery forced it into her head.

Additional support for this view would come from the alleged parallelism between loss of agency with respect to movements and loss of agency with respect to thoughts. When people suffer from alien hand syndrome, they claim that their hand moves independently of their will (sometimes, against their will). Subjects do not recognise themselves as those who initiated the movement, as if they were controlled by others or as if the hand had a will of its own. This experience has often been compared with some reports of thought insertion where the mind is described as a passive instrument in the grip of someone else's will, as a *medium* for thinking thoughts that are generated by other people or by external forces. In the loss-of-agency account, it is the *causal* element which is missing from the subject's awareness of her relation with the thought. The subject is aware of the content of the thought but she is not aware that she is responsible for producing the thought. To support this interpreta-tion, and the analogy between 'inserted' thoughts and alien movements, Gerrans (2001b) describes the experience of a subject as feeling like a mario-nette controlled by others. Campbell (2002) notices that loss of agency in thought insertion implies that there is no sense that the thought has been

---

[13] Bayne and Pacherie (2005, p. 176) notice that the view that thoughts are motor process can generate an infinite regress.

produced by the subject, it has just forcefully and intrusively appeared. Although it is an attractive option to account for a variety of delusions of passivity in a way that is sufficiently homogeneous, there are good reasons to keep disorders of thinking and disorders of activity apart in this context and to focus on the nature of the commitment to the thought that is regarded as 'inserted'.[14] I want to resist an account of thought insertion which rests primarily on a loss of the sense of agency, and propose that thought insertion should be analysed as a condition in which typically both the capacity of self ascription and authorship as endorsement fail with respect to the 'inserted' thought.

Let us assess the loss-of-agency account. First, the failure to experience a sense of agency does not discriminate between the phenomenon of the inserted thought and that of many ordinary beliefs. As Mullins and Spence (2003) argue, to offer an explanation of thought insertion which relies on the distinction between subjectivity and agency (Stephens and Graham 2000) or between sense of ownership and sense of agency (Campbell 2002) does not satisfactorily account for the peculiarity of the delusional experience. The unsolicited thoughts that come spontaneously to mind, without being preceded by explicit deliberative intention, do not typically give rise to delusional beliefs about others inserting or implanting thoughts. The sense of agency with respect to these beliefs is lacking as it is in the thought insertion case, but no such delusional explanation is reported. This suggests that the sense of passivity in belief formation cannot be the core element of the condition of thought insertion. If we talk about failure of acknowledgement and failure of authorship as the potential for justification and endorsement, the problem Mullins and Spence identify vanishes. Those ordinary thoughts that are not the outcome of explicit deliberation can still be acknowledged and even endorsed *post-hoc*. That is probably why they do not give rise to delusions of passivity. In our analysis of thought insertion in terms of a failure of acknowledgement and endorsement there is no need to make the controversial assumption that subjects *ordinarily* have a sense of agency with respect to their thoughts, where sense of agency amounts to a feeling that the thoughts have been *produced* by the subjects. In order to ascribe a thought to oneself and feel *entitled* to it, one does not need to have formed it as a result of explicit deliberation. As we saw, very few

---

[14] Moreover, it has been recently suggested (see Waters and Badcock 2008) that appealing to loss of agency in an explanation of disorders of passivity concerning bodily movements might also be unsatisfactory. The authors observe that the widely accepted distinction between loss of agency and loss of ownership with respect to bodily movements is not clear-cut.

thoughts are produced in this way and yet unsolicited thoughts do not ordinarily appear as alien to their subject. When we discussed the conditions for authorship, we found that deliberation is not a necessary condition for authorship of beliefs, because the commitment to the content of a thought can take the form of a reason-guided *post-hoc* justification.

Second, there are elements of discontinuity between disorders of thinking and of activity. The idea that subjects with thought insertion lack a sense of agency as thought production is the result of the forced analogy between thoughts and movements on which the loss-of-agency account rests. This analogy is very problematic, even when we compare basic descriptions of the phenomena. If you suffer from alien hand syndrome, the hand moves in a way that is not controlled by you, and you feel the movement is not yours, because you have not formed a prior intention to move your hand in that way. But in thought insertion you do not fail to acknowledge that the brain is yours because it has engaged in an act of thinking that was not willed by you. Rather, you take distance from the product of that thinking activity, and ascribe it to someone else. What matters to the ascription of the thought? That the thought is acknowledged and endorsed. Trying to establish whether there was a prior intention to produce the thought is irrelevant and slightly misleading: we do not typically form intentions to produce thoughts, although we might intend to engage in thinking activities that have as their objectives the solution of a problem or a deliberation. If we take introspection, self ascription and endorsement to be the central notions in the assessment of self knowledge for reported attitudes, then the analogy between 'inserted' thoughts and alien movements breaks down entirely. Movements themselves do not seem to be the appropriate object of introspection or justificatory exercises, although intentional actions can be authored to some extent, as they involve intentional attitudes that can be introspected, acknowledged and endorsed.

Third, the analysis of thought insertion that concentrates on the failure to experience a sense of agency does not allow for discriminations that are fine-grained enough to distinguish thought insertion from other delusions of passivity, such as thought-control. Recall the university student who believes that a lecturer is controlling her thoughts, and compare the case to that cited by Jaspers, where a thought is 'given electrically' to the subject that they should kill someone. The satisfaction of the spatiality and introspection conditions cannot discriminate between these two cases. But tracking the self ascription condition helps. In the case of the university lecturer, acknowledgement of the thoughts is preserved, but thoughts are controlled and possibly even produced by someone else. In the case of the murderous thought, there is no endorsement and no sense of agency. More importantly, there is no acknowledgement at all on behalf of the subject. It is this failure of self ascription that an observer perceives as a radical breakdown of self knowledge and that makes thought insertion distinct from thought control. It would be interesting to see whether the subject with 'inserted' thoughts ever acts on these thoughts. My understanding of the literature is that she does not. Thought insertion is one of the symptoms linked to violence in psychosis (e.g. Link and Stueve 1994)—however this may be due not to the fact that subjects act on the content of the 'inserted' thoughts but due to their acting on the content of the delusional explanation of the 'insertion' (especially acting against the person responsible for inserting the thought). Volavka (2002, p. 232) also argues that in the Link and Stueve study not enough attention was paid to the temporal relationships between psychotic symptoms and the violent act, so that it is possible that in some circumstances the symptoms developed only after the violent act. Stompe and colleagues (2004) found that control-override psychiatric symptoms (which include thought insertion) are not significantly correlated with violent acts.[15]

The difference between thought control and thought insertion is mirrored in the difference between anarchic hand and alien hand: these are cases in which the subject lacks agency—as she perceives the limb to move independently of her will—but only in the latter case the limb is described as *belonging to* someone else, or even as *being* someone else. In the anarchic hand case, the limb is recognised as the agent's own limb, and the movement is described as controlled by someone else, whereas in the alien hand case the limb is not recognised as the subject's own hand and is described as a separate entity with intentions. The notion of acknowledgement is doing the work here, as the preservation of the spatiality condition and the violation of the agency condition cannot discriminate between the two cases. Movements are outside the agent's control in both cases.

The experiences of having a thought broadcast externally or controlled by someone else are compatible with the preservation of the spatiality condition and in some cases even with the violation of the agency condition, but they differ from the experience of thought insertion. In thought broadcast and control, the thought can be acknowledged as the subject's own, self ascribed and even endorsed. What makes the 'inserted' thought different is the violation of the acknowledgement condition and (typically) a failure of authorship. One possible objection to this account is that some cases of thought insertion seem to suggest that the subject endorses the 'inserted' thought.

---

[15] Thanks to Matthew Broome for directing me to some of the relevant literature on thought insertion and violence.

A more careful consideration of these individual cases is needed before a response can be made. But here are some considerations. First, there are different types of thoughts. As we explained earlier, for some thoughts the notion of authorship as endorsement will not apply. If the 'inserted' thoughts are merely perceptual beliefs, then the question whether the subject endorses them will lose centrality and significance in the analysis of her condition, or the endorsement will be manifested only behaviourally and not via the exercise of reason-giving. If the 'inserted' thoughts are emotionally charged, and concern hating or intending to kill other people, then endorsement will play an important role, as such beliefs are those that, if acknowledged and integrated in a system of beliefs, would be central to the subject's self image.

Second, it is plausible to think that thoughts are not identified uniquely on the basis of their content. It is known that people recovering from thought insertion go through an intermediate phase of confusion but then end up acknowledging as their own the thoughts they once regarded as alien. Are those the same thoughts, first rejected and then acknowledged, or are we confronted with different thoughts that play a different role in one's belief system and self image, but that happen to have the same content? If a person with thought insertion is able to give reasons for a thought she reports as 'inserted', and endorses it as her own thought, one possible description of the situation is that there are really two thoughts. One is the 'inserted' one, disowned and rejected. The other is the thought which is acknowledged and endorsed. And they both have the same content.

I suggested at the start that this analysis of 'inserted' thought can do better justice to the phenomenon than alternative accounts, and it can also tell us something important about why certain thoughts are so puzzling that they resist interpretation. If the phenomenon of 'inserted' thoughts is described as a (radical) failure of ownership and authorship of thoughts, it is also an example of the role of self knowledge (of the agential type) in belief ascription. The disruption of self knowledge in subjects with thought insertion manifests itself not just as a false conception of their personal boundaries, but as a failure to ascribe to themselves and give reasons for a first-personally accessed and reported thought. Subjects with thought insertion do not have any difficulty in satisfying the introspection and spatiality condition, but they do not feel entitled to the thought they can introspect and struggle in making it an integral part of their own self narrative and self image. They come to believe that their personal boundaries have been breached and are horrified by the exception to the rule that, if something is in their head, then it is their thought. When something that is in their head turns out to be something that they do not recognise as one of their thoughts, they are very distressed and, as a consequence, might start doubting the ownership of other thoughts they can access first-personally.

## 5.3 **Self narratives**

I defended the claim that authorship gives rise to a form of self knowledge: by giving reasons for the content of their attitudes, subjects come to know that they have those attitudes in a way that differs from mere introspection or inference from previous behaviour. Subjects feel entitled to the beliefs they author and recognise themselves as people who endorse beliefs with those contents. In the case of 'inserted' thoughts, there is no entitlement: subjects do not ascribe those thoughts to themselves, nor do they endorse the thought contents with reasons. As a consequence, they don't see themselves as people who would entertain those thoughts. This has implications for belief ascription: the 'inserted' thoughts are not ascribed as beliefs to the subjects reporting them, as subjects do not seem to manifest any verbal or behavioural commitment to them.

Failures of rationality do not preclude the ascription of delusions as beliefs to the subjects reporting them: we saw in Chapters 2, 3, and 4 that delusions can play the role of beliefs in folk-psychological practices even if they turn out to be procedurally, epistemically or agentially irrational. Moreover, we saw that many instances of typical beliefs suffer from the same deviations from norms of rationality as delusions do. It might be seen as a substantial failure of the present project that I have not been able to single out what makes delusions special: they are irrational, as most other beliefs are. But I don't think that this result should be disappointing: it indicates that there is no categorical difference between (most) delusions and irrational beliefs. When reported thoughts seem to be so puzzling that they resist being ascribed as beliefs, their puzzling nature cannot be explained by reference to their irrationality. Ascribing disowned and un-authored thoughts as beliefs to the subjects reporting them would bring no benefits to interpreters, in terms of explanation and prediction of behaviour, because such thoughts would not be part of the subjects' own self narratives and would not feature in their deliberation of future thoughts and planning of future actions.

### 5.3.1 **Self narratives: truth or fiction?**

We tell stories about ourselves which help us recollect memories about our past experiences, identify certain patterns and a sense of direction in our life events and have some concept of who we are, what kind of persons we are, what we have achieved or failed to achieve, and what our next objectives are.[16] Philosophers, psychologists and psychiatrists alike[17] have studied narratives and conceptions of the self for some time, and recently the links between the capacity to develop a self narrative and thinking and acting autonomously have been identified—implications for normal and abnormal cognition have been explicitly drawn. It would be too ambitious to try and review the entire literature here, but I would like to suggest that the notions of ownership and authorship of thoughts play a role in self narratives, and thus in the production of autonomous thought and action.

> Generation of explanations about our perceptions, memories, and actions, and the relationships between them, leads to the construction of a personal narrative that ties together elements of our conscious experience into a coherent whole.
>
> (Roser and Gazzaniga 2004, p. 58)

I'll start from a debate that is still very lively, and perfectly relevant to the importance of giving reasons and authoring attitudes for obtaining knowledge of the self. Authoring an attitude can be seen as a means to integrate an isolated preference or an apparently insignificant belief into a coherent *whole* that delivers a conception of the self. This *whole* often has a narrative structure, but the question is whether the narrative is just a useful fiction or a true story. In an extremely influential paper, Daniel Dennett argues that the self is like the centre of gravity: it is a useful theoretical fiction, by which we can impose some order on complicated events. Appealing to Gazzaniga's research on the interpreter module, Dennett (1992) argues that the narrative in which the self is the leading character is produced by the brain. Gazzaniga (1985) describes the interpreter module as providing a running commentary and forming hypotheses to explain the subject's actions that are perceived as self-generated. One way of characterising Dennett's position is by reference to an instrumentalist view of interpretation, according to which we postulate the existence of abstract objects (such as beliefs) to account for observable events (such as bodily movements). For Dennett, the self narrative is the product of a constant activity of *self* interpretation where mental states are ascribed to the self in order to navigate the surrounding environment, predict future events and formulate

---

[16] The 'we' should not be interpreted always as a personal 'we'. Although the activity of autobiographical narration is often a fully conscious one, in most circumstances the narration does happen without the subject needing to pay special attention to it.

[17] For instance, see the work of Donna Addis, Dan McAdams, Aikaterini Fotopoulou, Martin Conway, David Velleman, Daniel Dennett, Peter Goldie, Tim Bayne and Elizabeth Pacherie, and Shaun Gallagher.

explanations for past events. In the narrative, there is one thing to which these mental states are ascribed, and one thing that perceives external objects and interacts with other individuals, a unified self as a *locus* of agency. But this is not necessarily how things are outside the fiction.

David Velleman (2005) partially agrees with Dennett's position that the self is the character of a fictive narrative, but argues that the narrative is not necessarily false, and thus the self may exist. Velleman's main objective is to square the insight in the fictionalist account of the self with the acknowledgement of a capacity that most humans have, that of self constitution. This is the capacity to invent or create oneself.[18]

> In Dennett's metaphor, the self is the non-existent author of a merely fictional autobiography composed by the human organism, which neither is nor embodies a real self.
>
> (Velleman 2005, p. 204)

> My only disagreement with Dennett will be that, whereas he regards an autobiography as fictive and consequently false in characterizing its protagonist, I regard it as both fictive and true. We invent ourselves, I shall argue, but we really are the characters whom we invent.
>
> (Velleman 2005, p. 206)

The key to Velleman's view is that the narrative can be produced unconsciously by a module in the agent's brain, but ultimately it reflects the behaviour of the agent and it is also able to produce changes in such behaviour. As he puts it, an autobiography and the behaviour that it narrates are mutually determining. We produce a narrative in order to interpret the events in our lives, but then also behave in such a way as to be faithful to the story we have been telling. This notion of mutual determination is what explains the phenomenon of self constitution, creating the self by making commitments about the future:

> As your hand hovers indecisively over the candy dish, you say, 'No, I won't,' not because you weren't about to take a candy, but because saying so may stop you from taking one.
>
> (Velleman 2005, p. 214)

According to Velleman, an autonomous agent is precisely an individual with the power of self constitution, and this suggests that judging whether a certain attitude is authored and integrated in a subject's self narrative can help us predict whether that attitude can affect the decisions made and the actions performed by that subject. Both the act of reason-giving by which subjects deliberate over

---

[18] See also Fernández (2009) for an exploration of the notion of self creation.

or justify the content of their beliefs, and the self-intimations of the type 'No, I won't' are expressions of what Moran called the 'deliberative stance'.

Can psychology adjudicate the dispute between Dennett and Velleman on whether the narrated self is a fiction? Two promising sources of information about the accuracy of self narratives are the literature on the reconstructive character of memory and the literature on confabulation in reason-giving. Tiberius, Gallagher and Zahavi explain how the narrative about the self is not (just) a faithful report of remembered events, but creates the context in which events can be remembered and a self concept be formed.

> A self-conception is not just the set of facts we might learn about ourselves; it is an interpretation of these facts within which values are prioritized, emotions are labeled, and attitudes are endorsed or rejected. Importantly, the process of organizing what we know about ourselves into a self-conception is partly a creative or constructive process.

> (Tiberius 2008, p. 116)

> In this sense the narrative (and self-narrative) process is not something that depends on the proper functioning of episodic (and autobiographical) memory, but in fact contributes to the functioning of memory. Just to the extent that the current contextual and semantic requirements of narrative construction motivate the recollection of a certain event, that recollection will be shaped, interpreted and reconstructed in the light of those requirements.

> (Gallagher 2003, p. 347)

> This narrative […] is not mainly a way of gaining insight into the nature of an already existing self. On the contrary, the self is first constructed in and through the narration. Who we are depends upon the story we (and others) tell about ourselves.

> (Zahavi 2003, p. 58)

Motivated reconstruction and interpretation shape memories and contribute to the creation of the self as a fictional character—but for Zahavi as for Velleman the fictional character exists outside the fiction, it is *created* by the fiction. However, narratives can be seen purely instrumentally, as a means to impose coherence on the disorganised material that we call 'self' (to use Dennett's language). As we are rarely rational, and always in evolution, achieving coherence can be done only at the cost of distorting the facts. This does not necessarily lead to pathological confabulation or delusional memories, but is a feature of normal cognition.

> [T]his value attached to narrativity in the representation of real events arises out of a desire to have real events display the coherence, integrity, fullness, and closure of an image of life that is and can only be imaginary.

> (White 1987, p. 24)

To some degree, and for the sake of creating a coherency to life, it is normal to confabulate and to enhance one's story. Self deception is not unusual; false memories are frequent.

(Gallagher 2003, p. 348)

People would go a long way to preserve a positive conception of themselves and there are everyday examples of behaviour that borders on self deception (we saw some examples of such behaviours in the previous chapters). When distortions are much more severe, not even perceptual information or general principles of plausibility serve as constraints on the narrative. Patients with anosognosia claim that their arms can move and do move, even if they should be able to see that their arms lay motionless at their sides. Such patients have not updated their narratives to include the presence of a serious impairment among their significant life events (see Section 1.4.4 for a detailed example).

The real reason for the evolution of these defense mechanisms (confabulations, rationalization), I suggest is to create a coherent system in order to impose stability in one's behaviour. [...] When something doesn't quite fit the script however, you very rarely tear up the entire story and start from scratch. What you do, instead, is to deny or confabulate in order to make the information fit the big picture.

(Ramachandran 1996, p. 351)

Patients with severe cognitive deficits often confabulate wildly in order to produce an explanation of the world that is consistent with their conscious experience. These confabulations include completely denying the existence of a deficit and probably result from interpretations of incomplete information [...]. Wild confabulations that seem untenable to most people, because of conscious access to information that contradicts them, probably seem completely normal to patients to whom only a subset of the elements of consciousness are available for integration.

(Roser and Gazzaniga 2004, p. 57)

Is there a straight-forward answer to the question whether the leading character in self narratives actually exists? I would like to go back to our discussion whether the process of authoring an attitude gives rise to self knowledge. If, at time t, I am mistaken about what my attitude towards something is, the fact that I can offer reasons for that attitude does not make it more representative of who I am. Suppose that I report having a negative attitude towards my partner, and predict that our relationship will soon be over, just because I can only think about instrumental reasons for dating him. People around me, instead, find that I'm happier since I have started going out with him and they notice that I am strongly attached to him. The narrative is false, but . . . the fact that I can offer plausible reasons for the negative attitude I report, and recognise myself in it, at time t, might contribute to changing the truth about what my attitude is. And at time $t_1$, I might have *become* a woman who is not happy with her partner as a consequence of genuinely believing that there are good reasons to be pessimistic about a relationship with him.

Self narratives can be true or false. They can be partial accounts of life events that are interpreted in a biased way and cannot take into account unconscious or preconscious behavioural dispositions. In the pathological cases memory impairments, motivational factors and limited access to personal information prevent the narrative from updating, and the narration is so insulated from the reality checks available to the narrator that it appears to others as blatantly false (e.g. Alzheimer's disease). But what is really interesting about narrations of this type is that, as Velleman suggests, they can start as being false and then become true, because in some circumstances they have the power to influence or determine behaviour. A bad singer can believe in herself to the point that her motivation to achieve success on the stage pushes her to train her voice and become the good singer she always thought she was.

### 5.3.2 Delusions: bad scientific theories or unreliable autobiographies?

How does the self narrative impact on the formation and explanation of delusions, and on their characterisation as beliefs? The literature on delusions has recently explored the possible connections between delusions as a breakdown of rationality and delusions as failures of self knowledge. Phil Gerrans (2009) criticises the inferential approach to the explanation of delusions, because it usually ignores the limitations of the capacity for mental time travel in subjects with delusions.

> The inferential conception of delusion treats the delusional subject as a scientist in the grip of an intractable confirmation bias. She recalls and attends selectively to evidence consistent with her biased hypothesis with the result that the delusions become ever more firmly woven into her Quinean web of beliefs [...]. I propose instead that processes of selective attention and recall exert their effects, not on a process of hypothesis confirmation but of autobiographical narrative. Someone with a delusion is not a mad scientist but an unreliable narrator.

(Gerrans 2009, p. 152)

Although for Gerrans two-factor accounts of delusions tend to under-emphasise the all-important role of abnormal experience in the formation of delusions, they may be correct in postulating the need for an additional factor. After all, there are people who have similar experiences as the experiences that give rise to delusions (e.g. hearing voices) but do not form or endorse any delusional hypothesis. This leads us to believe that abnormal experience cannot exhaustively explain the formation of a delusion. Instead of supporting the common suggestion that there may be a problem with probabilistic reasoning and the logic of confirmation, Gerrans proposes that the 'second factor' concerns the ability to engage in *mental time travel*. What distinguishes people who form the delusion from people who don't, is that the former attribute greater significance to their abnormal experiences. What might lead subjects to attribute excessive significance to experiences such as hearing voices? A plausible theory of hypersalience is found in Kapur (2003; 2004) who claims that an increased release of dopamine is responsible for contributing to the obsessive focus of subjects on their delusional thoughts.[19] Gerrans wants to explain why subjects pay too much attention to the content of their delusional thoughts, and does so by suggesting that mechanisms of salience operate on the construction of the subjects' autobiographies. To make this point, Gerrans introduces the notion of mental time travel previously used by Tulving (2002) and Gilbert (2004).

Mental time travel comprises the set of capacities that allow episodic autobiographies to be constructed according to constraints of narrative coherence. Episodic autobiographical memories are those that allow us to travel back in time and remember an event on the basis of what we saw, heard and felt at that time. When we have episodic memories, we do not remember an event from a third-personal point of view, but we live it again with its images, sounds and sensations. According to recent research on brain activity during memory and imagination, the hippocampus is largely responsible for gathering the relevant information stored in the brain and bringing the remembered event to life. When we imagine a possible future, the hippocampus does a similar job: it gathers information from past experience that is relevant to the future event to be imagined, and puts it together to form a representation of what that event will be like. There is abundant evidence suggesting a close relationship between episodic memory and imagination (e.g. Addis *et al.* 2007; Schacter and Addis 2008): in the ageing population, deterioration to the hippocampus results in impairments both in remembering specific events from a first-personal point of view, and imagining novel scenarios. Subjects with amnesia who have limited access to episodic memories find it harder to use their imagination to establish suggested links between events. The capacity to project the subject backwards in the past and forward in the future, and the constructive nature of memories of past events and acts of imaginations, are the main characteristics of mental time travel.

> Episodic recollection is a form of mental time travel allowing an individual to re-experience a prior experience. [...] Episodic memory is fundamentally tied to the

---

[19] See also Broome *et al.* (2005a).

self, in that it allows for the awareness of facts and events that are fused with the self's past and that provide guidance to the self's future.

(Keenan et al. 2003, p. 175)

According to Gerrans, it is relevant to the explanation of hypersalience in delusions that mental time travel allows retrieved experiences (which are either the object of memory or the bases for imagination) to come with an 'emotional tone' attached. The experiences are integrated in an autobiographical story which then partially determines what comes next in the story by guiding deliberation.

> When you remember or imagine skydiving or walking down the aisle, the emotional tone of the experience helps you decide to repeat or attempt it.

(Gerrans 2009, p. 157)

When only experiences with negative emotions attached are retrieved (as in depression), or when abnormal experiences are attributed excessive significance and weaved into the story as a dominant event (as in some delusions), the subjects' thought and their behaviour acquire pathological characteristics. According to Gerrans, the appeal to mental time travel in the explanation of delusions has some important advantages over competing models. First, it can explain data-gathering and attributional biases in subjects with delusions by focusing on the effects of attribution of salience, without presupposing independent cognitive deficits which may be difficult to detect with respect to ordinary irrationality. The factors which are likely to be responsible for reasoning biases (e.g. selective attention, and selective encoding and retrieval of information) are implicated in the construction of narratives as well. Second, the appeal to mental time travel in the explanation of delusions vindicates the apparent success of cognitive behavioural therapy in some cases, where subjects with delusions are encouraged to refocus attention on a different set of experiences from the ones that contribute to the delusional narrative, or to stop weaving the delusional experiences in their autobiographies by constructing scenarios in which such experiences would make sense even if the delusional state were false.

Gerrans tends to present mental time travel as opposed to weighing up possibilities by reasoning and suggests that we should distinguish the practice of developing autobiographies from that of formulating and testing scientific hypotheses. He compares two ways of making the decision whether to go surfing in the vicinity of dangerous-looking cliffs: either imagining what it would be like to go, or computing the probability of potential risks, such as that of a shark attack. The former method, achieved via mental time travel, can be misleading depending on the type of past experiences the agent has, which could be relevant to the present decision, or not. The latter method involves a calculus that does not involve the recall of past experiences.

> The point to emphasize is that the same cognitive processes influence both MTT and hypothetical reasoning. In the former case, however, they select or create an experience and insert it as an episode in an autobiography. In the latter, they select evidence and evaluate it for consistency with a theory according to a prescriptive theory of confirmation. There is no essential role for recalled or imagined experience except to suggest a hypothesis for testing.
>
> (Gerrans 2009, p. 162)

Why does there need to be a competition between the autobiographer and the scientist within us? I suggested earlier that for some thoughts, those thoughts that can be defended with reasons and are important to a conception of who we are, belief status is conditional on the subject being in a position to self ascribe the thought and provide reasons for it that she considers as good reasons. That is, it would not be beneficial to ascribe to a subject the belief that all songs on the radio are sung by him, unless the subject was able to defend that claim. The problem is not that the belief would be irrational, but that its attribution to the subject would not allow further explanation and prediction of behaviour in intentional terms—it would not be integrated in the subject's self narrative and thus it would not guide future action. My suggestion, which I see as entirely sympathetic to Gerrans' proposal but perhaps occupying a different position in the dialectic, would be that *for some thoughts* there is no clear-cut distinction between the stance of the scientist weighing up possibilities on the basis of past evidence, and the stance of the autobiographer trying (at the same time) to provide an accurate description of significant life events and to integrate these events into a coherent narrative. Some of the evidence that would be relevant to explaining my impression that all songs on the radio are sung by me is autobiographical and episodic in nature: Did I sign a deal with the radio station? Do I remember recording these songs? But background knowledge which does not need to be autobiographical or episodic could also provide a context for a judgement of plausibility: how likely is it that the station plays only songs performed by one (non-professional) singer? These considerations act together to constrain (or fail to constrain, in the case of delusion) the adoption of hypotheses about ourselves and the world around us.

### 5.3.3 Mental time travel and agency

In a recent paper discussing the effects of certain forms of psychopathology on autonomy and moral responsibility, Kennett and Matthews (2009) argue that one condition that is necessary for a person to be autonomous is the capacity to make choices and decisions which commit one's future self to certain courses of action (p. 329).[20] Summarising a report from Levine and colleagues (1998) and commenting on the role of mental time travel in planning, Kennett and Matthews make a case for the necessity of episodic memory for forward planning:

> M.L. suffered a severe brain injury and was in the immediate post-injury period amnesic both for events and persons as well as suffering impairments in semantic knowledge. He made a good recovery from his semantic deficits and he re-learned significant facts about his own past. However, his recall of events from his personal past remained fragmentary. Moreover and significantly, M.L. was unable to episodically re-experience *post*-injury events to the same extent as control subjects, although he could use familiarity or other non-episodic processes to distinguish events he had experienced from those he had not experienced. He continued to report a feeling of subjective distance from recall of events occurring *after* his recovery. He displayed errors of judgement and failures to understand his responsibilities as a parent that required supervision of his behaviour and structured routines. He was unable to secure paid employment [...]. Cases such as M.L. bring out the importance of the kind of access we have to past episodes for the purposes of planning and deliberation. An effective agent is the true author of the project, fully invested in its completion, and above all she has a knowledge of it that is part and parcel of her self knowledge.

> (Kennett and Matthews 2009, p. 340)

In conditions such as dissociative identity disorder[21], where people do not have complete access to their previous thoughts and actions, and do not have a sense of having been the author of these thoughts and actions, and in conditions similar to that of ML who cannot have episodic memories of events that occurred after his accident, deliberation and moral responsibility for action can be compromised. The person with dissociation who acts when in an alter state does not have the capacity to act on her previous commitments and values, or to deliberate on the basis of past experiences. People who have deficits in episodic memory such as ML cannot exercise deliberative control over the actions performed after their episodic memory was damaged.

The same conclusions Kennett and Matthews draw about certain conditions affecting memory could be drawn with respect to people with delusions, if they also suffered from an impairment in mental time travel, and their capacities for deliberation and self control were also shown to be absent or deficient. But there are other ways to bring home the fact that some delusions cannot be the basis for autonomous decision-making and action. These involve, once again,

---

[20] For an interesting account of the *stability* of the self, see Lenman (2009).
[21] This disorder was previously named 'multiple personality disorder'. For some historical background and interesting philosophical discussion of the conditions for this disorder, see Humphreys and Dennett (1989) and Hacking (1995).

the notion of ownership and authorship of thoughts, and their connection with ownership and authorship of decisions and actions.

Remember the example of Bonnie who claims she is going to move to Egypt, but she cannot give any reason why. The interpreter is in an uncomfortable position. If Bonnie had said that she wanted yellow shoes, but had not followed the expression of her desire with a reason, the interpreter would not have hesitated to take her report as a sufficient reason to ascribe to her a desire with that content. After all, people do desire strange things on a whim and some preferences for certain shapes, styles or colours might not be accompanied by any further explanation. But the claim that she wants to move to Egypt is different. It involves an important personal decision with far reaching consequences and it is the kind of decision that is usually made after careful consideration of the possible advantages and disadvantages of the move. If Bonnie cannot offer any reason for wanting to move to Egypt, then the interpreter might wonder whether Bonnie really wants to move to Egypt, whether her report has been meant, whether to take it seriously. The delusional reports we find most puzzling are not those that contradict some well-accepted opinion, or those that come with an elaborated and yet bizarre explanation. The reports that trouble interpreters, and often paralyse or compromise interpretation, are those that *sound like* the reports of beliefs that should be accompanied by some reasons, and should be the core feature of a chapter in the subject's autobiography, but are not defended with reasons, and the subject does not seem to identify with someone who has those beliefs.

In those circumstances, as when I say that someone has inserted into my head the thought 'Kill Lissie', the thought gives rise neither to autonomous decision, nor to autonomous action. There is no process of self constitution, on the basis of which a previous value or commitment of mine influences my behaviour. Rather, the thought remains on the surface, at the periphery of my autobiography.It has not been integrated and has not been rejected either: it simply floats there in my consciousness, occupying cognitive resources and having a disturbing effect, but generating no sense of ownership or authorship in myself.

Rarely do we have these clear-cut cases: delusional reports that are fully endorsed *versus* disowned thoughts. Most of the delusions we read about, and we come across, are integrated in the subject's narrative, to some extent, and with limitations. They may be excessively compartmentalised, for instance, or justified tentatively. That is what makes it so difficult to discuss the relationship between delusions, subjects' commitment to the content of the delusion, and autonomy. As authorship comes in degrees, so does the capacity to manifest the endorsement of the delusional thought in autonomous thought and action.

## 5.3.4 **Coherence *versus* correspondence**[22]

We seem to have a problem. On the one hand, self narratives that are cohesive and aim at integrating all the relevant conscious thoughts of the subject have clear epistemic benefits: they deliver a coherent self concept. On the other hand, when some of the thoughts are delusional, and thus likely to be both false and have a content that is distressing to the subject, cohesion might have epistemic disadvantages: by integrating delusional thoughts in a coherent narrative and finding reasons for them, the subject is less prone to revise her delusions in the presence of external challenges. Delusions that are the object of confabulation and rationalisation become *ingrained*.

The positive and negative aspects of confabulating and rationalising have been observed in other contexts: in normal cognition and in other psycho-pathologies. Finding reasons for a false and irrational belief cannot but give rise to more false and irrational beliefs, and thus be epistemically bad. But confabulations and rationalisations can have an adaptive function:

> The real reason for the evolution of these defense mechanisms (confabulations, rationalization), I suggest is to create a coherent system in order to impose stability in one's behaviour. [...] When something doesn't quite fit the script however, you very rarely tear up the entire story and start from scratch. What you do, instead, is to deny or confabulate in order to make the information fit the big picture.
>
> (Ramachandran 1996, p. 351)

Do any of these pragmatic benefits also have *epistemic* value? We shall explore the suggestion that confabulation is sometimes the only means by which people can maintain a unified and coherent sense of self—and ask whether this is beneficial in the case of delusions. Fotopoulou (2008) observes that after brain damage or memory loss, personal narratives can be disrupted, under-mining people's sense of coherence and making the future less predictable. This is often associated with increased anxiety and depression.

> Despite their poor correspondence with reality, confabulations represent attempts to define one's self in time and in relation to the world. Thus, they are subject to motiva-tional influences and they serve important identity formation functions.
>
> (Fotopoulou 2008, p. 542)

In the context of serious memory disorders, Fotopoulou argues that confabulators construct *distorted* or *false selves*. They may claim that they live in a different place, that they have a different profession, or a different family.

---

[22] Arguments in this section have been developed with Rochelle Cox. For more details, see Bortolotti and Cox (forthcoming).

The personal narrative confabulators construct is not 'anchored and constrained by reality' (2008, p. 548). These distortions are exaggerated by brain damage or memory loss, but are not different types of distortions from those present in normal subjects attempting to remember past events and making errors (see Burgess and Shallice 1996). Confabulators' narratives might also exhibit an exaggerated self-serving bias but the majority of people reconstruct memories that are consistent with their desired self-image.

> To some degree, and for the sake of creating a coherency to life, it is normal to confabulate and to enhance one's story. Self-deception is not unusual; false memories are frequent.
>
> (Gallagher 2003, p. 348)

It is what Fotopoulou calls the 'identity formation' of confabulation that interests us here. In dementia or amnesia, patients revisit their past and attempt to build a bridge with their premorbid self in order to make sense of their present experiences and feelings. Confabulations are instrumental for subjects to establish continuity between the image of themselves before the accident, the illness, or the memory loss, and the image of themselves afterwards. Confabulations are also an attempt to preserve a positive self image. These two functions of confabulation can also be observed in normal subjects (Wilson and Ross 2003) who tend to present their current selves in a way that is both coherent and largely favourable.

This reflection on the potential effects of confabulation suggests a tension between the aim of preserving coherence and the aim of being constrained by reality. According to Conway (2005), achieving a balance between coherence with self and correspondence with reality is one of the challenges faced by our autobiographical memory system. This balance allows us to maintain a coherent system where one's goals, beliefs, and self-images are consistent with autobiographical memories. Conway's model implies that if there is a change in self, there is also likely to be a change in the accessibility of autobiographical memories. To test this idea, Cox and Barnier asked high hypnotisable participants to generate memories in response to 10 cue sentences. Following a hypnotic induction, they gave participants a delusion suggestion to become one of their siblings. They then asked them to generate memories in response to another 10 cue sentences. This time, half of the sentences had been presented to participants before hypnosis and half of the sentences were new. Participants were informed that if the cue sentence was the same as one that had been previously presented, they should try to recall the same memory they had provided earlier. Cox and Barnier found that participants who experienced the suggested delusion had difficulty recalling the memories they had originally provided. Rather, they recalled different memories from the perspective of the deluded identity. This suggests that the original memories they had provided were no longer accessible to the deluded identity. For these participants, coherence with the deluded experience was prioritised over correspondence with reality.

'Normal' confabulators provide reasons for their attitudes that help them maintain coherence among their beliefs and preferences, although they are not aware of what prompted them to report those attitudes in the first place (Haidt 2001). In these situations, coherence trumps correspondence, as the real reasons for their attitudes (basic emotions or position effects driving judgements and choice) are not introspectively available. Consider also confabulators with dementia or brain damage. They act out a script that is roughly known to them, and that links their current experiences with common experiences lived by their previous selves and remembered in a superficial, fragmented and possibly even biased way. Again, coherence trumps correspondence, as the 'reality' to which their stories should make reference (their past lives and their connection to their present lives) is poorly (if at all) remembered, and poorly understood. Finally, consider subjects with delusions. They find themselves with a certain belief, or experience, and they support it with secondary confabulations that allow them to present a coherent and intelligible position, rather than crumble under the pressure of contradictions and challenges. Yet again coherence trumps correspondence, as the 'reality' they describe is coloured by beliefs whose process of acquisition is not necessarily introspectively available to them.

The obvious disadvantage of the preference for coherence over correspondence is that losing touch with reality can create a gulf between the person with delusions and confabulations and her interlocutors. Given that confabulations are made of ill-grounded statements about the present or the past, they do little to remedy the 'ignorance' (i.e. inaccessibility of information) which caused them in the first place, and they are not likely to be believed by others. Fotopoulou (2008, p. 560) remarks that in the most serious amnesic conditions there is often a lack of 'shared reality' between confabulators and the people who were once closest to them, which can be very distressing for patients and their families. Moreover, in the case of delusions, as I previously suggested, rationalisation can contribute to increasing the elaboration and the rigidity of delusions—this is likely to result in delusions becoming less sensitive to counterevidence or counterargument. However, confabulating can also have some pragmatic benefits that may lead to epistemic benefits: it allows people to keep constructing self narratives in situations where personal information is no longer available. As a result, it secures some psychological continuity with the confabulators' previous selves in the absence of reliable recollective capacities, and contributes to the preservation of psychological integration in absence of introspective access to the reasons for conscious mental states such as beliefs, desires and preferences. It also allows people to include new facts into previously developed narratives that have become fragmented.

When a delusion becomes integrated in a subject's self narrative and part of the self concept, giving up the delusion can generate lack of self esteem, confusion and depression in the subject. Suppose I have mistakenly believed for some time that I am a news presenter at the BBC. As a consequence of this delusion, I tell people in the pub about my life in the spotlight, always on TV, and about my good salary and my exotic holidays. But in real life I am jobless, I live on benefits, and I have no real friends. What will happen if I am 'cured of' my delusion? I will start doubting that I work for the BBC, but I will also appreciate that everything I thought to be true about myself was false. I will start seeing my life as it really is, empty. The effects of making one's self narrative correspond to reality can be devastating, and many subjects experience serious depression when they acquire insight into their illness.

## Summary of chapter 5

In this chapter I started by exploring the relationship between authorship, first-person authority and the intentionality of belief states. We ended Chapter 4 with the claim that the ascription of agentially irrational beliefs is perfectly possible, but in this chapter we wanted to know whether a state needs to be authored in order to be ascribed as a belief and in what way authorship of a thought gives rise to a type of first-person authority over that thought.

In Section 5.1, I argued that authorship contributes to self knowledge by creating for the subject an additional route to the knowledge that she has a certain belief. The literature on the epistemic faults of reason-giving reminds us that the processes of deliberation and justification which characterise authorship are often far from rational, and that the attitudes we author can also be irrational. However, there is no indication that authorship fails to contribute to first-person authority, unless we assume incredibly demanding conditions for first-person authority.

In Section 5.2, I consider a case in which thoughts are neither owned nor authored, and I observe that both first-person authority and belief ascription are compromised. The case is that of 'inserted' thoughts, a common phenomenon in schizophrenia, where subjects claim that some of the thoughts to which they have direct access have been inserted in their heads by someone else and are not theirs. Here we have a radical failure of ownership and authorship, which compromises the belief status of 'inserted' thoughts. There are no signs of the subject's commitment to the content of these thoughts, and no behavioural manifestation of their endorsement.

In Section 5.3, I asked what happens when authorship fails. Feeling entitled to the content of a belief allows the subject to write the belief into her personal narrative—the belief contributes to her concept of herself, and this self concept in turn has the potential to shape future behaviour. It is then unsurprising that some have described delusions as cases in which a subject becomes an unreliable autobiographer: what seems puzzling about delusions is not their being irrational, but their badly fitting with an overall narrative that affects the interpretation of the subject's personal history but also her capacities for decision-making and forward-planning.

# Chapter 6

## Conclusions

Let me summarise the key points of the present project.

### 6.1 **On delusions**

I hope I gave you reasons to take seriously the doxastic conception of delusions, and the view that there is considerable continuity between delusions and beliefs. The delusion that I am dead is very different from the belief that the supermarket will be closed on Sunday, but this does not show that there is a categorical difference between delusions and beliefs. Here is a challenge. For each delusion, I'll give you a belief that matches the type if not the degree of irrationality of the delusion. We saw some examples: paranoid beliefs are badly supported by the evidence, and sometimes also as resistant to counterevidence as delusions of persecution. The delusion that I'm dead is often justified in a viciously circular way, not dissimilar from the way in which prejudiced beliefs against a racial group are justified. The delusion that someone of a higher status loves me, or the delusion that my partner is unfaithful can be defended by mentioning facts that are apparently irrelevant. This is not so different from the strenuous defence of superstitious beliefs which seem to get confirmation no matter what happens. In many circumstances, the styles of reasoning that contribute to the irrationality of a delusion (externalisation and personalisation, self-serving biases, etc.) are common in groups of normal subjects, although normal subjects seem to have a better capacity to exercise reality checks on the beliefs they report.

One might suppose that a project aimed at clarifying the nature of delusions should deliver some wisdom on how delusions should be classified. I have done very little in this regard. But I have endorsed a negative thesis that I can emphasise here. What makes delusions different from other reported beliefs? The difference, if there is one, is not in their epistemic features. Thus a definition of delusions based exclusively on surface features of an epistemic kind (such as resisting counterevidence, being false, not being justified, etc.) will not demarcate successfully delusions from other irrational beliefs, and possibly from other manifestations of mental illness (e.g. confabulation, obsessions, etc.). What makes delusions pathological? Whatever it is, it is not their being irrational, because the irrationality of delusions is not different in kind from the irrationality of everyday beliefs. Delusions are on a continuum with irrational beliefs, and you are likely to find them towards the 'very irrational' end of the line, where the degree of rationality tracks both how much they deviate from norms of rationality for beliefs and how many norms of rationality they deviate from.

We assume there is a neat divide between people being mistaken about how much money they owe in their tax return, and people who bark like dogs. And it must seem wasteful, especially to clinical-orientated readers, to dedicate a full project to the nature of delusions and have nothing positive to say about what makes them pathological. So here are some suggestions worth exploring. One possibility is that delusions are pathological in that they negatively affect the well-being and the health of the subjects who report them (as many have already argued). Irrational beliefs that are not delusions seem less distressing, and don't seem to exhaust the cognitive resources of the subject in the same way that delusions do. Another possibility is that delusions are more puzzling than other irrational beliefs and this is how we instantly recognise that something is wrong when someone reports a delusion, even if we have no special training or experience. I doubt that it is true that *all* delusions are puzzling and easily detectable: delusions of jealousy or delusions about God revealing himself are not that puzzling in certain contexts and it might take some questioning to ascertain that the subject reporting them has a mental health issue. But this is not to deny that delusions such as Capgras and Cotard are very puzzling. Does this contribute to their being pathological? I don't think so. I am sure that it is a merely contingent fact (contingent on human history and culture) that we find the belief that a clone has replaced one's relative much more puzzling and disturbing than the belief that all Jewish people are after money, that black people are violent, or that women never make good scientists. The fact that something defies our expectations might signal something deep and important about the nature of that thing, or might just be due to its being statistically unusual and to its finding us unprepared. The puzzling content of some delusions is not an indication of their being pathological, it is just an effect of their being less common than other irrational beliefs. That is why, in the DSM-IV definition of delusions, there is that clause about delusions not being likely to be shared by the community to which the subject belongs. Sexist or racist beliefs are more common that beliefs about being dead.

Of course there are truly puzzling aspects of the reporting of delusional states, but these do not necessarily concern the content of the delusion, or at least, not the content in isolation from other things. What seems puzzling in some delusions is that the subject is not fully committed to the content of the delusion, and the most convincing arguments against the doxastic conception are those based on the observation of double-bookkeeping. If the subject is not in a position to ascribe the content of the delusion to herself, or to defend that content with reasons, we legitimately worry about delusions not being beliefs. Delusional moods and experiences which do not lead the subject to commit herself to the content of her reports may fail the belief test, not because they are irrational, but because they signal a failure of self knowledge.

## 6.2 **On beliefs**

In the book I also wanted to distinguish between the good and bad of interpretationism. It is good that we attempt to describe the nature of beliefs by looking at how the practice of belief ascription works. But it is bad that we idealise beliefs by supposing that belief ascription could not happen unless there was a general background of rationality. Thus, I offered reasons to reject the rationality constraint on belief ascription, and at the same time showed that there are still interesting things that we can say about the difference between beliefs and other intentional states and about the assumptions an interpreter relies on when she is out there, trying to make sense of what other speakers, infants and animals are doing. So, what can we say about the nature of beliefs, once we have rejected the rationality constraint? We can mention what their core features are—these features guide everyday interpretation, together with other generalisations, the interpreter's background knowledge, and relevant information about the environment and the subject. But are my 'core features' really different from rationality constraints? Let me draw some conclusions from the discussion so far by offering a sketchy guide to belief ascription. There won't be an exhaustive account of how *all* beliefs behave, because I don't think there can be one, but, after rejecting rationality constraints in chapters 2, 3 and 4, I want to emphasise the constructive side of the project.

The way in which interpreters ascribe beliefs changes depending on the shared environment, on the subject and on the context of interpretation. We know from our own daily practice of interpretation that there are no golden rules, and we have been reminded of it in the course of the previous chapters. It is to be expected, then, that some of the principles guiding the ascription of perceptual beliefs may not apply to the ascription of religious beliefs or metaphysical commitments; and the assumptions guiding the interpretation of a baby's first words are different from those guiding the interpretation of an old friend talking about his problems at work. Following the rough but convenient map drawn at the start, which captures the procedural, epistemic and agential dimensions of belief states, I want to provide a description of the core features of beliefs and an elucidation of the folk-psychological notion of belief.

### 6.2.1 Beliefs are integrated in a system and have some inferential relations with other intentional states

In Chapter 2, I asked whether procedural rationality can serve as a constraint on the ascription of beliefs, and argued that it cannot. It is too demanding to expect beliefs to be constrained by the norm of good integration, which is a norm of procedural rationality, but there are procedural aspects that are an important part of the notion of belief. Although badly integrated intentional states can be ascribed to subjects as beliefs, a belief-like state needs to have *some* inferential relations with other things the same subject believes, wishes, desires, and so on, in order to be usefully ascribed to that subject as a belief. 'Jonah doesn't let me get even close to his brand new car—he must think I'm a dangerous driver.' Here, I explain a subject's behaviour on the basis of a belief, the belief that I am not a good, reliable driver, which will affect other intentional states of the same subject, such as his preference for not letting me drive his car. If that belief did not have *any* connection *whatsoever* with *any* other intentional state of the subject, it would not be useful for the interpreter to ascribe it as a belief. Naturally, this does not rule out that some beliefs can be heavily compartmentalised and have sparse inferential relations to other intentional states. This will be partially determined by the nature of the belief and the level of commitment that the subject has to the content of the belief— how well the belief has been integrated in the subject's self narrative.

The feature I propose, that a subject's beliefs have *some* inferential relations with other intentional states, is not a rationality constraint. A belief can have some inferential relations with other intentional states without being procedurally rational. The belief that I won't lose my job in spite of a financial crisis may come from the conviction that many students want to read philosophy at university, but is not well-integrated in my belief system on the whole, and thus procedurally rational, if I also believe that fewer people will go to university as a consequence of the crisis.

### 6.2.2 Beliefs are sensitive to evidence or argument

In Chapter 3 we rejected responsiveness to evidence as a necessary condition for belief ascription, because it is an excessively demanding criterion. However, there is a sense in which considerations about evidence play a special role in the ascription of beliefs. Instead of demanding that beliefs be necessarily responsive to the available evidence, we can expect at least some beliefs to be at least *sensitive* to evidence. This feature might be irrelevant if we are interested in beliefs whose content is such that sensitivity to evidence is not expected or possible, such as beliefs about a supernatural world that is not directly experienced via the senses . Suppose that Francesco is convinced that he will reach Nirvana when he extinguishes greed, ignorance and hatred, and thus he embarks on a journey to obtain enlightenment, according to his Buddhist faith. To some extent, the content of Francesco's belief is insulated from empirical challenges. There will be times when he thinks that he has no greed, ignorance or hatred in himself, and yet he believes that he has not reached Nirvana yet. He can then come to believe that some other condition needs to be satisfied to get to that state of liberation from suffering; that he has not really ridden himself of greed, ignorance and hatred as he thought he did; or that he has reached Nirvana but he is not aware of having done so. Some of our beliefs are virtually unfalsifiable and our clinging to them may be regarded as a mark of irrationality, but even these beliefs display *some* sensitivity to evidence: they might not be rejected, but they are often revised or the inferential relations between them and other beliefs are revised in the light of new experiences.

Sensitivity to evidence is obviously a feature of perceptual beliefs, and of beliefs about the explanation and prediction of observable events. If Sunita believes that today there will be sunshine at lunchtime, and continues to believe so even when the sky gets darker and rain starts to fall, something is amiss. She does not need to abandon her belief outright: she might stubbornly come to believe that soon the rain will stop and the sun will return to shine. These slight revisions and adjustments to her beliefs about today's weather show that her beliefs are sensitive to how things are. Beliefs about the weather (or finance, health, crime, cinema, etc.) are fallible and are revised or adjusted as a consequence of further experiences, although they may be revised too slowly because we tend to be conservative, or may be insulated from contrary evidence if we invest them with emotional significance.

Notice that, although sensitivity to evidence has a better chance than responsiveness to evidence to work as a constraint on the ascription of beliefs, it is not a *rationality* constraint. A belief can be sensitive to evidence without being epistemically rational. For instance, I can come to revise my belief that recession has slowed down the housing market because I see that houses in London sell fast, ignoring that the house market is still slow, but the scarcity of houses on the market in an area where demand is constantly high causes the effect I have observed. Retaining an epistemic dimension in our account of beliefs vindicates the insight that the relationship between the content of an intentional state and the evidence available to the subject is central to whether that intentional state is a belief, and at the same time offers a guideline to belief ascription that can be met by most beliefs.

### 6.2.3 Beliefs can be manifested in behaviour

In Chapter 4 I distinguished between action guidance and behavioural manifestability. That distinction will come in handy now. Action guidance requires that beliefs lead to a specific action in the appropriate circumstances, so that the action performed can be seen as consistent with and explicable by the subject having that belief. Very few beliefs would satisfy this requirement of agential rationality, for different reasons. Some beliefs have contents that are not specific enough to be action guiding, as they cannot be seen to be the reason why the agent did something, in isolation from other beliefs or other intentional states ('The grass is green'). Moreover, attitude-behaviour consistency is a regulative ideal for real-life agents: expecting them to systematically act in a way that is consistent with their reported beliefs would lead to disappointment ('I should go to the gym more often').

Behavioural manifestability is a much looser notion than action guidance, but it is useful in the context of elucidating the folk-psychological notion of belief, as all beliefs have the potential to be manifested in behaviour, be this a mere verbal report, or a behavioural disposition of which the subject herself might not even be aware.

### 6.2.4 Beliefs can be self ascribed and some beliefs can be defended with reasons

As we saw in Chapters 4 and 5, judgements of ownership and authorship of thoughts seem to correlate with judgements about the intelligibility of belief reports. Intelligibility is a weaker notion than rationality. I can understand (sympathise with) behaviour that I do not regard as rational. If I expect people's behaviour to be *intelligible*, what I expect from them when they report belief states is that they are in a position to ascribe these beliefs to themselves and they have some relevant reason, some reason they regard as a good reason, for endorsing the content of their belief states. If I expect people's behaviour to be *rational*, I expect more (how much more depends on the type of belief): for instance, I might expect from people reporting beliefs that they have reasons in support of the content of their beliefs that are intersubjectively acknowledged as good reasons. These considerations helped us answer questions about the belief status of delusions: it is plausible to suggest that the more a subject is able to support the content of her delusion with reasons, the more the delusion is amenable to being characterised in intentional terms by an interpreter. By that I mean that it will be easier (and less indeterminate) to identify meaningful links between that delusional state and the subjects' (other) beliefs, and it will be easier to provide a satisfactory explanation and an accurate prediction of the subject's behaviour in intentional terms. Delusions whose content cannot be endorsed by the subject reporting them may not be usefully ascribed as beliefs to that subject.

Beliefs don't need to be rationally justified, but the subject reporting a belief needs to preserve the capacity to express some commitment to the content of that belief. Importantly, ownership and authorship are not sufficient for rationality. But they are conditions for a certain type of self knowledge, the agential authority that we sometimes exercise on the beliefs we have. This agential authority allows us to weave beliefs into a personal narrative which will guide future behaviour.

# Bibliography and reference list

Abelson, R.P. (1972). Are attitudes necessary? In B.T. King and E. McGinnies (eds.) *Attitudes, Conflict, and Social Change*. New York (NY): Academic Press; 19–32.

Abelson, R.P., Shank, R.C., and Langer, E.J. (eds.) (1994). *Beliefs, Reasoning, and Decision Making*. Hillsdale (NJ): Lawrence Erlbaum.

Addis, D.R. and Tippett, L.J. (2008). The contributions of autobiographical memory to the content and continuity of self: a social-cognitive neuroscience approach. In F. Sani (Ed.) *Self-Continuity: Individual and Collective Perspectives*. New York (NY): Psychology Press; 71–84.

Addis, D.R., Wong, A.T., and Schacter, D.L. (2007). Remembering the past and imagining the future: Common and distinct neural substrates during event construction and elaboration. *Neuropsychologia* 45(7): 1363–1377.

Ajzen, I. (2005). *Attitude, Personality and Behavior*. Maidenhead: McGraw-Hill.

Aimola, A.M. (1999). *Dark Side of the Moon: Studies in Unilateral Neglect*. PhD dissertation, University of Auckland.

Aimola Davies, A.M. and Davies, M. (2009). Explaining pathologies of belief. In M.R. Broome and L. Bortolotti (eds.) *Psychiatry as Cognitive Neuroscience: Philosophical Perspectives*. Oxford: Oxford University Press; chapter 14.

Aimola Davies, A.M., Davies, M., Ogden, J., Smithson, M., and White, R.C. (2008). Cognitive and motivational factors in anosognosia. In T. Bayne and J. Fernàndez (eds.) *Delusion and Self-deception: Affective and Motivational Influences on Belief Formation*. Hove: Psychology Press; 187–226.

Allen, C. and Bekoff, M. (1997). *Species of Mind: The Philosophy and Biology of Cognitive Ethology*. Cambridge (MA): MIT Press; chapter 5.

American Psychiatric Association (2000). *Diagnostic Statistical Manual of Mental Disorders*. (4th edn.), Text Revision (DSM-IV-TR).

Ames, D. (1984). Self shooting of a phantom head. *British Journal of Psychiatry* 145(2): 193–194.

Andreason, N.C. (2007). DSM and the death of phenomenology in America: An example of unintended consequences. *Schizophrenia Bulletin* 33(1): 108–112.

Appelbaum, P.S., Clark Robbins, P., and Monahan, J. (2000). Violence and delusion: Data from the MacArthur Violence Risk Assessment Study. *American Journal of Psychiatry*, 157(4): 566–572.

Aronson, E. (1999). Dissonance, hypocrisy and the self concept. In E. Harmon-Jones and J. Mills (eds.) *Cognitive Dissonance: Progress on a Pivotal Theory in Social Psychology*. Washington (DC): American Psychological Association; 103–126.

Barnier, A., Cox, R., O'Connor, A., Coltheart, M., Langdon, R., Breen, N., and Turner, M. (2008). Developing hypnotic analogues of clinical delusions: Mirrored-self misidentification. *Cognitive Neuropsychiatry* 13(5): 406–430.

Barnier, A.J. (2002). Posthypnotic amnesia for autobiographical episodes: A laboratory model of functional amnesia? *Psychological Science* 13(3): 232–237.

Barnier, A.J. and Council, J.R. (in press). Hypnotizability matters: The what, why, and how of measurement. In S.J. Lynn and I. Kirsch (eds.) *Handbook of Clinical Hypnosis* (2nd edn.). Washington (DC): American Psychological Association.

Barnier, A.J. and McConkey, K.M. (1999). Autobiographical remembering and forgetting: What can hypnosis tell us? *International Journal of Clinical and Experimental Hypnosis*, 47(4):346–365.

Barnier, A.J., McConkey, K.M., and Wright, J. (2004). Posthypnotic amnesia for autobiographical episodes: Influencing memory accessibility and quality. *International Journal of Clinical and Experimental Hypnosis* 52(3): 260–279.

Baumeister, R. (ed.) (1999). *The Self in Social Psychology: Key Readings.* Philadelphia (PA): Psychology Press.

Bayne, T. and Fernández, J. (2008)-(eds.) *Delusion and Self-deception: Affective and Motivational Influences on Belief Formation.* Hove: Psychology Press.

Bayne, T. and Pacherie E. (2004a). Bottom up or top down? *Philosophy, Psychiatry, & Psychology* 11(1): 1–11.

Bayne, T. and Pacherie, E. (2004b). Experience, belief, and the interpretive fold. *Philosophy, Psychiatry, & Psychology* 11(1): 81–86.

Bayne, T. and Pacherie, E. (2005). In defence of the doxastic conception of delusion. *Mind & Language* 20(2): 163–188.

Bayne, T. and Pacherie, E. (2007). Narrators and comparators: The architecture of agentive self-awareness. *Synthese* 159(3): 475–91.

Beck, A.T., Rector, N.A., Stolar, N., and Grant, P. (2008) *Schizophrenia: Cognitive Theory, Reseach and Therapy.* New York (NY): Guilford Press.

Bell, V., Halligan, P., and Ellis, H. (2003). Beliefs about delusions. *The Psychologist* 16(8): 418–423.

Bell, V., Halligan, P., and Ellis, H. (2006). Explaining delusions: a cognitive perspective. *Trends in Cognitive Science* 10(5): 219–226.

Bem, D.J. (1967). Self-Perception: An alternative interpretation of cognitive dissonance phenomena. *Psychological Review* 74(3): 183–200.

Bentall, R.P. (2003). The paranoid self. In T. Kircher and A. David (eds.) *The Self in Neuroscience and Psychiatry.* New York (NY): Cambridge University Press; 293–318.

Bentall, R.P. and Kaney, S. (1989). Content specific processing and persecutory delusions: an investigation using the emotional Stroop test. *British Journal of Medical Psychology* 62(4): 355–364.

Bentall, R.P. and Kaney, S. (1996). Abnormalities of self-representation and persecutory delusions: a test of cognitive model of paranoia. *Psychological Medicine* 26(6): 1231–1237.

Bentall, R.P., Corcoran, R., Howard, R., Blackwood, N., and Kinderman, P. (2001). Persecutory delusions: A review and theoretical integration. *Clinical Psychology Review* 21(8): 1143–1192.

Berg, N. and Gigerenzer, G. (2006). Unhappy inconsistencies in Kacelnik et al.'s many-happy-rationalities program. In L. Daston and C. Engel (eds.) *Is There a Value in Inconsistency?* Baden-Baden: Nomos; 423–433.

Berkowitz, L. (ed.) (1984). *Advances in Experimental Social Psychology*. New York (NY): Academic Press.

Berlyne, N. (1972). Confabulation. *British Journal of Psychiatry* 120(554): 31–39.

Bermúdez, J. (2001). Normativity and rationality in delusional psychiatric disorders. *Mind & Language*, 16(5): 493–457.

Berridge, K.C. and Robinson, T.E. (1998). What is the role of dopamine in reward: hedonic impact, reward learning, or incentive salience? *Brain Research Reviews* 28(3): 309–369.

Berrios, G.E. (1991). Delusions as 'wrong beliefs': a conceptual history. *British Journal of Psychiatry* 159 (suppl. 14): 6–13.

Berrios, G.E. (1998). Confabulations: a conceptual history. *Journal of the History of the Neurosciences* 7(3): 225–241.

Berrios, G.E. (2000). Confabulations. In G.E. Berrios and J.R. Hodges (eds.) *Memory Disorders in Psychiatric Practice*. New York (NY): Cambridge University Press; 348–368.

Berrios, G.E. and Luque, R. (1995a). Cotard's syndrome: analysis of 100 cases. *Acta Psychiatrica Scandinavica* 91(3): 185–188.

Berrios, G.E. and Luque, R. (1995b). Cotard's delusion or syndrome: a conceptual history. *Comprehensive Psychiatry* 35(3): 218–223.

Berti, A., Làvadas, E., Stracciari, A., Giannarelli, C., and Ossola, A. (1998). Anosognosia for motor impairment and dissociations with patients' evaluation of the disorder: Theoretical considerations. *Cognitive Neuropsychiatry* 3(1): 21–44.

Bettman, J.R., Luce, M.F., and Payne, J.W. (1998). Constructive consumer choice processes. *Journal of Consumer Research* 25(3): 187–217.

Binkofski, F., Buccino, G., Dohle, C., Seitz, R.J., and Freund, H.J. (1999). Mirror agnosia and mirror ataxia constitute different parietal lobe disorders. *Annals of Neurology* 46(1): 51–61.

Bisiach, E., Rusconi, M.L., and Vallar, G. (1991). Remission of somatoparaphrenic delusion through vestibular stimulation. *Neuropsychologia* 29(10): 1029–1031.

Blackwood, N.J., Howard, R., Bentall, R., and Murray, R. (2001). Cognitive neuropsychiatric models of persecutory delusions. *American Journal of Psychiatry* 158(4): 527–539.

Blakemore, S.J., Oakley, D.A., and Frith, C.D. (2003). Delusions of alien control in the normal brain. *Neuropsychologia* 41(8): 1058–1067.

Blaney, P.H. (1999). Paranoid conditions. In T. Millon, P.H. Blaney, and R.D. Davis (eds.) *Oxford Textbook of Psychopathology*. New York (NY): Oxford University Press; chapter 13.

Bleichrodt, H. and Pinto Prades, J. (2009). New evidence of preference reversals in health utility measurement. *Health Economics* 18(6): 713–726.

Bless, H., Betsch, T., and Franzen, A. (1998). Framing the framing effect. *European Journal of Social Psychology* 28(2): 287–291.

Bleuler, E. (1924). *Textbook of Psychiatry*. Transl. by A. Brill. New York (NY): Macmillan.

Bleuler, E. (1950). *Dementia Precox, or the Group of Schizophrenias*. New York (NY), International University Press.

Bloom, P. and German, T.P. (2000). Two reasons to abandon the false belief task as a test of theory of mind. *Cognition* 77(1): B25–B31.

Blum, G.S. (1975). A case study of hypnotically induced tubular vision. *International Journal of Clinical and Experimental Hypnosis* 23(2): 111–119.

Blum, L.A. (2002). *I'm not a racist, but . . . The Moral Quandary of Race*. Ithaca (NY): Cornell University Press.

Bolton, D. and Hill, J. (2003). *Mind, Meaning and Mental Disorder: the Nature of Causal Explanation in Psychology and Psychiatry*. New York (NY): Oxford University Press.

Bortolotti, L. (2002). Marks of irrationality. In S. Clarke and T. Lyons (eds.) *Scientific Realism and Common Sense: Recent Themes in the Philosophy of Science*. New York (NY): Kluwer; 157–174.

Bortolotti, L. (2003). Inconsistency and interpretation. *Philosophical Explorations* VI(2), 109–123.

Bortolotti, L. (2004). Can we interpret irrational behavior? *Behavior and Philosophy* 32(2): 359–375.

Bortolotti, L. (2005a). Delusions and the background of rationality. *Mind & Language* 20(2): 189–208.

Bortolotti, L. (2005b). Intentionality without rationality. *Proceedings of the Aristotelian Society* CV(3): 385–392.

Bortolotti, L. (2009). The epistemic benefits of reason giving. *Theory & Psychology* 19(5): 1–22.

Bortolotti, L. and Broome, M.R. (2007). If you didn't care, you wouldn't notice: recognition and estrangement in psychopathology. *Philosophy Psychiatry, and Psychology*, 14(1): 39–42.

Bortolotti, L. and Broome, M.R. (2008). Delusional beliefs and reason giving. *Philosophical Psychology* 21(3): 1–21.

Bortolotti, L. and Broome, M.R. (2009). A role for ownership and authorship in the analysis of thought insertion. *Phenomenology and the Cognitive Sciences* 8(2): 205–224.

Bortolotti, L. and Cox, R. (forthcoming). 'Faultless' ignorance: strengths and limitations of epistemic accounts of confabulation. *Consciousness and Cognition*.

Bortolotti, L., Cox, R., and Barnier, A. (submitted). Can we create delusions in the laboratory?

Bowden, W. (1993). The onset of paranoia. *Schizophrenia Bulletin* 19(1): 165–167.

Brakoulias, V., Langdon, R., Sloss, G., Coltheart, M., Meares, R., and Harris, A. (2008). Delusions and reasoning: a study involving cognitive behavioural therapy. *Cognitive Neuropsychiatry* 13(2): 148–165.

Breen, N., Caine, D., and Coltheart, M. (2000). Models of face recognition and delusional misidentification: A critical review. *Cognitive Neuropsychology* 17(1–3), 55–71.

Breen, N., Caine, D., and Coltheart, M. (2001). Mirrored-self misidentification: Two cases of focal onset dementia. *Neurocase* 7(3), 239–254.

Breen, N., Caine, D., Coltheart, M., Hendy, J., and Roberts, C. (2000). Towards an understanding of delusions of misidentification: four case studies. In M. Coltheart and M. Davies (eds.) *Pathologies of Belief*. Oxford: Blackwell; 74–110.

Brett-Jones, J., Garety, P., and Hemsley, D. (1987). Measuring delusional experiences: a method and its application. *British Journal of Clinical Psychology* 26(4): 257–277.

Broome, M.R. (2004). Rationality in psychosis and understanding the deluded. *Philosophy, Psychiatry, & Psychology* 11(1): 35–41.

Broome, M.R., Johns L.C., Valli, I., Woolley, J.B., Tabraham, P., Valmaggia, L., Peters, E., Garety, P., and McGuire, P. (2007). Delusion formation and reasoning biases in those at clinical high risk for psychosis. *British Journal of Psychiatry* 191(51): s38–42.

Broome, M.R., Woolley, J.B., Tabraham, P., Johns, L., Bramon, E., Murray, G., Pariante, C., McGuire, P., and Murray, R. (2005a). What causes the onset of psychosis? *Schizophrenia Research* 79(1): 23–34.

Broome, M.R., Woolley, J.B., Johns, L.C., Valmaggia, L., Tabraham, P., Gafoor, R., Bramon, E., and McGuire, P. (2005b). Outreach and support in South London (OASIS): implementation of a clinical service for prodromal psychosis and the at risk mental state. *European Psychiatry* 20(5–6): 372–378.

Broome, M.R., Bortolotti, L., and Mameli, M. (forthcoming). Moral responsibility and mental illness: a case study. *Cambridge Quarterly of Healthcare Ethics*.

Brüne, M. (2005). 'Theory of mind' in schizophrenia: A review of the literature. *Schizophrenia Bulletin* 31(1): 21–42.

Bryant, R.A. and McConkey, K.M. (1989a). Hypnotic blindness, awareness, and attribution. *Journal of Abnormal Psychology* 98(4): 443–447.

Bryant, R.A. and McConkey, K.M. (1989b). Visual conversion disorder: A case analysis of the influence of visual information. *Journal of Abnormal Psychology* 98(3): 326–329.

Buehner, M. and Cheng, P. (2005). Causal learning. In K.J. Holyoak and R.G. Morrison (eds.) *Cambridge Handbook of Thinking and Reasoning*. New York (NY): Cambridge University Press; chapter 7.

Burge, T. (1988). Individualism and self-knowledge. *Journal of Philosophy*, 85(11): 649–663.

Burgess, P.W. and Shallice, T. (1996). Confabulation and the control of recollection. *Memory* 4(4): 359–341.

Burn, C., Barnier, A.J., and McConkey, K.M. (2001). Information processing during hypnotically suggested sex change. *International Journal of Clinical and Experimental Hypnosis* 49(3): 231–242.

Burns, B. and Reyher, J. (1976). Activating posthypnotic conflict: Emergent uncovering psychopathology repression, and psychopathology. *Journal of Personality Assessment* 40(5): 492–501.

Butler, P. (2000). Reverse Othello syndrome subsequent to traumatic brain injury. *Psychiatry: Interpersonal and Biological Processes* 63(1): 85–92.

Call, J. and Tomasello, M. (1999). A nonverbal false belief task: The performance of children and great apes. *Child Development* 70(2): 381–395.

Campbell, J. (1999). Schizophrenia, the space of reasons and thinking as a motor process. *The Monist* 82(4): 609–625.

Campbell, J. (2001) Rationality, meaning and the analysis of delusion. *Philosophy, Psychiatry, &Psychology* 8(2–3): 89–100.

Campbell, J. (2002). The ownership of thoughts. *Philosophy, Psychiatry, & Psychology* 9(1): 35–39.

Campbell, J. (2009). What does rationality have to do with psychological causation? Propositional attitudes as mechanisms and as control variables. In M. Broome and L. Bortolotti (eds.) *Psychiatry as Cognitive Neuroscience: Philosophical Perspectives*. Oxford: Oxford University Press; chapter 7.

Carman, T. (2003). First persons: On Richard Moran's Authority and Estrangement. *Inquiry* 46(3): 395–408.

Carruthers, P. (1989). Brute experience. *The Journal of Philosophy* 86(5): 258–269.

Carruthers, P. (2005). *Consciousness: Essays from a Higher-Order Perspective*. Oxford: Oxford University Press.

Ceci, S. (1995). False beliefs: some developmental and clinical considerations. In D. Schacter (ed.) *Memory Distortions*. Cambridge (MA): Harvard University Press; 91–125.

Chadwick, P. and Lowe, C. (1990). Measurement and modification of delusional beliefs. *Journal of Consulting and Clinical Psychology* 58(2): 225–232.

Chaiken, S., Giner-Sorolla, R., and Chen, S. (1996). Beyond accuracy: Defense and impression motives in heuristic and systematic information processing. In P.M. Gollwitzer and J.A. Bargh (eds.) *The Psychology of Action: Linking Motivation and Cognition to Behavior*. New York (NY): Guilford Press; 553–578.

Charlton, B.G. (2000). *Psychiatry and the Human Condition*. Oxford: Radcliffe Medical.

Charlton, B.G. (2003). Theory of mind delusions and bizarre delusions in an evolutionary perspective: psychiatry and the social brain. In M. Brune, H. Ribbert, and W. Schiefenhovel (eds.) *The Social Brain - Evolution and Pathology*. Chichester: Wiley; 315–338.

Cherniak, C. (1986) *Minimal Rationality*. Cambridge Mass: MIT Press.

Child, W. (1994). *Causality, Interpretation and the Mind*. Oxford: Clarendon Press.

Chinn, C.A. and Brewer, W. (2001). Models of data: A theory of how people evaluate data. *Cognition and Instruction* 19(3): 323–393.

Clarke, S. (2008). SIM and the City: Rationalism in psychology and philosophy and Haidt's account of moral judgment. *Philosophical Psychology* 21(6): 799–820.

Colbert, S.M., Peters, E.K., and Garety, P.A. (2006). Need for closure and anxiety in delusions: A longitudinal investigation in early psychosis. *Behaviour Research and Therapy* 44(10): 1385–1396.

Coliva, A. (2002). Thought insertion and immunity to error through misidentification. *Philosophy, Psychiatry, & Psychology* 9(1): 27–34.

Coltheart, M. (2005a). Delusional belief. *Australian Journal of Psychology* 57(2): 72–76.

Coltheart, M. (2005b). Conscious experience and delusional belief. *Philosophy, Psychiatry & Psychology* 12(2): 153–157.

Coltheart, M. (2007). The 33rd Sir Frederick Bartlett Lecture: Cognitive neuropsychiatry and delusional belief. *The Quarterly Journal of Experimental Psychology* 60(8): 1041–1062.

Coltheart, M., Langdon, R., and McKay, R. (2007). Schizophrenia and monothematic delusions. *Schizophrenia Bulletin* 33(3): 642–647.

Combs, D. and Penn, D. (2008). Social cognition in paranoia. In D. Freeman, R. Bentall, and P. Garety (eds.) (2008). *Persecutory Delusions. Assessment, Theory and Treatment*. Oxford: Oxford University Press; 175–204.

Conway, M.A. (2005). Memory and the self. *Journal of Memory and Language* 53(4): 594–628.

Conway, M.A. and Tacchi, P.C. (1996). Motivated confabulation. *Neurocase* 2(4): 325–339.

Cooper, J. (2007). *Cognitive Dissonance: Fifty Years of a Classic Theory*. London: Sage.

Cooper, R. (2007). *Psychiatry and Philosophy of Science*. Stocksfield: Acumen.

Cox, R.E. and Barnier, A.J. (2003). Posthypnotic amnesia for a first romantic relationship: forgetting the entire relationship versus forgetting selected events. *Memory* 11(3): 307–318.

Cox, R.E. and Barnier, A.J. (2009a). Hypnotic illusions and clinical delusions: A hypnotic paradigm for investigating delusions of misidentification. *International Journal of Clinical and Experimental Hypnosis* 57(1): 1–32.

Cox, R.E. and Barnier, A.J. (2009b). Selective information processing in hypnotic identity delusion: The impact of time of encoding and retrieval. *Contemporary Hypnosis* 26(2): 65–79.

Cox, R.E. and Bryant, R.A. (2008). Advances in hypnosis research: Methods, designs, and contributions of intrinsic and instrumental hypnosis. Invited chapter in M.R. Nash and A.J. Barnier (eds.), *The Oxford Handbook of Hypnosis: Theory, Research and Practice* Oxford: Oxford University Press; 311–336.

Currie, G. (2000). Imagination, delusion and hallucinations. In M. Coltheart and M. Davies (eds.) *Pathologies of Belief*. Oxford: Blackwell; 167–182.

Currie, G. and Jureidini, J. (2001). Delusions, rationality, empathy. *Philosophy, Psychiatry, &Psychology* 8(2–3): 159–162.

Currie, G. and Ravenscroft, I. (2002). *Recreative Minds: Imagination in Philosophy and Psychology*. New York (NY): Oxford University Press.

Dalla Barba, G. (1993a). Confabulation: Knowledge and recollective experience. *Cognitive Neuropsychology* 10(11): 1–20.

Dalla Barba, G. (1993b). Different patterns of confabulations. *Cortex* 29(4): 567–581.

Davidson, D. (1973). Radical interpretation. *Dialectica* 27: 314–28. Reprinted in D. Davidson (1984) *Inquiries into Truth and Interpretation*. Oxford: Clarendon Press; 125–140.

Davidson, D. (1974a). On the very idea of a conceptual scheme. *Proceedings and Addresses of the American Philosophical Association* 47: 5–20. Reprinted in D. Davidson (1984) *Inquiries into Truth and Interpretation*. Oxford: Clarendon Press; 183–198.

Davidson, D. (1974b). Psychology as philosophy. In S.C. Brown (ed.) *Philosophy of Psychology*. London: Macmillan. Reprinted in D. Davidson (1982) *Essays on Actions and Events*. Oxford: Oxford University Press; 229–238.

Davidson, D. (1975) Thought and talk. In S. Guttenplan (ed.) *Mind and Language*, Oxford: Oxford University Press; 7–23. Reprinted in D. Davidson (1984) *Inquiries into Truth and Interpretation*. Oxford: Clarendon Press; 155–170.

Davidson, D. (1982). Paradoxes of irrationality. In R. Wollheim (ed.) *Philosophical Essays on Freud*. London: Cambridge University Press; 289–305. Reprinted in D. Davidson (2004). *Problems of Rationality*. Oxford: Clarendon Press; 169–188.

Davidson, D. (1985a). Incoherence and irrationality. *Dialectica* 39: 345–354. Reprinted in D. Davidson (2004). *Problems of Irrationality*. Oxford: Clarendon Press; 189–198.

Davidson, D. (1985b). Deception and division. In J. Elster (ed.) *The Multiple Self*. Cambridge: Cambridge University Press. Reprinted in D. Davidson (2004) *Problems of Rationality*. Oxford: Clarendon Press; 199–212.

Davidson, D. (2001) What thought requires. In J. Branquinho (ed.) *The Foundations of Cognitive Science*. Oxford: Clarendon Press; 121–32. Reprinted in D. Davidson (2004) *Problems of Rationality*. Oxford: Clarendon Press; 135–150.

Davies, M. (2008). Delusion and motivationally biased belief: self deception in the two factor framework. In T. Bayne and J. Fernàndez (eds.) *Delusion and Self-deception: Affective and Motivational Influences on Belief Formation*. Hove: Psychology Press; 71–86.

Davies, M. and Coltheart, M. (2000). Introduction. In M. Coltheart and M. Davies (eds.) *Pathologies of Belief*. Oxford: Blackwell; 1–46.

Davies, M., Coltheart, M., Langdon, R., and Breen, N. (2001). Monothematic delusions: Towards a two-factor account. *Philosophy, Psychiatry, &Psychology* 8(2/3): 133–158.

De Paul, M.R. and Ramsey, W.M. (eds.) (1998). *Rethinking Intuition: The Psychology of Intuition and Its Role in Philosophical Inquiry*. Lanham (MD): Rowman & Littlefield.

Delespaul, P. and van Os, J. (2003). Jaspers was right after all – delusions are distinct from normal beliefs: Against. *British Journal of Psychiatry* 183(4): 285–286.

DeLuca, J. (2004). Commentary on 'The Pleasantness of False Beliefs'. *Neuro-Psychoanalysis* 6(1): 20–22.

Dennett, D.C. (1979a). Intentional systems. In D.C. Dennett (ed.) *Brainstorms: Philosophical Essays on Mind and Psychology*. Montgomery (VT): Bradford Books; 3–22.

Dennett, D.C. (1979b). True believers. In D. Dennett (1987) *The Intentional Stance*. Cambridge (MA): MIT Press; 13–36.

Dennett, D.C. (1981). Making sense of ourselves. In D. Dennett (1987) *The Intentional Stance*. Cambridge (MA): MIT Press; 83–101.

Dennett, D.C. (1987). Reflections: real patterns, deeper facts and empty questions. In D. Dennett (1987) *The Intentional Stance*. Cambridge (MA): MIT Press; 37–42.

Dennett, D.C. (1992). The self as a center of narrative gravity. In F. Kessel, P. Cole and D. Johnson (eds.) *Self and Consciousness: Multiple Perspectives*. Hillsdale (NJ): Lawrence Erlbaum; 103–115.

Dennett, D.C. (1995). Do animals have beliefs? In H.L. Roitblat and J.-A. Meyer (eds.) *Comparative Approaches to Cognitive Science*. Cambridge (MA): MIT Press; 111–118.

Dickinson, A. and Balleine, B. (2000) Causal cognition and goal-directed action. In C. Heyes and L. Huber (eds.) *Evolution of Cognition*. Cambridge (MA): The MIT Press; 185–204.

Diez-Alegria, C., Vazquez, C., Nieto-Moreno, M., Valiente, C., and Fuentenebro, F. (2006). Personalizing and externalizing biases in deluded and depressed patients: Are attributional biases a stable and specific characteristic of delusions? *British Journal of Clinical Psychology* 45(4): 531–544.

Dretske, F. (2006). Minimal rationality. In S. Hurley and M. Nudds (eds.) *Rational Animals?* Oxford: Oxford University Press; 107–115.

Drury, V., Birchwood, M. and Cochrane, R. (2000). Cognitive therapy and recovery from acute psychosis: a controlled trial (3. Five year follow up). *British Journal of Psychiatry* 177(1): 8–14.

Dudley, R.E. and Over, D. (2003). People with delusions jump to conclusions. *Clinical Psychology and Psychotherapy* 10(5): 263–274.

Edwards, W. (1982). Conservatism in human information processing. In D. Kahneman, P. Slovic, and A. Tversky (eds.) *Judgements under Uncertainty: Heuristics and Biases*. New York (NY): Cambridge University Press; 359–369.

Egan, A. (2008). Imagination, delusion, and self deception. In T. Bayne and J. Fernández (eds.) *Delusion and Self-deception: Affective and Motivational Influences on Belief Formation.* Hove: Psychology Press; 263–280.

Eilan, N. (2000). On understanding schizophrenia. In D. Zahavi (ed.) *Exploring the self.* Amsterdam: John Benjamins; 97–113.

Elkin, G.D. (1999). *Introduction to Clinical Psychiatry.* Columbus (OH): McGraw-Hill Professional.

Ellis, H. (1998). Cognitive neuropsychiatry and delusional misidentification syndromes: an exemplary vindication of a new discipline. *Cognitive Neuropsychiatry* 3(2): 81–89.

Ellis, H. and Szulecka, T.K. (1996). The disguised lover: a case of Frégoli delusion. In P. Halligan and J. Marshall (eds.) *Method in Madness.* Exeter: Psychology Press; 39–50.

Ellis, H., Young, A.W., Quayle, A.H., and De Pauw, K.W. (1997) Reduced autonomic responses to faces in Capgras delusion. *Proceedings Biological Sciences* 264(1384): 1085–1092.

Emmons, S., Geiser, C., and Kaplan, K. (1997) *Living with Schizophrenia.* London: Taylor and Francis.

Evnine, S. (2008). *Epistemic Dimensions of Personhood.* New York (NY): Oxford University Press.

Fabrigar, L.R., MacDonald, T.K., and Wegener, D.T. (2005). The structure of attitudes. In D. Albarraccin, B.T. Johnson, and M.P. Zanna (eds.) *The Handbook of Attitudes.* Mahwah (NJ): Lawrence Erlbaum; 79–124.

Fabrigar, L.R., Petty, R.E., Smith, S.M., and Crites, S.L. (2006). Understanding knowledge effects on attitude-behavior consistency: the role of relevance, complexity, and amount of knowledge. *Journal of Personality and Social Psychology* 90(4): 556–77.

Fargas, J. and Williams, K. (2002). *Social Influence: Direct and Indirect Processes.* Philadelphia (PA): Psychology Press.

Fazio, R.H. and Zanna, M.P. (1981). Direct experience and attitude-behavior consistency. In L. Berkowitz (ed.) *Advances in Experimental Social Psychology.* New York (NY): Academic Press; 162–193.

Fear, C. and Healy, D. (1995). Obsessive compulsive disorders and delusional disorders: notes on their history, nosology and interface. *Journal of Serotonin Research* 1(1): 1–13.

Feinberg, T.E., Deluca, J., Giacino, J.T., Roane, D.M., and Solms, M. (2005). Right hemisphere pathology and the self: Delusional misidentification and reduplication. In T.E. Feinberg and J.P. Keenan (eds.) *The Lost Self: Pathologies of the Brain and Identity.* Oxford: Oxford University Press.

Feist, G.J. (2006). *The Psychology of Science and the Origins of the Scientific Mind.* New Haven (CT): Yale University Press.

Fernández, J. (2003). Privileged access naturalized. *The Philosophical Quarterly* 53(212): 352–372.

Fernández, J. (2009). Happiness and life choices: Sartre on desires, deliberation and action. In L. Bortolotti (ed.) *Philosophy and Happiness.* Houndmills, Basingstoke: Palgrave Macmillan; 200–214.

Fernández, J. (forthcoming). Thought insertion and self knowledge. *Mind & Language.*

Ferrero, L. (2003). An elusive challenge to the authorship account. *Philosophical Psychology* 16(4): 565–567.

Festinger, L. (1957). *A Theory of Cognitive Dissonance.* Stanford (CA): Stanford University Press.

Festinger, L. and Carlsmith, J.M. (1959). Cognitive consequences of forced compliance. *Journal of Abnormal and Social Psychology* 58(2): 203–210.

Fine, C., Craigie, J., and Gold, I. (2005). Damned if you do, damned if you don't: The impasse in cognitive accounts of the Capgras delusion. *Philosophy, Psychiatry, & Psychology* 12: 143–151.

Fine, C., Gardner, M., Craigie, J., and Gold, I. (2007). Hopping, skipping or jumping to conclusions? Clarifying the role of the JTC bias in delusions. *Cognitive Neuropsychiatry* 12(1): 46–77.

Fisher, S. and Fisher, R. (1993). *The Psychology of Adaptation to Absurdity: Tactics of Make-believe*. Hillsdale (NJ): Lawrence Erlbaum.

Fiske, S.T. (2000). Stereotyping, prejudice, and discrimination at the seam between the centuries: evolution, culture, mind, and brain. *European Journal of Social Psychology* 30(3): 299–322.

Fiske, S.T. (2004). Intent and ordinary bias: Unintended thought and social motivation create casual prejudice. *Social Justice Research* 17: 117–127.

Fiske, S.T. and Taylor, S.E. (1984). *Social Schemata in Social Cognition*. Reading (MA): Addison-Wesley.

Fletcher, P.C. and Frith, C.D. (2009). Perceiving is believing: a Bayesian approach to explaining the positive symptoms of schizophrenia. *Nature Reviews Neuroscience* 10(1): 48–58.

Foley, R. (1998). Rationality and intellectual self-trust. In M. De Paul and W. Ramsey (eds.) *Rethinking Intuition: The Psychology of Intuition and Its Role in Philosophical Inquiry*. Lanham (MD): Rowman & Littlefield; 241–256.

Förstl, H., Almeida, O.P., and Iacoponi, E. (1991). Capgras delusion in the elderly: the evidence for a possible organic origin. *International Journal of Geriatric Psychiatry* 6(12): 845–852.

Förstl, H., Almeida, O.P., Owen, A.M., Burns, A., and Howard, R. (1991). Psychiatric, neurological and medical aspects of misidentification syndromes: A review of 260 cases. *Psychological Medicine* 21(4): 905–910.

Fotopoulou, A. (2008) False-selves in neuropsychological rehabilitation: The challenge of confabulation. *Neuropsychological Rehabilitation* 18(5/6): 541–565.

Fotopoulou, A. and Conway, M. (2004). Confabulation: pleasant and unpleasant. *Neuro-Psychoanalysis* 6(1): 26–33.

Fotopoulou, A., Conway, M.A., Solms, M., Kopelman, M., and Tyrer, S. (2008a). Self-serving confabulation in prose recall. *Neuropsychologia* 46(5): 1429–1441.

Fotopoulou, A., Conway, M.A., Solms, M., Birchall, D., and Tyrer, S. (2008b). Is the content of confabulation positive? An experimental study. *Cortex* 44(7): 764–772.

Fotopoulou, A., Conway, M.A., and Solms, M. (2007a). Confabulation: motivated reality monitoring. *Neuropsychologia* 45(10): 2180–90.

Fotopoulou, A., Conway, M.A., Birchall, D., Griffiths, P., and Tyrer, S. (2007b). Confabulation: revising the motivational hypothesis. *Neurocase* 13(1): 6–15.

Fotopoulou, A., Solms, M., and Turnbull, O. (2004). Wishful reality distortions in confabulation: a case report. *Neuropsychologia* 42(6): 727–744.

Fowler, D., Garety P., and Kuipers (1995). *Cognitive Behaviour Therapy for Psychosis: Theory and Practice*. New York (NY): Wiley.

Frankish, K. (2009). Delusions: a two-level framework. In M.R. Broome and L. Bortolotti (eds.) *Psychiatry as Cognitive Neuroscience: Philosophical Perspectives.* Oxford: Oxford University Press; chapter 14.

Frazer, S.J. and Roberts, J.M. (1994). Three cases of Capgras' syndrome. *British Journal of Psychiatry* 164(4): 557–559.

Freeman, D. (2007). Suspicious minds: the psychology of persecutory delusions. *Clinical Psychology Review* 27(4): 425–457.

Freeman, D. (2008). The assessment of persecutory ideation. In D. Freeman, R. Bentall, and P. Garety (eds.) *Persecutory Delusions. Assessment, Theory and Treatment.* Oxford: Oxford University Press; 23–52.

Freeman, D. and Freeman, J. (2008). *Paranoia: The 21st-century fear.* New York (NY): Oxford University Press.

Freeman, D. and Garety, P. (2004). *Paranoia: The Psychology of Persecutory Delusions.* Hove: Psychology Press.

Freeman, D., Bentall, R., and Garety, P. (eds.) (2008). *Persecutory Delusions. Assessment, Theory and Treatment.* Oxford: Oxford University Press.

Freeman, D., Garety, P., and Kuipers, E. (2001). Persecutory delusions: developing the understanding of belief maintenance and emotional distress. *Psychological Medicine* 31(7): 1293–1306.

Freeman, D., Garety, P., Kuipers, E., Colbert, E., Jolley, S., Fowler, D., Dunn, G., and Bebbington, P. (2006). Delusions and decision-making style: Use of the Need for Closure Scale. *Behaviour Research and Therapy* 44(8): 1147–1158.

Freud, S. (1917). *Delusion and Dream.* Transl. by H. Downey. New York (NY): Moffat Yard.

Frith, C. (1992). *The Cognitive Neuropsychology of Schizophrenia.* Hove: Lawrence Erlbaum.

Fulford, K.W.M. (1993). Mental illness and the mind-brain problem: Delusion, belief and Searle's theory of intentionality. *Theoretical Medicine and Bioethics* 14(2): 181–194.

Fulford, K.W.M. (1998). Completing Kraepelin's psychopathology: Insight, delusion and the phenomenology of illness. In X.F. Amador and A. David (eds.) *Insight and Psychosis.* New York (NY): Oxford University Press; 47–65.

Fulford, K.W.M., Thornton, T., and Graham, G. (2006). *Oxford Textbook of Philosophy and Psychiatry.* New York (NY): Oxford University Press.

Gallagher, S. (2000). Philosophical conceptions of the self: implications for cognitive science. *Trends in Cognitive Science* 4(1): 14–21.

Gallagher, S. (2003). Self-narratives in schizophrenia. In T. Kircher and A. David (eds.) *The Self in Neuroscience and Psychiatry.* New York (NY): Cambridge University Press; 336–357.

Gallagher, S. (2004). Neurocognitive models of schizophrenia: A neurophenomenological critique. *Psychopathology* 37(1): 8–19.

Gallagher, S. (2007). Sense of agency and higher-order cognition: Levels of explanation for schizophrenia. *Cognitive Semiotics* 0 : 32–48.

Gallagher, S. (2009). Delusional realities. In M.R. Broome and L.Bortolotti (eds.) *Psychiatry as Cognitive Neuroscience: Philosophical Perspectives.* Oxford: Oxford University Press; chapter 13.

Gamble, C. and Brennan, G. (2006). *Working with Serious Mental Iillness: a Manual for Clinical Practice*. London: Elsevier.

Garety, P.A. (1991). Reasoning and delusions. *British Journal of Psychiatry* 159(14): 14–18.

Garety, P.A. and Freeman, D. (1999). Cognitive approaches to delusions: A critical review of theories and evidence. *British Journal of Clinical Psychology* 38(2): 113–154.

Garety, P.A. and Hemsley, D. (1987). Characteristics of delusional experience. *European Archives of Psychiatry and Neurological Sciences* 236: 294–298.

Garety, P.A. and Hemsley, D. (1997). *Delusions: Investigations into the Psychology of Delusional Reasoning*. Hove: Psychology Press.

Garety, P.A., Bebbington, P., Fowler, D., Freeman, D., and Kuipers, E. (2007). Implications for neurobiological research of cognitive models of psychosis. *Psychological Medicine* 37(10): 1377–1391.

Garety, P.A., Bentall, R. and Freeman, D. (2008). Research evidence of the effectiveness of cognitive behavioural therapy for persecutory delusions: more work is needed. In D. Freeman, R. Bentall and P. Garety (eds.) *Persecutory Delusions: Assessment, Theory, and Treatment*. Oxford: Oxford University Press; 329–350.

Garety, P.A., Freeman, D., Jolley, S., Dunn, G. Bebbington, P.E., Kuipers, E., Fowler, D.G., and Dudley, R. (2005). Reasoning, emotions, and delusional conviction in psychosis. *Journal of Abnormal Psychology* 114(3): 373–384.

Garety, P.A, Kuipers, E., Fowler, D.G, Freeman, D., and Bebbington, P.E. (2001). A cognitive model of the positive symptoms of psychosis. *Psychological Medicine* 31(2): 189–195.

Gazzaniga, M. (1985). *The Social Brain: Discovering the Networks of the Mind*. New York (NY): Basic Books.

Gerrans, P. (2000). Refining the explanation of the Cotard delusion. *Mind & Language* 15(1): 111–122.

Gerrans, P. (2001a). Delusions as performance failures. *Cognitive Neuropsychiatry* 6(3): 161–173.

Gerrans, P. (2001b). Authorship and ownership of thoughts. *Philosophy, Psychiatry and Psychology* 8(2–3): 231–237.

Gerrans, P. (2002a). A one-stage explanation of the Cotard delusion. *Philosophy, Psychiatry, & Psychology* 9(1): 47–53.

Gerrans, P. (2002b). Multiple paths to delusion. *Philosophy, Psychiatry, & Psychology* 9(1): 65–72.

Gerrans, P. (2009). Mad scientists or unreliable autobiographers? Dopamine dysregulation and delusion. In M.R. Broome and L. Bortolotti (eds.) *Psychiatry as Cognitive Neuroscience: Philosophical Perspectives*. Oxford: Oxford University Press; chapter 8.

Gibbs, P.J. (2000). Thought insertion and the inseparability thesis. *Philosophy, Psychiatry, & Psychology* 7(3): 195–202.

Gigerenzer, G. (2008). *Rationality for Mortals*. New York (NY): Oxford University Press.

Gigerenzer, G., Todd, P., and ABC group (2000). *Simple Heuristics that Make Us Smart*. New York (NY): Oxford University Press.

Gilbert, D. (2004). Affective forecasting . . . or . . . the big wombassa: what you think you're going to get, and what you don't get, when you get what you want. Interview: *The Edge*, *the Third Culture*, 13th February. Available at: http://www.edge.org/3rd_culture/ gilbert03/gilbert_index.html accessed in January 2009.

Gilleen, J. and David, A. (2005). The cognitive psychiatry of delusions: from psychopathology to neuropsychology and back again. *Psychological Medicine* 35(1): 5–12.

Glowinski, R., Payman, V., and Frencham, K. (2008). Confabulation: a spontaneous and fantastic review. *Australian and New Zealand Journal of Psychiatry* 42(11): 932–940.

Glymour, C. (2007). Statistical jokes and social effects: intervention and invariance in social relations. In A. Gopnik and L. Schulz (eds.) *Causal Learning: Psychology, philosophy, and Computation.* New York (NY): Oxford University Press; 294–300.

Gold, I. and Hohwy, J. (2000). Rationality and schizophrenic delusion. *Mind & Language* 15(1): 146–167.

Goldman, A.I. (1992). Interpretation psychologized. In *Liaisons.* Cambridge (Mass.): MIT Press; 9–35.

Goldman, A.I. (1993). *Philosophical Applications of Cognitive Science.* Boulder: Westview Press.

Goleman, D. (1989). Delusion, benign and bizarre, is recognised as common. *New York Times,* June 27th.

Graham, G. (2004). Self-ascription: Thought insertion. In J. Radden (ed.) *The Philosophy of Psychiatry: a Companion.* New York (NY): Oxford University Press; 89–105.

Graham, G. and Stephens, G.L. (1994). Mind and mine. In G. Graham and G.L. Stephens (eds.) *Philosophical Psychology.* Cambridge (Mass.): MIT Press; 91–109.

Gray, J.A. (1995). The contents of consciousness: A neuropsychological conjecture. *Behavioral and Brain Sciences* 18(4): 659–672.

Hacking, I. (1995). *Rewriting the Soul: Multiple Personality and the Sciences of Memory.* Princeton (NJ): Princeton University Press.

Haggard, P., Cartledge, P., Dafydd, M., and Oakley, D. A. (2004). Anomalous control: When 'free will' is not conscious. *Consciousness and Cognition* 13(3): 646–654.

Haidt, J. (2001). The Emotional Dog and its Rational Tail: a social intuitionist approach to moral judgement. *Psychological Review* 108(4): 814–834.

Haidt, J., and Bjorklund, F. (2008). Social intuitionists answer six questions about moral psychology. In W. Sinnott-Armstrong (ed.) *Moral Psychology, Volume 2: The Cognitive Science of Morality: Intuition and Diversity.* Cambridge (MA): MIT Press; 181–217.

Halligan, P.W. and Marshall, J.C. (1996). The wise prophet makes sure of the event first: Hallucinations, amnesia, and delusions. In P.W. Halligan and J.C. Marshall (eds.) *Method in Madness.* Exeter: Psychology Press; 235–266.

Halligan, P.W., Athwal, B.S., Oakley, D.A., and Frackowiak, R.S.J. (2000). Imaging hypnotic paralysis: Implications for conversion hysteria. *The Lancet* 355(9208): 986–987.

Halligan, P.W., Bass, C., and Wade, D.T. (2000). New approaches to conversion hysteria. *British Medical Journal* 320(7248): 1488–1489.

Halligan, P.W., Marshall, J.C., and Wade, D.T. (1995). Unilateral somatoparaphrenia after right hemisphere stroke: A case description. *Cortex* 31(1): 173–182.

Hamilton, A. (2007). Against the belief model of delusion. In M.C. Chung, K.W.M. Fulford and G. Graham (eds.) *Reconceiving Schizophrenia.* Oxford: Oxford University Press; 217–34.

Harman, G. (1999). *Reasoning, Meaning and Mind*. Oxford: Clarendon Press.

Harrington, L., Siegert, R.J., and McClure, J. (2005). Theory of mind in schizophrenia: a critical review. *Cognitive Neuropsychiatry* 10(4): 249–286.

Heal, J. (1998). Understanding other minds from the inside. In A. O'Hear (ed.) *Current Issues in Philosophy of Mind*. Cambridge: Cambridge University Press; 83–100.

Heil, J. (1988). Privileged access. *Mind*, 97(386): 238–235.

Heine, S.J. and Hamamura, T. (2007). In search of East Asian self-enhancement. *Personality and Social Psychology Review* 11(1): 1–24.

Hertwig, R. and Gigerenzer, G. (1999). The conjunction fallacy revisited: how intelligent inferences look like reasoning errors. *Journal of Behavioral Decision Making* 12(4): 275–305.

Higgins, E.T. and Kruglanski A.W. (eds.) *Motivational Science: Social and Personality Perspectives*. Philadelphia (PA): Psychology Press.

Hirstein, W. (2005). *Brain Fiction: Self deception and the Riddle of Confabulation*. Cambridge (MA): MIT Press.

Hirstein, W. (2009) (ed.) *Confabulation: Views from Neuroscience, Psychiatry, Psychology and Philosophy*. New York (NY): Oxford University Press.

Hoerl, C. (2001). On thought insertion. *Philosophy, Psychiatry, & Psychology* 8(2–3): 189–200.

Hohwy, J. (2004). Top-down and bottom-up in delusion formation. *Philosophy, Psychiatry, & Psychology* 11(1): 65–70.

Hohwy, J. (2007). The sense of self in the phenomenology of agency and perception. *Psyche* 13(1). Available at http://psyche.csse.monash.edu/symposia/siegel/Hohwy.pdf. and accessed in January 2009.

Hohwy, J. and Rosenberg, R. (2005). Unusual experiences, reality testing and delusions of alien control. *Mind & Language* 20(2): 141–162.

House, A. and Hodges, J. (1988). Persistent denial of handicap after infarction of the right basal ganglia: A case study. *Journal of Neurology, Neurosurgery, and Psychiatry* 51(1): 112–115.

Humphreys, N. and Dennett, D. (1989). Speaking for our selves. An assessment of multiple personality disorder. *Raritan* 9(1): 68–98.

Huq, S., Garety, P., and Hemsley, D. (1988). Probabilistic judgements in deluded and non-deluded subjects. *Quarterly Journal of Experimental Psychology* 40A(4): 801–812.

Hyman, I.E., Husband, T.H., and Billings, F.J. (1995). False memories of childhood experiences. *Applied Cognitive Psychology* 9(3): 181–197.

Insel, T. and Akiskal, H. (1986). Obsessive-compulsive disorder with psychotic features: A phenomenologic analysis. *American Journal of Psychiatry* 143(12): 1527–1533.

Jaspers, K (1963). *General Psychopathology*. Transl. by J. Hoenig and M. Hamilton. Manchester: Manchester University Press. Originally published as *Allgemeine Psychopathologie*, Berlin, Springer 1959.

Jeannerod M. and Pacherie E. (2004). Agency, simulation and self-identification. *Mind & Language* 19(2): 113–146.

Johns, L.C. and van Os, J. (2001). The continuity of psychotic experiences in the general population. *Clinical Psychology Review* 21(8): 1125–1141.

Johnson, M.K. (2006). Memory and reality. *The American Psychologist* 61(8): 760–771.

Johnson, M.K., Hashtroudi, S., and Lindsay, S. (1993). Source monitoring. *Psychological Bulletin* 114(1): 3–28.

Johnstone, E., Cooling, N., Frith, C., Crow, T., and Owens, D. (1988). Phenomenology of organic and functional psychoses and the overlap between them. *British Journal of Psychiatry* 153(6): 770–776.

Jones, H. (2003). Jaspers was right after all – delusions are distinct from normal beliefs: For. *British Journal of Psychiatry* 183(4): 285–286.

Jordan, H.W., Lockert, E.W., Johnson-Warren, M., Cabell, C., Cooke, T., Greer, W., and Howe, G. (2006) Erotomania revisited: Thirty-four years later. *Journal of the National Medical Association* 98(5): 787–793.

Junginger, J., Parks-Levy, J., and McGuire, L. (1998). Delusions and symptom-consistent violence. *Psychiatric Services* 49(2): 218–220.

Kahneman, D., Slovic, P., and Tversky, A. (eds.) (1982). *Judgements under Uncertainty: Heuristics and Biases.* New York (NY): Cambridge University Press.

Kapur, S. (2003). Psychosis as a state of aberrant salience: a framework for linking biology, phenomenology and pharmacology in schizophrenia. *American Journal of Psychiatry* 160(1): 13–23.

Kapur, S. (2004). How antipsychotics become anti-'psychotic' - from dopamine to salience to psychosis. *Trends in Pharmacological Sciences* 25(8): 402–406.

Kapur, S., Mizrahi, R., and Li, M. (2005a). From dopamine to salience to psychosis - linking biology, pharmacology and phenomenology of psychosis. *Schizophrenia Research* 79(1): 59–68.

Kapur, S., Arenovich, T., Agid, O., Zipursky, R., Lindborg, S., and Jones, B. (2005b). Evidence for onset of antipsychotic effects within the first 24 hours of treatment. *American Journal of Psychiatry* 162(5): 939–946.

Keenan, J.P., Wheeler, M., and Ewers, M. (2003). The neural correlates of self-awareness and self-recognition. In T. Kircher and A. David (eds.) *The Self in Neuroscience and Psychiatry.* New York (NY): Cambridge University Press; 166–179.

Kelly, T. (2003). Epistemic rationality as instrumental rationality: a critique. *Philosophy and Phenomenological Research* LXVI (3): 612–640.

Kemp, R., Chua, S., McKenna, P., and David, A. (1997). Reasoning and delusions. *British Journal of Psychiatry* 170(5): 398–405.

Kendler, K. (1980). Are there delusions specific for paranoid disorders vs. schizophrenia? *Schizophrenia Bulletin* 61(1): 1–3.

Kendler, K. and Parnas, J. (2008) (eds.) *Philosophical Issues in Psychiatry: Explanation, Phenomenology, and Nosology.* Baltimore (MD): Johns Hopkins University Press.

Kennett, J. and Matthews, S. (2002). Identity, control and responsibility: the case of dissociative identity disorder. *Philosophical Psychology* 15(4): 509–526.

Kennett, J. and Matthews, S. (2003). Delusion, dissociation and identity. *Philosophical Explorations* VI(1): 31–49.

Kennett, J. and Matthews, S. (2009). Mental time travel, agency and responsibility. In M.R. Broome and L. Bortolotti (eds.) *Psychiatry as Cognitive Neuroscience: Philosophical Perspectives.* Oxford: Oxford University Press; chapter 16.

Kenny, A. (1976). Human abilities and dynamic modalities. In J. Manninen and R.Tuomela (eds.) *Essays on Explanation and Understanding.* Dordrecht: Springer.

Kihlstrom, J.F. and Hoyt, I.P. (1988). Hypnosis and the psychology of delusions. In T.F. Otlmanns and B.A. Maher (eds.) *Delusional beliefs*. Oxford: Wiley; 66–109.

Kinderman, P. and Bentall, R. (1997) Causal attributions in paranoia and depression: Internal, personal, and situational attributions for negative events. *Journal of Abnormal Psychology* 106(2): 341–345.

Kingdon, D. and Turkington, D. (2004). *Cognitive Therapy for Schizophrenia*. New York (NY): Guilford Press.

Kingdon, D., Ashcroft, K., Turkington, D. (2008). Cognitive behavioural therapy for persecutory delusions: three case examples. In D. Freeman, R. Bentall, and P. Garety (eds.) *Persecutory Delusions. Assessment, Theory and Treatment*. Oxford: Oxford University Press; 393–410.

Kircher, T. and David, A. (eds.) (2003). *The Self in Neuroscience and Psychiatry*. New York (NY): Cambridge University Press.

Knobe, J. (2003). Intentional action and side effects in ordinary language. *Analysis* 63(3): 190–193.

Knobe, J. (2005). Theory of mind and moral cognition: explaining the connections. *Trends in Cognitive Science* 9(8): 357–359.

Komiyama, M. (1989). Fictionality of schizophrenic delusions. *Japanese Journal of Psychiatry and Neurology* 43(1): 13–18.

Kopelman, M.D. (1987). Two types of confabulation. *Journal of Neurology, Neurosurgery and Psychiatry* 50(11): 1482–1487.

Kopelman, M.D. (1999). Varieties of false memories. *Cognitive Neuropsychology* 16(3–5): 197–214.

Kopelman, M.D. (2002). Disorders of memory. *Brain* 125(10): 2152–2190.

Kopelman, M.D., Guinan, E., and Lewis, P. (1995). Delusional memory, confabulation and frontal lobe dysfunction. In R. Campbell and M. Conway (eds.) *Broken Memories: Case Studies in Memory Impairment*. Oxford: Blackwell; 137–153.

Kopelman, M.D., Ng, N., and van Den Boruke, O. (1997). Confabulation extending across episodic, personal and general semantic memory. *Cognitive Neuropsychology* 14(5): 683–712.

Krabbendam, L., Myin-Germeys, I., Bak, M., and van Os, J. (2005). Explaining transitions over the hypothesized psychosis continuum. *Australian and New Zealand Journal of Psychiatry* 39(3): 180–186.

Krafft-Ebing, R. von (2007). *Textbook of Insanity: Based On Clinical Observations For Practitioners And Students Of Medicine*. Transl. by C. Chaddock. Kessinger Publishing. Originally published in 1879 as: *Lehrbuch der Psychiatrie auf klinischer Grundlage für practische Ärzte und Studirende*. Stuttgart: F. Enke.

Kruglanski, A.W. (1989). *Lay Epistemics and Human Knowledge: Cognitive and Motivational Bases*. New York (NY): Plenum.

Kühberger, A. (1998). The influence of framing on risky decisions: A meta-analysis. *Organizational Behaviour and Human Decision Processes* 75(1): 23–55.

Lagnado, D.A, Waldman, M.R., Hagmayer, Y., and Sloman, S.A. (2007). Beyond Covariation: Cues to Causal Structure. In A. Gopnik and L. Schulz (eds.) *Causal*

*Learning: Psychology, Philosophy, and Computation.* New York (NY): Oxford University Press; 154–172.

Lagnado, D.A. and Sloman, S.A. (2006). Time as a guide to cause. *Learning & Memory* 32(3): 451–460.

Langdon, R. and Coltheart, M. (2000). The cognitive neuropsychology of delusions. In M. Coltheart and M. Davies (eds.) *Pathologies of Belief.* Oxford: Blackwell; 183–216.

Langdon, R., Corner, T., McLaren, J., Ward, P., and Colheart, M. (2006). Externalising and personalising biases in persecutory delusions: The relationship with poor insight and theory-of-mind. *Behaviour Research and Therapy* 44(5): 699–713.

Langdon, R., McKay, R., and Coltheart, M. (2008a). The cognitive neuropsychological understanding of persecutory delusions. In D. Freeman, R. Bentall, and P. Garety (eds.) *Persecutory Delusions. Assessment, Theory and Treatment.* Oxford: Oxford University Press; 221–236.

Langdon, R., Ward, P., and Coltheart, M. (2008b). Reasoning anomalies associated with delusions in schizophrenia. *Schizophrenia Bulletin.* Available online at: http://schizo-phreniabulletin.oxfordjournals.org/cgi/reprint/sbn069v1. DOI: 10.1093/schbul/sbn069.

Laruelle, M. and Abi-Dargham, A. (1999) Dopamine as the wind of the psychotic fire: new evidence from brain imaging studies. *Journal of Psychopharmacology* 13(4): 358–371.

Lawlor, K. (2003). Elusive reasons: a problem for first-person authority. *Philosophical Psychology* 16(4): 549–564.

Leary, M.R. (2007). Motivational and emotional aspects of the self. *Annual Review of Psychology* 58: 317–344.

Lee, E., Meguro, K., Hashimoto, R., Meguro, M., Ishii, H., Yamaguchi, S., and Mori, E. (2007). Confabulations in episodic memory are associated with delusions in Alzheimer's Disease. *Journal of Geriatric Psychiatry and Neurology* 20(1): 34–40.

Leeser, J. and O'Donohue, W. (1999). What is a delusion? Epistemological dimensions. *Journal of Abnormal Psychology* 108(4): 687–694.

Lenman, J. (2009). The politics of the self: stability, normativity and the lives we can live with living. In L. Bortolotti (ed.) *Philosophy and Happiness.* Houndmills, Basingstoke: Palgrave Macmillan; 183–199.

Leslie, A.M. (1987). Pretense and representation: The origins of 'theory of mind'. *Psychological Review* 94(4): 412–426.

Levine, B., Black, S.E., Cabeza, R., Sinden, M., Mcintosh, A.R, Toth, J.P., Tulving, E., and Stuss, D.T. (1998). Episodic memory and the self in a case of isolated retrograde amnesia. *Brain* 121(10): 1951–1973.

Levy, N. (2008). Self deception without thought experiments. In T. Bayne and J. Fernández (eds.) *Delusions and Self-deception: Affective and Motivational Influences on Belief Formation.* Hove: Psychology Press; 227–242.

Lewis, D. (1982) Logic for equivocators. *Noûs* 1(6): 431–441.

Lewis, S. and Guthrie, E. (2002). *Master Medicine: Psychiatry.* Philadelphia (PA): Elsevier.

Li, S. and Xie, X. (2006). A new look at the 'Asian disease' problem: A choice between the best possible outcomes or between the worst possible outcomes? *Thinking & Reasoning* 12(2): 129–143.

Lichtenstein, S. and Slovic, P. (1971). Reversals of preference between bids and choices in gambling decisions. *Journal of Experimental Psychology* 89(1): 46–55.

Link, B.G. and Steuve, A. (1994). Psychotic symptoms and the violent/illegal behaviour of mental patients compared to community controls. In J. Monahan and H.J. Steadman (eds.) *Violence and Mental Disorder: Developments in Risk Assessment*. Chicago (IL): University of Chicago Press; 137–159.

Loewer, B. (1997). A guide to naturalizing semantics. In B. Hale and C. Wright (eds.) *A Companion to the Philosophy of Language*. Oxford: Blackwell; 108–126.

Lord, C.G., Ross, L., and Lepper, M.R. (1979). Biased assimilation and attitude polarization: The effects of prior theories on subsequently considered evidence. *Journal of Personality and Social Psychology* 37(11): 2098–2109.

Lucchelli, F. and Spinnler, H. (2007). The case of lost Wilma: a clinical report of Capgras delusion. *Neurological Science* 28(4): 188–195.

Lukes, S. (1982) Relativism in its place. In M. Hollis and S. Lukes (eds.) *Rationality and Relativism*. Oxford: Blackwell; 261–305.

MacIntyre, A. (1999) *Dependent Rational Animals: Why Human Beings Need the Virtues*. Peru (IL): Open Court.

Maher, B.A. (1974). Delusional thinking and perceptual disorder. *Journal of Individual Psychology* 30(1): 98–113.

Maher, B.A. (1988). Anomalous experience and delusional thinking: The logic of explanations. In T.F. Oltmann and B.A. Maher (eds.) *Delusional Beliefs*. New York (NY): Wiley; 15–33.

Maher, B.A. (1992). Models and methods for the study of reasoning in delusions. *European Review of Applied Psychology* 42(22): 97–102.

Maher, B.A. (1999). Anomalous experience in everyday life: Its significance for psychopathology. *The Monist* 82(4): 547–70.

Maher, B.A. (2003). Schizophrenia, aberrant utterance and delusions of control: The disconnection of speech and thought, and the connection of experience and belief. *Mind & Language* 18(1): 1–22.

Malle, B.F. (2004). *How the Mind Explains Behavior: Folk Explanations, Meaning, and Social Interaction*. Cambridge (MA): MIT Press.

Malle, B.F. (2006). Of windmills and strawmen: Folk assumptions of mind and action. In S. Pockett, W.P. Banks, and S. Gallagher (eds.) *Does Consciousness Cause Behavior? An Investigation of the Nature of Volition*. Cambridge (MA): MIT Press; 207–231.

Mameli, M. and Bortolotti, L. (2006). Animal rights, animal minds, and human mindreading. *Journal of Medical Ethics* 32(2): 84–89.

Marchetti, C. and Della Sala, S. (1998). Disentangling the alien and anarchic hand. *Cognitive Neuropsychiatry* 3(3): 191–207.

Marshall, J.C. and Halligan, P.W. (1996). Introduction. In P.W. Halligan and J.C. Marshall (eds.) *Method in Madness*. Exeter: Psychology Press; 3–11.

McAdams, D.P. (1999). Personal narratives and the life story. In L. Pervin and O. John (eds.) *Handbook of Personality: Theory and Research* (2nd ed.). New York (NY): Guilford Press; 478–500.

McAdams, D.P. (2001). *The Person: An integrated Introduction to Personality Psychology* (3rd ed.). Fort Worth(TX): Harcourt.

McAllister-Williams, R. (1997). The description of primary delusions: confusions in standard texts and among clinicians. *Psychiatric Bulletin* 21(6): 346–349.

McConkey, K.M. (2008). Generations and landscapes of hypnosis: Questions we've asked, questions we should ask. In M.R. Nash and A.J. Barnier (eds.) *The Oxford Handbook of Hypnosis: Theory, Research and Practice*. Oxford: Oxford University Press; 53–77.

McConkey, K.M., Szeps, A., and Barnier, A.J. (2001). Indexing the experience of sex change in hypnosis and imagination. *International Journal of Clinical and Experimental Hypnosis* 49(2): 123–138.

McDowell, J. (1985). Functionalism and anomalous monism. In B. McLaughlin and E. Lepore (eds.) *Actions and events*. Oxford: Blackwell; 387–398.

McKay, A.P., McKenna, P.J., and Laws, K. (1996). Severe schizophrenia: what is it like? In P. Halligan and J. Marshall (eds.) *Method in Madness*. Exeter: Psychology Press; 95–122.

McKay, R. and Cipolotti, L. (2007). Attributional styles in a case of Cotard delusion. *Consciousness and Cognition* 16(2): 349–359.

McKay, R., Langdon, R., and Coltheart, M. (2005b). Paranoia, persecutory delusions and attributional biases. *Psychiatry Research* 136(2–3): 233–245.

McKay, R., Langdon, R., and Colheart, M. (2007). Models of misbelief: Integrating motivational and deficit theories of delusions. *Consciousness and Cognition* 16(4): 932–941.

McKay, R., Langdon, R., and Coltheart, M. (2005a). 'Sleights of mind': Delusions, defences, and self deception. *Cognitive Neuropsychology* 10(4): 305–326.

Mele, A. (1997). Real self deception. *Behavioral and Brain Sciences* 20(1): 91–136.

Mele, A. (2001). *Self deception Unmasked*. Princeton (NJ): Princeton University Press.

Mele, A. (2007). Self deception and three psychiatric delusions. In M. Timmons and J. Greco, A. Mele (eds.) *Rationality and the Good*. New York (NY): Oxford University Press; 163–176.

Mele, A. (2008). Self deception and delusions. In T. Bayne and J. Fernández (eds.) *Delusions and Self-deception: Affective and Motivational Influences on Belief Formation*. Hove: Psychology Press; 55–70.

Metcalf, K., Langdon, R., and Coltheart, M. (2007). Models of confabulation: A critical review and a new framework. *Cognitive Neuropsychology* 24(1): 23–47.

Milgram, S. (1974). *Obedience to Authority: An Experimental View*. New York (NY): Haper & Row.

Miller, D.T. and Ross, M. (1975). Self-serving biases in the attribution of causality: Fact or fiction? *Psychological Bulletin* 82(2): 213–225.

Miller, E. and Karoni, P. (1996). The cognitive psychology of delusions: a review. *Applied Cognitive Psychology* 10(6): 487–502.

Millon, T., Blaney, P.H., and Davis, R.D. (eds.) (1999). *Oxford Textbook of Psychopathology*. New York (NY): Oxford University Press.

Moran, R. (2001). *Authority and Estrangement: an Essay on Self knowledge*. Princeton (NJ): Princeton University Press.

Moran, R. (2004). Précis of Authority and Estrangement. *Philosophy and Phenomenological Research* LXIX(2): 423–426.

Moritz, S. and Woodward, T.S. (2005). Jumping to delusions in delusional and non-delusional schizophrenic patients. *British Journal of Clinical Psychology* 44(2): 193–207.

Moscovitch, M. (1995). Confabulation. In D. Schacter (ed.) *Memory Distortions.* Cambridge (MA): Harvard University Press; 226–253.

Moulin, C., Conway, M., Thompson, R., James, N., and Jones, R. (2005). Disordered memory awareness: recollective confabulation in two cases of persistent déjà vecu. *Neuropsychologia* 43(9): 1362–1378.

Moyal-Sharrock, D. (2004). *Understanding Wittgenstein's 'On Certainty'.* Basingstoke: Palgrave Macmillan.

Mullen, R. (2003). Delusions: the continuum versus category debate. *Australian and New Zealand Journal of Psychiatry* 37(5): 505–511.

Mullins, S. and Spence, S. (2003). Re-examining thought insertion. *British Journal of Psychiatry* 182(4): 293–298.

Muramoto, Y. and Yamaguchi, S. (1997). Another type of self-serving bias: Coexistence of self-effacing and group-serving tendencies in attribution in the Japanese culture. *Japanese Journal of Experimental Social Psychology* 37(1): 65–75.

Murphy, D. (2006). *Psychiatry in the Scientific Image.* Cambridge (MA): MIT Press.

Nedjam, Z., Dalla Barba, G., and Pillon, B. (2000). Confabulation in a patient with fronto-temporal dementia and a patient with Alzheimer's Disease. *Cortex* 36(4): 561–577.

Nelson, H. (2005). *Cognitive Behavioural Therapy with Delusions and Hallucinations. A Practice Manual.* Cheltenham: Nelson Thornes.

Nisbett, R. and Ross, L. (1980). *Human Inference: Strategies and Shortcomings of Social Judgment.* Englewood Cliffs (NJ): Prentice-Hall.

Nisbett, R. and Wilson, T. (1977). Telling more than we can know: Verbal reports on mental processes. *Psychological Review* 84(3): 231–259.

Noble, J. and McConkey, K.M. (1995). Hypnotic sex change: Creating and challenging a delusion in the laboratory. *Journal of Abnormal Psychology* 104(1): 69–74.

O'Brien, G. and Opie, J. (2003). The Multiplicity of Consciousness and the Emergence of the Self. In T. Kicher and A. Davids (eds.) *The Self in Neuroscience and Psychiatry.* New York (NY): Cambridge University Press; 107–120.

O'Dwyer, A. and Marks, I. (2000). Obsessive-compulsive disorder and delusions revisited. *British Journal of Psychiatry* 176(3): 281–284.

Oakley, D.A. (2006). Hypnosis as a tool in research: Experimental psychopathology. *Contemporary Hypnosis* 23(1): 3–14.

Örulv, L. and Hydén, L-C. (2006). Confabulation: sense-making, self-making and world-making in dementia. *Discourse Studies* 8(5): 647–673.

Oxford English Dictionary (2007). Entry 'Ownership'. Oxford University Press. Available at: http://dictionary.oed.com/. Entry and accessed in January 2009.

Oyebode, F. and Sargeant, R. (1996). Delusional misidentification syndromes: a descriptive study. *Psychopathology* 29(4): 209–14.

Oyebode, F. and Sims, A. (2008). *Sims' Symptoms in the Mind: An Introduction to Descriptive Psychopathology (Made Memorable).* Philadelphia (PA): Elsevier.

Pacherie, E. (2008). Perception, Emotions, and Delusions. The Case of the Capgras Delusion. In T. Bayne and J. Fernàndez (eds.), *Delusions and Self deception: Affective and Motivational Influences on Belief Formation*. Hove: Psychology Press; 105–123.

Pacherie, E., Green, M., and Bayne, T. (2006). Phenomenology and delusions: Who put the 'alien' in alien control? *Consciousness and Cognition* 15(3): 566–577.

Paglieri, F. (2009). Acceptance as conditional disposition. In H. Leitgeb and A. Hieke (eds.) *Reduction and Elimination in Philosophy of Mind and Philosophy of Neuroscience*. Berlin: Ontos-Verlag.

Paglieri, F. and McKay, R. (2006). Believing without accepting: The doxastic conception of delusions revised (abstract). In *Cervelli, persone e società. Atti del VII congresso nazionale SIFA* Università Vita-Salute: Cesano Maderno (MI); 113–115.

Parnas, J. and Handset, P. (2003). Phenomenology of self-experience in early schizophrenia. *Comprehensive Psychiatry* 44(2): 121–134.

Parnas, J. and Sass, L.A. (2001). Self, solipsism, and schizophrenic delusions. *Philosophy, Psychiatry & Psychology* 8(2–3): 101–120.

Park, R.L. (2008). *Superstition: Belief in the Age of Science*. Princeton (NJ): Princeton University Press.

Payne, R.L. (1992). First person account: My Schizophrenia. *Schizophrenia Bulletin* 18(4): 725–728.

Peacocke, C. (1998). Conscious attitudes, attention, and self-knowledge. In C. Wright, B. Smith, and C. Macdonald (eds.) *Knowing our Own Minds*. Oxford: Clarendon Press; 63–98.

Perkins, K.A. and Reyher, J. (1971). Repression, psychopathology and drive representation: An experimental hypnotic investigation of impulse inhibition. *American Journal of Clinical Hypnosis* 13(4): 249–258.

Pettit, P. and Smith, M. (1990). Backgrounding desire. *The Philosophical Review* 99(4): 565–592.

Phillips, J. (2003). Psychopathology and the narrative self. *Philosophy, Psychiatry, & Psychology* 10(4): 313–328.

Phillips, M.L. and David, A.S. (1997). Visual scan paths are abnormal in deluded schizophrenics. *Neuropyschologia* 35(1): 99–105.

Pickup, G. (2008). Relationship between theory of mind and executive function in schizophrenia: A systematic review. *Psychopathology* 41(4): 206–213.

Putwain, D. and Sammons, A. (2002). *Psychology and Crime: An Introduction to Criminological Psychology*. London and New York: Routledge.

Quattrone, G. and Tversky, A. (1984). Causal *versus* diagnostic contingencies: On self deception and on the voter's illusion. *Journal of Personality and Social Psychology* 46(2): 237–248.

Quine, W.V.O. (1960). *Word and object*. Cambridge (MA): MIT Press.

Quine, W.V.O. and Ullian, J.S. (1978). *The Web of Belief* (2nd edn.). Columbus (OH): McGraw-Hill Higher Education.

Radden, J. (2004). *The Philosophy of Psychiatry*. New York (NY): Oxford University Press.

Ramachandran, V.S. (1996). The evolutionary biology of self deception, laughter, dreaming and depression: some clues from anosognosia. *Medical Hypotheses* 47(5): 347–362.

Ramachandran, V.S. and Blakeslee, S. (1998). *Phantoms in the Brain: Human Nature and the Architecture of the Mind*. Fourth Estate: London.

Ratcliffe, M. (2004). Interpreting delusions. *Phenomenology and Cognitive Sciences* 3(1): 25–48.

Repacholi, B. and Slaughter, V. (eds.) (2003). *Individual Differences in Theory of Mind*. New York (NY): Psychology Press.

Rescher, N. and Brandom, R. (1979). *The Logic of Inconsistency: a Study in Non-standard Possible-world Semantics and Ontology*. Oxford: Blackwell.

Reyher, J. (1961). Posthypnotic stimulation of hypnotically induced conflict in relation to psychosomatic reactions and psychopathology. *Psychosomatic Medicine* 23(5): 384–391.

Reyher, J. (1962). A paradigm for determining the clinical relevance of hypnotically induced psychopathology. *Psychological Bulletin* 59(4): 344–352.

Reyher, J. (1969). Comment on 'Artificial induction of posthypnotic conflict'. *Journal of Abnormal Psychology* 74(4): 420–422.

Reyher, J. and Basch, J.A. (1970). Degree of repression and frequency of psychosomatic symptoms. *Perceptual and Motor Skills* 30(2): 559–562.

Rhodes, J. and Gipps, R. (2008). Delusions, certainty, and the background. *Philosophy, Psychiatry, & Psychology* 15(4): 295–310.

Roessler, J. (2001). Understanding delusions of alien control. *Philosophy, Psychiatry, & Psychology* 8(2–3): 177–187.

Roser, M. and Gazzaniga, M. (2004). Automatic brains- interpretive minds. *Current Directions in Psychological Science* 13(2): 56–59.

Rosset, E. (2008). It's no accident: our bias for intentional explanations. *Cognition* 108(3): 771–80.

Rusche, S.E. and Brewster, Z.W. (2008). 'Because they tip for shit!': The social psychology of everyday racism in restaurants. *Sociology Compass* 2(6): 2008–2029.

Rutten, B., van Os, J., Dominguez, M., and Krabbendam, L. (2008). Epidemiology and social factors: findings from the Netherlands Mental Health Survey and Incidence Study (NEMESIS). In D. Freeman, R. Bentall, and P. Garety (eds.) *Persecutory Delusions. Assessment, Theory and Treatment*. Oxford: Oxford University Press; 53–71.

Samuels, R. (2009). Delusions as a natural kind. In M.R. Broome and L. Bortolotti (eds.) *Psychiatry as Cognitive Neuroscience: Philosophical Perspectives*. Oxford: Oxford University Press; chapter 3.

Samuels, R., Stich, S., and Bishop, M. (2002). Ending the Rationality Wars: How to make disputes about human rationality disappear. In R. Elio (ed.) *Common Sense, Reasoning, and Rationality*. New York (NY): Oxford University Press; 236–268.

Sass, L. (1994). *The Paradoxes of Delusion: Wittgenstein, Schreber, and the Schizophrenic Mind*. New York (NY); Cornell University Press.

Sass, L. (2001). Self and world in schizophrenia: Three classic approaches. *Philosophy, Psychiatry, & Psychology* 8(4): 251–270.

Sass, L. (2004). Some reflections on the (analytic) philosophical approach to delusion. *Philosophy, Psychiatry, & Psychology* 11(1): 71–80.

Scepkowski, L. and Cronin-Golomb, A. (2003). The alien hand: Cases, categorizations, and anatomical correlates. *Behavioral and Cognitive Neuroscience Reviews* 2(4): 261–277.

Schacter, D.L. (ed.) (1995). *Memory Distortions*. Cambridge (MA): Harvard University Press.

Schacter, D.L. and Addis, D.R. (2008). The cognitive neuroscience of constructive memory: Remembering the past and imagining the future. In J. Driver, P. Haggard, and T. Shallice (eds.) *Mental Processes in the Human Brain*. Oxford: Oxford University Press; 27–47.

Schacter, D.L., Addis, D.R., and Buckner, R.L. (2008). Episodic simulation of future events: concepts, data, and application. *Annals of the New York Academy of Sciences (Special Issue: The Year in Cognitive Neuroscience 2008)* 1124(1): 39–60.

Schacter, D.L., Kagan, J., and Leichtman, M. (1995). True and false memories in children and adults: a cognitive neuroscience perspective. *Psychology, Public Policy & Law* 1(2): 411–428.

Schacter, D.L., Verfaellie, M., and Anes, M.D. (1997). Illusory memories in amnesic patients: conceptual and perceptual false recognition. *Neuropsychology* 11(3): 331–342.

Schnider, A. (2001). Spontaneous confabulation, reality monitoring, and the limbic system – a review. *Brain Research Reviews* 36(2–3): 150–160.

Schnider, A., Von Daniken, C., and Gutbrod, K. (1996). The mechanisms of spontaneous and provoked confabulations. *Brain* 119(4): 1365–1375.

Schwitzgebel, E. (2006). 'Belief'. In E. Zalta (ed.) *The Stanford Encyclopedia of Philosophy*. Available at: http://plato.stanford.edu/entries/belief and accessed in January 2009.

Schwitzgebel, E. (forthcoming). Do ethicists steal more books? *Philosophical Psychology*.

Schwitzgebel, E. and Rust, J. (forthcoming). The moral behaviour of ethicists: peer opinion. *Mind*.

Sedikides, C., Gaertner, L., and Toguchi, Y. (2003). Pancultural self-enhancement. *Journal of Personality and Social Psychology* 84(1): 60–79.

Sedikides, C., Gaertner, L., and Vevea, J.L. (2005). Pancultural self-enhancement reloaded: A meta-analytic reply to Heine. *Journal of Personality and Social Psychology* 89(4): 539–551.

Sharfetter, C. (2003). The self-experience of schizophrenics. In T. Kircher and A. David (eds.) *The Self in Neuroscience and Psychiatry*. New York (NY): Cambridge University Press; 272–289.

Sheehan, P.W. (1991). Hypnosis, context, and commitment. In S.J. Lynn and J.W. Rhue (eds.) *Theories of Hypnosis: Current Models and Perspectives*. New York (NY): Guilford Press; 520–541.

Sheehan, P.W. and McConkey, K.M. (1982). *Hypnosis and Experience: The Exploration of Phenomena and Process*. Hillsdale (NJ): Lawrence Erlbaum.

Shepperd, J., Malone, W., and Sweeny, K. (2008). Exploring causes of the self-serving bias. *Social and Personality Psychology Compass* 2(2): 895–908.

Shor, R.E. and Orne, E.C. (1962). *The Harvard Group Scale of Hypnotic Susceptibility, Form A*. Palo Alto (CA): Consulting Psychologists Press.

Siddle, R., Haddock, G., Tarrier, N., and Faragher, E.B. (2002). Religious delusions in patients admitted to hospital with schizophrenia. *Social Psychiatry and Psychiatric Epidemiology* 37(3): 130–138.

Silva, J.A., Leong, G.B., Weinstock, R., and Boyer, C.L. (1994). Delusional misidentification syndromes and dangerousness. *Psychopathology* 27(3–5): 215–219.

Silva, J.A., Leong, G.B., Weinstock, R., and Klein, R.L. (1995). Psychiatric factors associated with dangerous misidentification delusions. *Bulletin of the American Academy of Psychiatry & the Law* 23(1): 53–61.

Simpson, J. and Done, D. (2002). Elasticity and confabulation in schizophrenic delusions. *Psychological Medicine* 32(3): 451–458.

Sims, A. (2003). *Symptoms in the Mind* (3rd edn.)Philadelphia (PA): Elsevier.

Skodol, A. (1998). *Psychopathology and Violent Crime*. Washington (DC): American Psychiatric Publishing.

Sloman, S.A. (2008). Thinking about action. The logic of intervention in reasoning and decision making. *Interdisciplines*. Available at: http://www.interdisciplines.org/ causality/papers/4 and accessed in January 2009.

Sloman, S.A. and Fernbach, P.M. (2008). The value of rational analysis: An assessment of causal reasoning and learning. In N. Chater and M. Oaksford (eds.) *The Probabilistic Mind: Prospects for Rational Models of Cognition*. Oxford: Oxford University Press; chapter 21.

Slovic, P. and Lichtenstein, S. (1983). Preference reversals: a broader perspective. *American Economic Review* 73(4): 596–605.

Snyder, M. (1984). When beliefs create reality. In L. Berkowitz (ed.) *Advances in Experimental Social Psychology*. New York (NY): Academic Press; 248–299.

Sokolov, E.N. (1969). The modeling properties of the nervous system. In I. Maltzman and K. Coles (eds.) *Handbook of Contemporary Soviet Psychology*. New York (NY): Basic Books; 670–704.

Solyom, L., Di Nicoal, V., Phil, M., Sookman, D., and Luchinis, D. (1985). Is there an obsessive psychosis? Aetiological and prognostic factors of an atypical form of obsessive-compulsive neurosis. *Canadian Journal of Psychiatry* 30(5): 372–379.

Spelman, B.A. and Mandel, D.R. (2002). Psychology of Causal Reasoning. In L. Nadel (ed.) *Encyclopedia of Cognitive Science*. New York (NY): Wiley.

Stalmeier, P., Wakker, P., and Bezembinder, T. (1997). Preference reversals: violations of unidimensional procedure invariance. *Journal of Experimental Psychology: Human Perception and Performance* 23(4): 1196–1205.

Stanovich, K.E. (1999). *Who is Rational? Studies of Individual Differences in Reasoning*. Mahwah (NJ): Lawrence Erlbaum.

Stein, E. (1996). *Without Good Reasons*. New York (NY): Oxford University Press.

Stephens, G.L. and Graham, G. (2000). *When Self-Consciousness Breaks: Alien Voices and Inserted Thoughts*. Cambridge (MA): MIT Press.

Stephens, G.L. and Graham, G. (2004). Reconceiving delusions. *International Review of Psychiatry* 16(3): 236–241.

Stephens, G.L. and Graham, G. (2006). The delusional stance. In M. Cheung Chung, W. Fulford, G. Graham (eds.) *Reconceiving Schizophrenia* Oxford: Oxford University Press; 193–216.

Sternberg, R.J. and Smith, E.E. (eds.) (1988). *The Psychology of Human Thought*. New York (NY): Cambridge University Press.

Sternberg, R.J., Roediger, H.L., and Halpern, D.F. (2007). *Critical Thinking in Psychology*. New York (NY): Cambridge University Press.

Stich, S. (1979). Do animals have beliefs? *Australasian Journal of Philosophy* 57(1): 15–28.

Stich, S. (1981). Dennett on intentional systems. *Philosophical Topics* 12(1): 39–62.

Stich, S. (1990). *The Fragmentation of Reason*. Cambridge (MA): MIT Press.

Stompe, T., Ortwein-Swoboda, G., and Shanda, H. (2004). Schizophrenia, delusional symptoms, and violence: The threat/control-override concept reexamined. *Schizophrenia Bulletin* 30(1): 31–44.

Stone, T. and Young, A.W. (1997). Delusions and brain injury: the philosophy and psychology of belief. *Mind & Language* 12(3–4): 327–364.

Sutcliffe, J.P. (1961). 'Credulous' and 'skeptical' views of hypnotic phenomena: Experiments in esthesia, hallucination and delusion. *Journal of Abnormal and Social Psychology* 62(2): 189–200.

Swann, W.B. Jr. (1990). To be adored or to be known? The interplay of self-enhancement and self-verification. In E.T. Higgins and R. M. Sorrentino (eds.), *Motivation and Cognition: Foundations of Social Behavior* (Vol. 2). New York (NY): Guilford; 408–448.

Tavris, C. and Aronson, E. (2008). *Mistakes Were Made (but not by me)*. London: Pinter and Martin.

Taylor, P. (1985). Motives for offending among violent and psychotic men. *British Journal of Psychiatry* 147(5): 491–498.

Taylor, P. (1998). When symptoms of psychosis drive serious violence. *Social Psychiatry and Psychiatric Epidemiology* 33 (suppl.1): 47–54.

Taylor, S.E. and Brown, J.D. (1988). Illusion and well-being: A social psychological perspective on mental health. *Psychological Bulletin* 103(2): 193–210. Reprinted in A.W. Kruglanski, and E. T. Higgins (eds.) (2003) *Social Psychology: A General Reader*. New York (NY): Psychology Press.

Thagard, P. and Nisbett, R. (1983). Rationality and charity. *Philosophy of Science* 50 (2): 250–267

Thornton, T. (2002). Thought insertion, cognitivism, and inner space. *Cognitive Neuropsychiatry* 7(3): 237–249.

Thornton, T. (2008). Why the idea of framework propositions cannot contribute to an understanding of delusion. *Phenomenology and the Cognitive Sciences* 7(2): 159–175.

Tiberius, V. (2008). *The Reflective Life: Living Wisely with our Limits*. Oxford: Oxford University Press.

Tirole, J. (2002). Rational irrationality: some economics of self-management. *European Economic Review* 46(4–5): 633–655.

Tolman, E. (1932). *Purposive behavior in animals and men*. New York (NY): Century.

Tranel, D. and Damasio, A.R. (1985). Knowledge without awareness: an autonomic index of facial recognition by prosopagnosics. *Science* 228(4706): 1453–1454.

Tranel, D. and Damasio, A.R. (1988). Non-conscious face recognition in patients with face agnosia. *Behavioral Brain Research* 30(3): 235–249.

Tulving, E. (2002). Episodic memory: from mind to brain. *Annual Review of Psychology* 53: 1–25.

Turnbull, O., Jenkins, S., and Rowley, M. (2004). The pleasantness of false beliefs: an emotion-based account of confabulation. *Neuro-Psychoanalysis* 6(1): 5–45 (including commentaries).

Tversky, A. and Kahneman, D. (1973). Availability: A heuristic for judging frequency and probability. *Cognitive Psychology* 5(2): 207–232.

Tversky, A. and Kahneman, D. (1974). Judgment under uncertainty: Heuristics and biases. *Science* 185(4157): 1124–1131.

Tversky, A. and Kahneman, D. (1981). The framing of decisions and the psychology of choice. *Science* 211(4481): 453–458.

Tversky, A. and Kahneman, D. (1982a). Judgments of and by representativeness. In D. Kahneman, P. Slovic and A. Tversky (eds.) *Judgment under Uncertainty: Heuristics and Biases.* Cambridge (UK): Cambridge University Press; chapter 6.

Tversky, A. and Kahneman, D. (1982b). Evidential impact of base rates. In D. Kahneman, P. Slovic and A. Tversky (eds.) *Judgment under Uncertainty: Heuristics and Biases.* Cambridge (UK): Cambridge University Press; chapter 10.

Tversky, A. and Kahneman, D. (1983). Extensional vs. intuitive reasoning: The conjunction fallacy in probability judgment. *Psychological Review* 90(4): 293–315.

Tversky, A. and Kahneman, D. (1986). Rational choice and the framing of decisions. *Journal of Business* 59 (suppl. 4): 251–278.

Tversky, A. and Shafir, E. (2004). *Preference, Belief, & Similarity: Selected Writings.* Cambridge (MA): MIT Press.

Tversky, A. and Thaler, R. (1990). Anomalies: preference reversals. *Journal of Economic Perspectives* 4(2): 201–11.

Van der Gaag, M. (2006). A neuropsychiatric model of biological and psychological processes in the remission of delusions and auditory hallucinations. *Schizophrenia Bulletin* 32 (suppl. 1): 113–122.

Velleman, D. (2005). The self as narrator. In J. Christman and J. Anderson (eds.) *Autonomy and the Challenges to Liberalism: New Essays.* New York (NY): Cambridge University Press; 56–76. Reprinted in D. Velleman (2005) *Self to Self.* New York (NY): Cambridge University Press; 203–223.

Volavka, J.(2002). *Neurobiology of Violence.* Washington (DC): American Psychiatric Publishing.

Vosgerau, G. and Newen, A. (2007). Thoughts, motor actions, and the self. *Mind & Language* 22(1): 22–43.

Vyse, S.A. (1997). *Believing in Magic: The Psychology of Superstition.* New York (NY): Oxford University Press.

Ward, N.S., Oakley, D.A., Frackowiak, R.S.J., and Halligan, P.W. (2003). Differential brain activations during intentionally simulated and subjectively experienced paralysis. *Cognitive Neuropsychiatry* 8(4): 295–312.

Waters, F. and Badcock, J. (2008). First-rank symptoms in schizophrenia: Reexamining mechanisms of self-recognition. *Schizophrenia Bulletin.* Doi:10.1093/schbul/sbn112.

Watson, P.C. and Johnson-Laird, P.N. (1965). *Psychology of reasoning: Structure and content.* London: Batsford.

Wegner, D.M. (2002). *The Illusion of Conscious Will.* Cambridge (MA): MIT Press.

Wegner, D.M. (2004). Précis of The Illusion of Conscious Will. *Brain and Behavioral Sciences* 27(5): 649–682.

Wegner, D.M. and Sparrow, B. (2004). Authorship processing. In M. Gazzaniga (ed.), *The Cognitive Neurosciences.* Cambridge (MA): MIT Press; 1201–1209.

Wegner, D.M. and Wheatley, T. (1999). Apparent mental causation. *American Psychologist* 54(7): 480–492.

Weinstein, E. (1991). Anosognosia and denial of illness. In G. Progatano and D. Schacter (eds.) *Awareness of Deficit after Brain Injury*. New York (NY): Oxford University Press; 240–257.

Weinstein, E. (1996). Reduplicative misidentification syndromes. In P. Halligan and J. Marshall (eds.) *Method in Madness*. Exeter: Psychology Press; 13–36.

Weitzenhoffer, A.M. and Hilgard, E.R. (1962). *Stanford Hypnotic Susceptibility Scale, Form C*. Palo Alto (CA): Consulting Psychologists Press.

Wessely, S., Buchanan, A., Reed, A., Cutting, J., Everitt, B., Garety, P., and Taylor, P. (1993). Acting on delusions: (I) Prevalence. *British Journal of Psychiatry* 163(1): 69–76.

White, H. (1987). *The Content of the Form*. Baltimore (MD): John Hopkins University Press.

Wicker, A.W. (1969). Attitudes versus actions: the relationship of verbal and overt behavioural responses to attitude objects. *Journal of Social Issues* 25(4): 41–78.

Wilson, A.E. and Ross, M. (2003). The identity function of autobiographical memory: Time is on our side. *Memory* 11(2): 137–149.

Wilson, T.D. (2002). *Strangers to ourselves: Discovering the Adaptive Unconscious*. Cambridge (MA): Harvard University Press.

Wilson, T.D. and Dunn, D.S. (1986). Effects of introspection on attitude-behavior consistency: Analyzing reasons *versus* focusing on feelings. *Journal of Experimental Social Psychology* 22(3): 249–263.

Wilson, T.D. and Dunn, E. (2004). Self knowledge: Its limits, value, and potential for improvement. *Annual Review of Psychology* 55(1): 493–518.

Wilson, T.D. and Hodges, S.D. (1994). Effects of analyzing reasons on attitude change: the moderating role of attitude accessibility. *Social Cognition* 11(4): 353–366.

Wilson, T.D. and Kraft, D. (1993). Why do I love thee?: Effects of repeated introspections about a dating relationship on attitudes toward the relationship. *Personality and Social Psychology Bulletin* 19(4): 409–418.

Wilson, T.D. and Schooler, J. (1991). Thinking too much: Introspection can reduce the quality of preferences and decisions. *Journal of Personality and Social Psychology* 60(2): 181–192.

Wilson, T.D., Hodges, S.D., and LaFleur, S.J. (1984). Effects of analyzing reasons on attitude-behavior consistency. *Journal of Personality and Social Psychology* 47(1): 5–16.

Wilson, T.D., Kraft, D., and Dunn, D.S. (1989). The disruptive effects of explaining attitudes: the moderating effect of knowledge about the attitude object. *Journal of Experimental Social Psychology* 25(5): 379–400.

Wilson, T.D., Lindsey, S., and Schooler, T.Y. (2000). A model of dual attitudes. *Psychological Review* 107(1): 101–126.

Wilson, T.D., Lisle, D., Schooler, J., Hodges, S.D., Klaaren, K.J., and LaFleur, S.J. (1993). Introspecting about reasons can reduce post-choice satisfaction. *Personality and Social Psychology Bulletin* 19(5): 331–339.

Wimmer, H. and Perner, J. (1983). Beliefs about beliefs: Representation and constraining function of wrong beliefs in young children's understanding of deception. *Cognition* 13(1): 103–128.

Wittgenstein, L. (1969). *On Certainty*. (eds.) by G.E.M. Anscombe, G.H.Wright, and D.Paul. Transl. by G.E.M. Anscombe, and D. Paul. Oxford: Blackwell.

Woolfolk, R.L., Doris, J.M., and Darley, J.M. (2006). Identification, situational constraint, and social cognition: Studies in the attribution of moral responsibility. *Cognition* 100(2): 283–301.

Word, C.O., Zanna, M.P., and Cooper, J. (1974). The nonverbal mediation of self-fulfilling prophecies in interracial interaction. *Journal of Experimental Social Psychology* 10(2): 109–120.

Yager, J. and Gitlin, M.J. (2005). Clinical manifestations of psychiatric disorders. In B.J. Sadock and V.A. Sadock (eds.) *Kaplan and Sadock's Comprehensive Textbook of Psychiatry Eighth Edition*, vol. 1. Philadelphia (PA): Lippincott Williams and Wilkins; 964–1002.

Yan, W. and Gaier, E.L. (1994). Causal attributions for college success and failure: An Asian-American comparison. *Journal of Cross-cultural Psychology* 25(1): 146–158.

Yinger, J. (1995). *Closed Doors, Opportunities Lost: The Continuing Costs of Housing Discrimination*. New York(NY): Russell Sage Foundation.

Young, A.W. (2000) Wondrous strange: The neuropsychology of abnormal beliefs. In M. Coltheart and M. Davies (eds.) *Pathologies of Belief*. Oxford: Blackwell; 47–73.

Young, A.W. and de Pauw, K.W. (2002). One stage is not enough. *Philosophy, Psychiatry, & Psychology* 9(1): 55–59.

Young, A.W. and Leafhead, K. (1996). Betwixt life and death: Case studies of the Cotard delusion. In P. Halligan and J. Marshall (eds.) *Method in Madness: Case Studies in Cognitive Neuropsychiatry*. Hove: Psychology Press; chapter 8.

Young, A.W., Reid, I., Wright, S., and Hellawell, D.J. (1993). Face-processing impairments and the Capgras delusion. *British Journal of Psychiatry* 162(5): 695–698.

Young, G. (2007). Clarifying 'Familiarity': Examining differences in the phenomenal experiences of patients suffering from prosopagnosia and Capgras delusion. *Philosophy, Psychiatry, & Psychology* 14(1): 29–37.

Young, G. (2008). Capgras delusion: An interactionist model. *Consciousness and Cognition* 17(3): 863–876.

Young, H.F. and Bentall, R.P. (1997). Probabilistic reasoning in deluded, depressed and normal subjects: Effects of task difficulty and meaningful *versus* non-meaningful material. *Psychological Medicine* 27(2): 455–465.

Yung, A.R., Phillips, L.J., Yuen, H.P., Francey, S.M., McFarlane, C.A., Hallgren, M. and McGorry, P.D. (2003). Psychosis prediction: 12-month follow up of a high-risk ('prodromal') group. *Schizophrenia Research* 60(1): 21–32.

Zahavi, D. (2003). Phenomenology of self. In T. Kircher and A. David (eds.) *The Self in Neuroscience and Psychiatry*. New York (NY): Cambridge University Press; 56–75.

Zanna, M.P., Olson, J.M., and Fazio, R.H. (1981). Self-perception and attitude-behavior consistency. *Personality and Social Psychology Bulletin* 7(2): 252–256.

Zimbardo, P.G. (1999). Discontinuity theory: Cognitive and social searches for rationality and normality may lead to madness. In M.P. Zanna (ed.) *Advances in Experimental Social Psychology*. London: Academic Press; 345–486.

Zimbardo, P.G., Andersen, S.M., and Kabat, L.G. (1981). Induced hearing deficit generates experimental paranoia. *Science* 212(4502): 1529–1531.

# Index